HANDBOOK OF NUTRITION, HEALTH, AND AGING

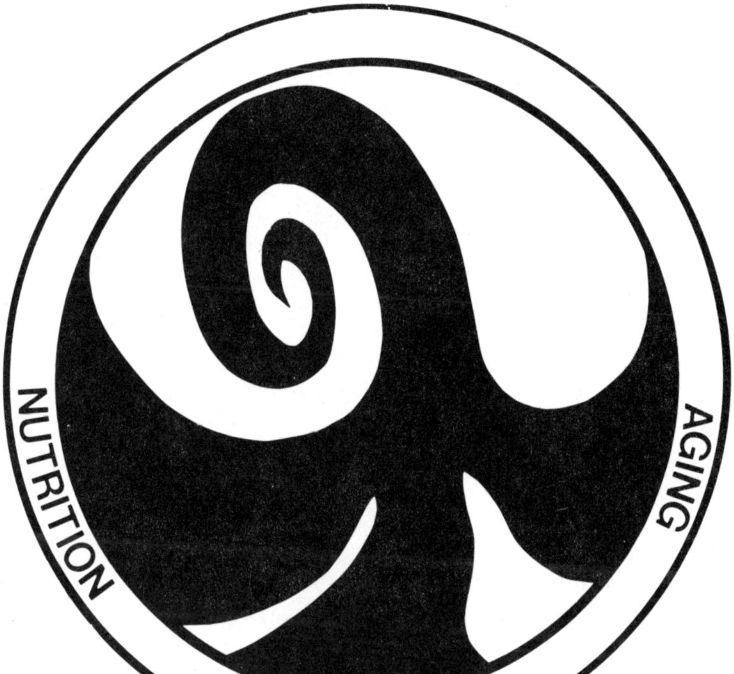

Three great watersheds of knowledge converge in a vortex representing the inevitable intense mutual relationships among components of the triad of nutrition, health, and aging.

HANDBOOK OF NUTRITION, HEALTH, AND AGING

by

Donald M. Watkin, M.D., M.P.H., F.A.C.P.

Chief, Occupational Health Division
Federal Aviation Administration
United States Department of Transportation

and

School of Medicine and Health Sciences
The George Washington University
Washington, D.C.

Foreword by Arthur S. Flemming, Former U.S. Commissioner on Aging and Secretary of Health, Education and Welfare

np

NOYES PUBLICATIONS
Park Ridge, New Jersey, USA

Library of Congress Catalog Card Number: 82-14450
ISBN: 0-8155-0929-4
Printed in the United States

Published in the United States of America by
Noyes Publications
Mill Road, Park Ridge, New Jersey 07656

10 9 8 7 6 5 4 3 2

Library of Congress Cataloging in Publication Data

Watkin, Donald M.
Handbook of nutrition, health, and aging.

Bibliography: p.
Includes index.
1. Aging--Nutritional aspects. 2. Age factors in
disease. 3. Health. I. Title.
QP86.W37 1983 612'.67 82-14450
ISBN 0-8155-0929-4

Foreword

During my period of service as U.S. Commissioner on Aging I was fortunate to have Dr. Donald M. Watkin as one of my associates. As a result, I found myself being reminded time and again of the interrelationships between nutrition, health and aging. It became clear to me that in the development and implementation of policies in any one of these areas it is very easy to overlook these interrelationships and that when this happens it is the older persons who are the losers.

I am delighted that Dr. Watkin decided to write this book. His decision to do so means that many persons in the fields of nutrition, health and aging will benefit from his insights and will be reminded in a forceful and effective manner of the interactions that should take place between these areas.

Dr. Watkin, who brings to the writing of this book a unique background of training and experience in the Nutrition, Health, and Aging (NHA) Triad, makes an excellent case for fundamental research if, as he puts it, ". . . mysteries of the nutrition-health-aging relationships are to be unravelled."

At the same time he makes it clear that ". . . sufficient information is now available enabling American society to catalyze the application of this knowledge to present problems."

I feel that we are particularly indebted, however, to Dr. Watkin for recognizing that present-day deficiencies in the management of the health and nutrition of older Americans result ". . . not from absolute unavailability of health services or food but rather from an appalling ignorance on the part of many elderly about how, when, where, and why to take advantage of health services and nutrition services available to them." In other words, here are areas where increased investments of time, energy and resources in information and referral and outreach services will help bring about the interactions between health, nutrition and aging which Dr. Watkin's book demonstrates can mean so much to the well-being of the older persons of our nation.

Dr. Watkin has coupled invaluable insights growing out of years of research and experience with a call for action in behalf of older Americans.

Arthur S. Flemming
U.S. Commissioner on Aging, 1973-78
Secretary, Health, Education and Welfare, 1958-61

Preface

Nutrition, health and aging are topics receiving unprecedented space and time in all media. Although health and aging have been concerns of human beings throughout recorded history, the modern era is the first during which scientists, health care providers, leaders of industry and legislators and executives of governments have begun to focus on the role nutrition may play in the pathogeneses of diseases and in determining the rate at which the relentless process of physiologic aging occurs. Since nutrition has been found to be one of the very few factors under human control which increases the oldest age to which lower animals survive, it has become such an object of concern that the true nature of its impact on both diseases and the process of aging has often been obscured by misplaced enthusiasm if not by outright fraud. This book is designed to serve as a guide not only for the scientists who seek references to work already performed but also for others who desire to know the state of the art and how knowledge of the nutrition-health-aging triad may be applied to lives of individuals and to groups.

Finding colleagues who have had a comparable breadth of experience in dealing with the nutrition-health-aging triad has been difficult. Many nutritional biochemists are not physicians and have had relatively little concern for application of nutrition principles to human beings. Most physicians have a poor understanding of biochemical and applied nutrition principles. Those few who do are often concerned only with nutritional aspects of specific diseases or with application of nutrition principles to certain age categories such as infancy and childhood and to physiological conditions such as pregnancy. Very few physicians acknowledge the important role nutrition *in utero* and throughout infancy, childhood and youth has on biologic aging and the diseases which characterize old age. Many physicians who are professionally concerned with the elderly have little conception of aging as a biologic process beginning at conception and continuing until death. Very few have had experience in applying what is already known about nutrition and gerontology to population groups.

The vast majority of persons with professional training in nutrition are nonmedical nutritionists and nonmedical dietitians. While they play highly significant roles in the health industry, few have had the experience required to design research needed to augment understanding of the mechanisms underlying the relationships between nutrition and aging *per se*. However, they are the backbone of all professional efforts to deliver nutrition services to persons in the older age group. Many also contribute effectively to the education in nutrition of younger persons. Unfortunately, few of these nonmedical nutritionists and nonmedical dietitians have sufficient backgrounds in biochemistry or sufficient exposure to the problems of clinical medicine to enable them to become charismatic leaders among health-oriented professionals. Nurses, while much more familiar with applied clinical medicine, usually have had little training in the biochemistry of nutrition and the basic sciences underlying modern approaches to gerontology.

This book is intended to hew a course between the complexities of scientific research at one extreme and the monumental problems of application of present knowledge to individuals and population groups at the other.

Credits are deserved by the many who have provided substrates upon which the ideas in this volume have been nurtured. Among these are my colleagues at the Harvard Medical School and the Harvard School of Public Health, at the Gerontology Research Center of the National Institute on Aging in Baltimore, at the National Cancer Institute in Bethesda, from the Interdepartmental Committee on Nutrition for National Defense worldwide, in the Pan-American Health Organization, at the Massachusetts Institute of Technology, in the United States Veterans Administration, on the Panel on Aging of the White House Conference on Food Nutrition and Health and of the Section on Nutrition at the White House Conference on Aging. I am particularly indebted to my colleagues in the United States Administration on Aging both in Washington and in the Regional Offices and in the State Agencies on Aging and in the State Health Departments who have contributed so many of the concepts on which this book is structured. Much credit is also deserved by my "Partners in Research" of the Coronary Primary Prevention

Trial's Lipid Research Clinic at George Washington University's School of Medicine and Health Sciences. Finally, I am indebted to my fellow staff members at the Federal Aviation Administration who daily face the issues arising from aging as an inexorable process.

For their assistance in the preparation of this manuscript, I am indebted to John Schlorholtz, Hamilton College, 1980; Cynthia Craig Olds, University of Pennsylvania, 1978; and my favorite attorney, Virginia G. Watkin, a partner of Covington and Burling, Washington, D.C.

My gratitude also extends to Mary Ellen Watkin and Jerry Monteith, Artists-in-the-Schools of the Montana Arts Council for their conception in the Frontispiece of the mutual relations of aging, health and nutrition. Perhaps most of all I am grateful to Dr. Arthur S. Flemming, my mentor for many years both before and during his tenure as U.S. Commissioner on Aging, for preparing the Foreword. Finally, I am indebted to the estate of Carlota Perez for significant aid given to support preparation of this book.

Donald M. Watkin, M.D., M.P.H., F.A.C.P.
Washington, D.C., U.S.A.
December 1982

The opinions expressed in this book are those of the author and do not necessarily reflect those of the Department of Transportation, the Department of Health and Human Services or the George Washington University.

Contents

Part I

THE NUTRITION - HEALTH - AGING TRIAD

-1-

State of the Art

The nutrition-health-aging triad in its relation to man and animals is a topic of incredible complexity. Each of its three components is in itself an agglomerate.

Nutrition, for example, covers such diverse sciences as agronomy, meteorology, animal husbandry, genetics, biochemistry, anthropology, molecular biology, pathology, pharmacology, physiology and all of the multitude of clinical sciences. In addition, it also is concerned with education, population, economics, politics, transportation, warehousing, distribution, retailing, catering, education, sociology, psychology and the individual's ability to find, prepare, digest and metabolize specific foods and their component nutrients.

Health as defined by the World Health Organization[1] is that "state of complete physical, mental and social well being and not merely the absence of disease and infirmity". Even in the absence of such an all-encompassing definition, the health agglomerate includes such a range of topics as genetics, obstetrics, perinatology, growth and development, drug and alcohol abuse, reproduction, diseases, disabilities, education, institutional care, scientific instrumentation, rehabilitation and thanatology. Furthermore, the health agglomerate also is involved in politics, economics, manpower resources, and the development and construction of physical plant and equipment.

The aging third of the triad, as with the other two thirds, involves all living things. It, too, is concerned with genetics, biochemistry, molecular biology, diseases and disabilities. Aging also concerns itself with such matters as income maintenance, retirement, housing, transportation, the family constellation, community services, institutions, education, legal services and crime prevention.

Combining each of these agglomerates into a single triad where each element of each agglomerate may react jointly and independently with each element of each other agglomerate produces a level of complexity which can only be explained by giving each agglomerate an exponent and representing the triad as an entity raised to a power represented by the sum if not the product of those exponents.[2]

Since modern nutrition had its genesis between the two great wars, since modern aspects of health have evolved in the same era, and since aging as a science had its genesis during and shortly after World War II, the nutrition-health-aging triad is still in the very early stages of development. An understanding of what is already known about the triad is an essential infrastructure upon which newly discovered information in the future may be assembled in an orderly fashion. Since investigations of unknown realms tend to repeat themselves in cyclic fashion, understanding of what has transpired in the past often saves investigators immeasurable time and increases the efficiency of new investigations. For the non-scientist, the history of the nutrition-health-aging triad may in itself serve as a shield protecting the one who absorbs the information from the barbs and arrows of outrageous promotion, faddism and quackery.

WHY CONCERN?

Ubiquitous Desire for Longevity

The Biblical genealogy of Methuselah[3] and George Bernard Shaw's classic play "Back to Methuselah"[4] are two bits of literature temporally separated by thousands of years which indicate that old age itself has been a long-standing desirable commodity in world markets. Quests for the sources of eternal youth have not been confined to adventurers like Ponce de Leon. Scientists, pseudoscientists and far larger numbers of utter charlatans have searched in vain for the secret of Methuselah's 969 years. Among those whose labors have produced believable results are actuarials of major insurance companies who have found positive correlations between obesity and high prevalence rates of disease, disability and death.[5] By inference from these and data from animal investigations,[6,7] many medical authorities[8,9] suggest that persons remaining slender throughout their lifetimes will probably live to older ages than those who become obese. Others seeking longevity via almost everything else from diets and spas to music and meditation are less scientifically convincing but still garner adherents by the thousands.

In the interval between the wars and in the period following World War II, studies in geographic pathology[10,11] suggested that certain diseases were less common among population groups traditionally ingesting foods qualitatively different from those commonly ingested in the United States and other technically advanced countries. The absence of these diseases was often correlated with an advanced age at death.

In recent years, reports through news media of population groups, the majority of whom seem to be far older than mean ages for other populations, have led to numerous reports and expeditions to examine possible explanations for the older average ages at death. A classic among such explorations was that of Alexander Leaf reported in 1973 in the National Geographic[12] and subsequently elsewhere.[13] While the reported advanced ages of some of these populations are rarely probably accurate, there seems to be little question that many of these groups, such as Leaf found in Ecuador, in Hunza and in the Trans-Caucasian Republics in the Soviet Union, are in excess of 90 years and, therefore, well beyond the average age at death of persons in the United States at the same time. An analysis of Leaf's reports suggests that frugal nutrition and intense physical work, either combined or independently, may be factors responsible for the longevity of these particular population groups.

In the post-World War II era, numerous longitudinal studies of specific individuals had been performed in the United States. Classic among these are the Framingham Heart Study,[14] the study of Johns Hopkins University Medical Students,[15] the studies in Tecumseh, Michigan,[16] the studies in the Boston Veterans Administration Outpatient Clinic,[17] and the studies performed at the Gerontology Research Center of what is now the National Institute of Aging in Baltimore, Maryland.[18] Data from these studies do not conclusively implicate good nutrition as a desirable route to advanced old age, since nutrition practices frequently summarize other behavioral characteristics which in themselves have decided influences on longevity. Nonetheless, data from the longitudinal studies are suggestive enough to stimulate interest on the part of scientific community as well as of the public who are aware of them. They tend to confirm the suggestions previously derived from actuarial statistics.

The news media rarely overlook an opportunity to report without pretenses of great accuracy the existence of individuals who claim to be very old and who attribute longevity to various diets. An example of this was a report appearing in the Miami publication *Diario Las Americas* which described a man found in the interior of Brazil who claimed to be over 140 and who had spent most of his life on a diet composed of roots and berries.[19] Unfortunately the cause and effect relationship between such regimens and old age has not been scientifically proven, and the damage to health from such regimens makes their use without strict supervision by knowledgeable professionals extremely dangerous.

More scientific approaches to the nutrition-health-aging triad began with studies beginning almost 50 years ago by McCay and various colleagues.[6,20-25] These demonstrated that first trout and then rats fed diets adequate in nutrients but restricted in Calories outlived by highly significant increments in time similar species fed *ad libitum.* Comparable studies were performed later by Widdowson and McCance[26] by Berg and Sims[27-29] and by Ross[7,30-33] and Ross and Bras.[34-36]

Although McCay's initial work was published over 5 decades ago, and although its authenticity has been verified many times, the mechanism by which restriction of Calories leads to prolongation of life in rats has yet to be revealed. A recent review of scientific literature published in the 11-year interval 1965 through 1975 in English, Russian, Spanish, or Czech dealing with the mechanism of action of such Caloric restriction revealed, out of 291 references detected by the Medlars II system at the National Library of Medicine, only three articles which in any way dealt with possible mechanisms of action.[37] None of these represented experimental designs directed at the particular issue referred to above.

Nutrition's Role in the Prevention and Management of Disease and Disability

Far more attention has been paid to the interrelationships between nutrition and disease. The importance of diet in the management of pre-insulin era diabetes was a classic example of this interdependency. More recently the use of special diets to manage individuals with certain inborn errors of metabolism has become routine. The management of patients with gout by a combination of diet and drug therapies has protected many with hyperuricemia from the complications of this ancient disease. One school of thought on the management of patients with osteoporosis suggests that dietary increments in daily calcium intake may modify its course.[38]

In the cardiovascular realm, dietary management of patients with hypertension was popular in the pre-drug therapy era. Such regimens as the rice diet[39-41] succeeded in large measure as a result of their extremely low salt content. Dietary management of patients with atherosclerosis, particularly that of the coronary arteries, has focussed on control of dietary cholesterol and fat. In spite of well over half a century of investigations in this particular area, the role of diet in the management of atherosclerosis is still a matter of considerable controversy.[42-49]

Interrelationships among neoplastic diseases and nutrition have received considerable attention in the past and are now undergoing a resurgence of interest as a result of the acknowledgement by the National Cancer Institute[50] that nutrition, an environmental factor directly under man's control, may be responsible for many of the observations revealed by geographic pathology in which certain population groups appear to be afflicted by specific types of neoplasia.[51-58]

In the field of hemotology, anemias have been attributed to deficiencies in iron,[59] folic acid,[60] vitamin B_{12}, [61] vitamin E,[62,63] other B complex vitamins,[56,64] trace elements,[66-69] and proteins.[70]

Certain neuropsychiatric conditions have long been recognized as having origins in disordered nutrition. Such alcohol-related syndromes as those named for Korsakoff[71] and Wernicke[72] as well as peripheral neuritis,[73] are attributable to thiamin deficiency. Much concern has recently been given to reports[74,75] that many persons institutionalized for chronic brain syndrome in reality are victims of malnutrition and show remarkable improvement in affect when fed appropriate dietary regimens.

The skin and the nails have long been used by nutritional pathologists in identifying deficiency diseases in man and animals. Classic among these is the dermatitis associated with pellagra[76] caused by deficiency of niacin.

Dental caries have been related[77] to plaque formation aggravated in the presence of high carbohydrate diets.

Malabsorption syndromes may lead to deficiencies of various vitamins[78] which may be treated effectively by appropriate vitamin therapy where indicated. Malabsorption syndromes may be treated also by the incorporation of medium chain triglycerides into the dietary regimens of those patients unable to absorb conventional triglycerides.[79] Various diseases of the liver, particulary Laennec's cirrhosis, have been treated for years by special regimens incorporating appropriate vitamins with adequate protein. More advanced liver disease, however, especially that involving hepatic coma, may be successfully treated by reducing the total dietary protein and utilizing in the diet only those proteins of highest biological value.[377]

Diseases of the genito-urinary system have been successfully treated even before the days of hemodialysis by utilizing diets low in protein of high biological value.[80] Various types of renal and vesicle lithiasis may be effectively managed by appropriate control of dietary ingredients.[81,82]

All of these advances in the field of medicine as they relate to nutrition have heightened the awareness of potential disease sufferers, as well as those already afflicted, with nutrition's vital role in the prevention and/or therapy of disease.

Arising from the growing concern with the interrelations of nutrition and disease, several efforts in the 1960's were directed at testing the hypothesis that specific diets could ameliorate clinical symptoms of disease, or, prospectively, could reduce the incidence of clinically evident diseases during the intervals of the studies. Foremost among these were the National Diet Heart Study sponsored by the National

Heart Institute of the National Institutes of Health;[43,44] the Veterans Administration (VA) Diet Heart Study conducted at the VA Center in Los Angeles;[83,84] and the Anti-Coronary Club program conducted by the New York City Health Department.[85] While these investigations revealed the ability of diets to reduce serum cholesterol levels, they did not succeed in providing statistically significant evidence supporting the concept that diets of the kind used had high correlations with reductions in the incidence of vascular disease. The VA study, in fact, raised the question of whether diets such as those utilized increased the incidence of neoplastic disease in the persons under study.

INTEREST IN DELIVERY OF NUTRITION SERVICES

While medical scientists have had some difficulty resolving questions raised by disease-oriented studies, social scientists and others not specifically concerned with disease have devised meal delivery systems which have been initiated and expanded and which continue to flourish bathed in the light of intense popularity on the part of both providers and consumers.

Although home delivered meal systems, commonly referred to as "Meals-on-Wheels," had been in operation for a number of years,[86] interest in nutrition for the elderly took a new and positive turn in 1966 when an experimental project was established in Miami, Florida.[87] This was structured not on the delivery of meals to home bound elderly, but rather on the congregation of elderly at sites where meals meeting specific standards could be served and where other supportive services could be made available. The almost instant success of this demonstration project led in 1968 to an expansion of the program to a series of over 30 demonstration projects located throughout the United States and designed to test the effectiveness of various service delivery systems.[88] These projects, as was true for the initial project in Miami, were extremely popular. By 1969, at the time of the White House Conference on Food, Nutrition and Health, they provided data on which were based the recommendations[89,90] proposed by that Conference's Panel on Aging which led directly to introduction in the House of Representatives and in the Senate of bills culminating in Public Law 92-258 (March 22, 1972). This law amended the Older Americans Act of 1965 by incorporating into the Act a Title VII authorizing the Nutrition Program for Older Americans (NPOA).

Although delayed in implementation for one and one-half years by various Presidential vetoes or threats thereof, the Nutrition Program for Older Americans (NPOA) was implemented nationally in September of 1973 and has been a growing, very popular, highly visible activity operating in 56 jurisdictions through over 1100 projects and over 12,000 sites.[2] In principle, the delivery of nutrition services provides a center of gravity[37] which attracts persons age 60 and over to specific sites which also serve as loci where participants may receive certain health services and education and counselling in regard to a large number of problem areas related to the nutrition-health-aging triad. The NPOA fulfills needs perceived by the elderly themselves and perceived with considerable understanding by the public at large. In this capacity, the NPOA has done more than anything to date to increase the concern of the general public for, and the willingness of the general public to support, further explorations among the interrelationships of the nutrition-health-aging triad.

WHAT HAS EVOLVED FROM THIS CONCERN AND INTEREST?

Science

Over the course of the past four decades, a few investigators have attempted through metabolic balance studies to establish whether or not nutrient requirements were correlated with chronologic age. The vast majority of these were performed in "aged" who ranged in age from 60 to 80 years. The methodology applied in these studies was essentially that described by Reifenstein, Albright and Wells[91] and was used to study small groups of elderly persons under a wide variety of experimental conditions. Quite predictably, in retrospect, some studies reported increases, some decreases and the majority no differences in nutrient requirements among young and old. Numerous surveys of food consumption have indicated one or more deficiencies in the nutrient intake of older population groups. However, interpretations of these deficiencies depended entirely upon the standards used. If a standard was quantitatively high, the deficiency was great; if a standard was not high, the deficiency was small or nonexistent.

Investigators using animals have confirmed the work of McCay but have failed to come up with any mechanistic approach which would explain why Caloric under-nutrition prolongs the life of the animals under study.[37]

As noted above, considerable attention has been paid to nutrition-disease interrelationships with some success, but also with results defying interpretation.

Nonscience

In spite of the absence of hard data demonstrating cause and effect relationships between nutrition and health and nutrition and successful aging, the presumed logic of such relationships especially among nonscientists often seems overwhelming. The acceptance of such logic is manifest in the extreme popularity of the Nutrition Program for Older Americans (NPOA). It even has led to negation of the Congressionally mandated requirement that an effective evaluation of program impact be performed. Furthermore, the popularity of the presumed logic has been exploited by the food and drug industries who fill the media with promotional material suggesting the virtues of certain products in carefully contrived messages which stop just short of violating regulations laid down by the Food and Drug Administration and the Federal Trade Commission. Exploitation of an even more sadistic nature is practiced by the faddists whose publications, broadcasts and personal appearances imply that health may be guaranteed and aging prevented by ingestion of certain specific foods or food products.

Health

Although there is a lack of hard data, the accumulated soft data of the past century is sufficient to suggest that nutrition is the bedrock upon which other measures involving the prevention of disease, disability and premature physiological aging are structured. Unfortunately, the public has a lack of understanding of the fact that time is involved in deriving positive results from good nutrition. This is particularly true in regard to the prevention of the diseases and disabilities of old age and of premature physiological aging. Over the past century, little attention has been focussed on providing young mothers and fathers and young children with nutrition education which would relate their intake of food while *in utero* or while young to what will happen during the latter half of their lives.

But those who are already old also have nutritional needs which have not yet been fully acknowledged. The main difference between old and young persons lies in the lowered reserves of the older individuals. In view of these lowered reserves, it is extremely important that old persons have constancy of nutrient intake regardless of their state of health or the state of their finances. To insure such constancy many old persons need assistance in the procurement of food, in the preparation of meals, and in meal service. Many actually need assistance in being fed. Many require medical supervision to insure adequate metabolism and excretion of the food products ingested. Finally, all need to be reminded on a regular basis that physical work is indeed an "eighth nutrient group" without which even the ingestion of the best combination of nutrients will not produce the most desirable end results.

WHAT IS THE BEST ADVICE AT THIS TIME?

Individualized Regimens

Evidence is overwhelming that chronological age is not a criterion characterizing a need for any particular form of nutrition. Regardless of the age of the person for whom a dietary regimen is designed, that regimen must be individualized to meet the particular needs of that person. In the latter part of life this is even more important than among younger individuals, since the prevalence of bizarre histories of disease and disability is far higher among those in older age groups.

Education of All Age Cohorts

Education of those already old and through them of those who are not yet old is essential if present knowledge of the nutrition-health-aging triad is to be used to benefit mankind. For those who are young, the role of nutrition in the prevention of disease and disabilities and of premature physiologic aging must be stressed. For those who are already old, the relation of nutrition to the management of diseases and disabilities and of nutrition to health promotion and to the necessity of maintaining at the highest possible level the lowered reserves characteristic of old age cannot be overemphasized.

Prompt Treatment of Illness

Prompt intervention by health industry personnel is needed to keep minor problems from snowballing to the point where limited reserves are exhausted. Prompt therapy for all remediable illnesses and prompt attention to the impact these illnesses have on nutritional status are essential.

1980 Recommended Dietary Allowances (RDA)

In the light of what is now known, it would appear that the Recommended Dietary Allowances (RDA) as promulgated by the Food and Nutrition Board of the National Research Council — National Academy of Sciences[92a] provide reasonable bases upon which to plan nutritional regimens for older adults. The RDA are not immutable standards based on hard data. Rather, they are guidelines issuing from consensus among members of the Food and Nutrition Board whose opinion reflects broadly based knowledge not only of nutrient requirements and interrelationships, but also of the dietary preferences, socioeconomic conditioners and health-related nutritional needs of the American public. With respect to the aged, the RDA require judicious interpretation by knowledgeable professionally trained health industry providers if their application is to have meaningful significance.

More than Foods and Nutrients

In modern nutrition, foods and their contained nutrients are not the only considerations, especially when older persons are involved. Persons 60 years of age and over account for more than half of the over

$200 billion in health costs in the United States, even though they represent only 13% of the total population. One survey[93] of ambulatory free living persons in this age category has indicated that half of the numbers examined had from one to five chronic diseases but that only one-fifth were aware that they suffered from even one of these illnesses.

Detection and Management of Disease

Such statistics strongly suggest that nutrition for the elderly must of necessity be combined with extensive health screening covering far more items than would be required in younger aged cohorts.[94] Abnormalities uncovered by the screening process need to be managed promptly by appropriately trained health industry personnel. Only when health problems — physical, emotional, attitudinal — are managed in such a way as to optimize the health status of a particular individual will that individual be able to benefit from appropriate nutrition.

Modern medicine designed to improve the health of the elderly frequently involves administration of drugs, hormones and physical agents such as radiotherapy which themselves increase the need during therapy for specific nutrients. Roe has recently reviewed[95] the wealth of information available on known drug-nutrition interrelationships. Dudrick[96] had demonstrated the remarkable influence compensatory nutrition has in improving the effectiveness of cancer chemotherapy. What is often overlooked, however, is the fact that many illnesses, normally self-limiting in younger age groups, may have a devastating effect on older individuals unless special attention is paid to insuring the fact that those individuals receive nutrition appropriate to their illness from the moment of onset of the disease or disability. Reserves in older people are low, and, therefore, their ability to withstand dehydration and Calorie, protein, vitamin and mineral undernutrition is reduced.

Ingestion and Retention of Fluid and Food

These factors impose upon those concerned with the health of older persons the responsibility not only of providing them with fluid and food, but also of assuring that the fluid and food provided are actually ingested and retained. Fluid and food do no good if they are not ingested and retained. This implies need not only for education of family and friends who may care at home for older persons during illness and disability, but also for the education of those in hospitals and other health-related institutions responsible for the health care, including nutrition, of older patients therein.

The Double Threat of Alcohol

Alcohol, considered by many to be a drug and by some to be a way of life, is no respector of age. Many elderly for variety of reasons acquire the alcohol habit to the extent of endangering their health, not to mention depleting their economic resources.[97] While drinking alcohol in moderation can be just as pleasant for the elderly as it is for younger persons, many elderly threatened with isolation and feelings of abandonment turn to alcohol as a panacea-type drug. Alcohol, by providing truly empty Calories and by draining the economic resources of the individual contributes directly to many nutritional deficiency states which are relatively uncommon in the United States among non-alcholoic elderly. The management of chronic alcoholism in the elderly requires knowledge not only of the health status of older drinkers, but also of the factors underlying the alcoholic state. Here again nutrition, while essential to improving the health of chronic alcoholics, is but one factor among many which must be heeded in the management of elderly alcoholics.

Tobacco Proscribed

Tobacco is another drug-like substance which adversely affects the nutritional and health status of older persons. Not only does it drain the purse and burn the clothes, to quote an old verse, but it also jades the taste buds of the already taste-impaired elderly, aggravates existing pulmonary and cardiovascular ailments and, in many, has adverse effects on the function of the gastrointestinal tract.[98] Many life long smokers are able to justify their habit in younger years by saying it prevented excessive intake of Calories. In the older age group, however, excessive Calorie intake is not common even among non-smokers. Longitudinal data suggest that weight reduction occurs in the elderly starting at about age 60 and continues throughout the rest of life.[18] Considering the fact that smoking is a physically dangerous habit, at home, at work, in the automobile, or in the hospital and that the injuries derived from smoking-related accidents create serious health problems, including nutritional problems, the use of tobacco should be proscribed for all elderly persons as well as for those in younger age groups.

Supplements Only Under Supervision

Food intake studies in the elderly[99,100] suggest that a large percentage of older people take one or more dietary supplements. Whether these be in the form of a liquid vitamin-mineral supplement or a multivitamin pill containing minerals and trace elements, care need be exercised to assure that elderly persons use low potency compounds in appropriate amounts. Therapeutic vitamin preparations have specific indications but should not be used on a self-medication basis. Even low potency compounds need supervision of the number consumed daily and of other dimensions of the dietary intake for each individual. Particularly dangerous are excessive intakes of fat-soluble vitamins A and D. As a general rule, good nutrition at any age consists of appropriate intakes of a wide variety of properly prepared foods. Dietary supplements which are often costly should be used only when specific indications exist.

ORGANIZATION OF THIS BOOK

This book is organized in four parts:

Part I. The Nutrition-Health-Aging (NHA) Triad:

This section has already dealt with the state of the art and now will deal with the questions (a) What is Aging?; (b) What is Nutrition?; (c) What is Health?; and (d) How do these Interact?

Part II. Specific Nutrients and Their Relationships to Aging:

Protein, fat and carbohydrate will be reviewed separately and as contributors to total energy intake. Their interactions will be examined. Minerals and trace elements will be reviewed. Specific fat-soluble and water-soluble vitamins will be discussed. The important role of water in relation to aging will be examined. Calories (energy) will be re-examined. Finally, the importance of physical work — potentially an "eighth nutrient group" — will be emphasized.

Part III. Present Federally-Sponsored Service Programs:

This section deals with the history and development of those programs designed to provide nutrition and health services to those already old and to the remainder of the population, all of whom are aging from conception onward. These services include not only the delivery of meals but also such matters as the delivery of emergency rations when indicated, the delivery of education and counselling not only in regard to nutrition but also in regard to all aspects of modern life which have an impact on nutrition, and the potential of other service delivery programs not now oriented toward aging which may serve as vehicles of improvement in the nutrition, health and life expectancy of those who are not yet old.

Part IV. The Administration on Aging (AoA):

This section will concentrate on the United States Administration on Aging as the Federal agency foremost in focusing on nutrition and aging and their interrelationships with health. It will also concentrate on the need for the development of better modes of the delivery of services to those who are eligible to participate in AoA programs.

Appendix

The Table of Recommended (Daily) Dietary Allowances (RDA), Revised 1980, of the Food and Nutrition Board, National Academy of Sciences-National Council.

Bibliography

These document the text but also provide sources, many of which are difficult to locate through conventional library and computerized search channels, for those readers who may wish to pursue certain matters in depth.

-2-

What Is Aging?

MEANING PROTEAN

Despite its ubiquity, the meaning of aging is protean, depending in large measure on the background of the definer. For the economist, aging usually suggests a phase of life associated with declining income, often to the point where not only a previously enjoyed standard of living but also life itself may be seriously threatened. For the sociologist, aging represents that phase of life when the individual is abandoned by offspring, saddened and frightened by ever-increasing mortality of other relatives and of friends, terrified by the environmental changes about him, and withdrawn into an unreal world inimical to his mental and physical health, his attitudes toward others, and to life itself. For the physician, aging is a phase of life characterized by the prevalence of many diseases, chronic and acute, and particularly by the culmination of symptomatology attributable to lifelong increments from life styles, environmental hazards, diseases and trauma. For professionals of any persuasion concerned with nutrition, aging is a period of life during which the maintenance of ideal nutritional status is complicated often to the point of being impossible by the many matters which concern the economists, the sociologists and the physicians.

AS PERCEIVED BY THE BIOLOGICAL SCIENTIST

For the biological scientist, however, aging is not that euphemistic term for old age found in the titles of Federal, State and local government agencies and of well known organizations representing the interests of those already old. The biological scientist is truly a gerontologist rather than a geriatrist, devoting himself or herself to the scientific study of the physiological, biochemical, and pathologic phenomena associated with aging. In addition, the biological scientist perceives aging as a process in man beginning no later than conception and persisting until death. For him or her, the essence of aging is that aggregation of changes of biochemical processes engendering those structural and functional alterations with age in cells and acellular tissues which ultimately produce the visible and tangible changes associated with aging of the whole organism.

HOW OLD IS AGED?

The question naturally arises as to when the changes associated with aging cumulate to the extent that the cumulator may be designated aged. Assuming the life span (technically, the oldest age to which any member of a given species has survived) for human beings (TLS[h]) to be approximately 114 years,[100] an aged person was defined as late as 1973 as one in whom at least 65 per cent of the changes associated with biologic aging had already occurred.[101] Such a philosophy placed the golden door at age 74. Recent changes in mortality rates,[101a-101c] altering attitudes toward retirement, and the ever increasing percentages of those over 60 in the older age cohorts[101d] suggest that new terminology is desirable for both scientific and sociological purposes. Such a terminology[101e,101f] is based on the assumption that the TLS[h] provides an appropriate denominator.

The term *aged** is reserved for those who have survived through at least three-quarters of the TLS,[h] *i.e.,* persons equal to or greater than 86 years of age. From a scientific standpoint, practically nothing is known of the nutrient requirements of persons in this category because very, very few have been the subjects of any, let alone nutritional, investigations. Medical studies[101g,101j] suggest that persons in this category are genetically unique. Epidemiologic studies[101k] suggest that those who have followed seven health practices — five of which are nutrition related — throughout life have health status equivalent to those 35 years of age who have followed from zero to two. Here it must be pointed out that health status, whether quantified by the Cumulative Illness Rating Scale (C.I.R.S.)[101h] or by the "ridit" (relative to an identified distribution),[101k] is not the only factor influencing death rates among today's aged. While death rates from the fourth through the eighth decade still follow the straight-line semi-log plot of Gompertz,[101l] doubling every eight years, those persons 86 and older (a group increasing in numbers more rapidly than any of the cohorts over age 60[101d]) appear to have doubling times for mortality which are far, far longer[101e] than predictable from the Gompertz plot.[101l] These considerations suggest that longevity of the aged is determined by genetic constitution with environmental factors (including nutrition) perceived to play a relatively small role.[101m] The increasing numbers of the old are occasioned by the fact that environmental sanitation and industrial hygiene practices, the absence of epidemics and famine, a reasonable standard of living and, in the last half century, the diminution of deaths from acute infectious diseases resulting in part from the introduction of antimicrobial agents have enabled those with elite genetic constitutions to survive long enough to be categorized as aged.

This current perception has not been tested by any prospective or, for that matter, any well-planned restrospective investigations. Therefore, *the aged,** defined as those who have survived through at least three-quarters of the TLS,[h] deserve a very high priority in studies of the mutual relations of nutrition and aging.

The term *the elderly** is applied to those who have survived at least two-thirds of the TLS,[h] *i.e.* those equal to or greater than 76 but equal to or less than 85 years of age.[101e,101f] Persons in this category are the oldest to have shown an epidemiologic association between health practices and mortality.[101n] Many continue to work in their chosen vocations. They too represent a genetically unique group who have managed to survive many onslaughts of acute diseases but who tend to be more afflicted with chronic illnesses than the aged. Among them, the doubling of mortality every eight years continues to confirm the widely held adage that age is the greatest risk factor of all.

The term *the aging** (used here in recognition of its common use as a collective noun, as in the Administration on [the] Aging, the State Agency for [the] Aging, *etc.*, not as the participle indicating a process which is continuous from at least as early as conception until death) identifies those who have survived at least three-fifths of the TLS,[h] *i.e.*, those equal to or greater than 68 and equal to or less than 75 years of age.[101e,101f]

A change in the minimum age for receipt of Social Security payments from 62 and 65 to 68 seems inevitable. Compulsory retirement for Federal civil servants which for years was set at 70 has been abolished. Although organized labor has continued to press for lower retirement ages, their attitude reflects concern for the large numbers of unemployed youth and is no reflection on the abilities or performance of older workers. As noted above[101a-101c] death rates from cardiovascular and other causes of mortality have been falling precipitously in the last

*These definitions have evolved so recently that they are not generally used in publications dealing with older persons. Hence, in this book, the terms "the aging", "elderly", and "aged" are used in the conventional generic sense without reference to the specific age categories which appear in these paragraphs.

two decades. It seems logical, therefore, to defer the earliest accolades of seniority to 68 years from the 60 years or less as presently mandated in regulations governing programs of the United States Administration on Aging.[1061]

THE CHALLENGE NOW: LIVE OUT THE HUMAN LIFE SPAN

If one makes the not unwarranted assumption *(v.i.)* that the lifespan of a species as technically defined above is determined by immutable genetics required for species survival, one can readily recognize that the foremost challenge facing all scientists today is the maintenance of life of high quality until a few days, weeks, or at most months, before a specific individual attains that chronological age defining the lifespan of man. For most, attainment of this age is a very remote possibility. Estimates by Medvedev[102] suggest that, of all four billion persons alive today, only two will attain the lifespan of man. The remainder will all die well before that chronologic age by virtue of disease or accident. It is obvious, therefore, that a major effort need be made to eliminate preventable causes of death among men of any age. High on this list must be all forms of accidental demise. Since accidents often produce serious disabilities which in themselves ultimately cause death, accident prevention by itself can be a major contributor to increasing the average age at death of mankind. Prevention of the birth of individuals with genetic and congenital eventually fatal metabolic and physical defects represents another measure which would increase the average age at death. Perhaps most importantly, those measures which may be taken throughout life to prevent entirely or to defer to a later age the onset of chronic diseases which devastate young and old alike deserve the attention not only of scientists now immersed in the solution of such problems but also of those who influence public opinion which, in turn, influences the behavior, and therefore the average age at death, of all mankind. Among these diseases the most obvious are atherosclerosis and neoplasia.

THE MEANS: CONTROL LIFE STYLE AND NUTRITIONAL ENVIRONMENT

In achieving the goal of life of high quality continuing until shortly before the lifespan of man, mankind must assault formidable bastions of ignorance, prejudice, negative attitudes, and irrational behavior. Even if such an assault could be mounted promptly, years, decades, and generations might elapse before significant data indicating change could be acquired. Unfortunately, mounting such an assault on a large scale is not now possible. What is within the reach of each individual, however, is that person's ability to govern his own life and the lives of those in his immediate sphere of influence in such a way as to achieve in his own microuniverse the best possible odds against congenital and genetic defects, accidents, and chronic illnesses.

To achieve such odds, the individual needs to provide himself and those close to him with the best environment possible. In trying to do so, he may find that certain environmental factors literally are far beyond his own control. At this time, it is impossible for an individual to control the weather or his exposure to community-wide environmental pollutants. However, he can learn to drive safely, drink alcohol with moderation, avoid self pollution with tobacco and drugs, seek medical advice which may prevent the birth of persons with congenital and genetic defects and, significantly, control the nutrition of himself and those under his purview. In the United States, nutrition is an environmental factor directly under the control of each individual old enough to forage for himself. For those too young to care for their own nutritional requirements, parents or guardians, whether specific persons or public agencies, have the responsibility and the authority to control the nutritional environment of those in their charge.

Such environmental control needs to be exercised with respect to aging not only after retirement but literally from conception to death. Regardless of the genetic background of the individual family unit, control of the nutritional environment throughout life affords a practicable, tangible, acceptable method of preventing diseases and disabilities which often lead to premature demise.

The importance of the application of all such measures is emphasized by considering the facts that the average age at death in the United States in 1971 for males was 61 years and for females, 66. These are not the ages usually reported through the media where a decade is added to the ages given above. The reported ages represent the life expectancies of males and females born this year and are derived by a formula based on many assumptions.

NUTRITION AND PHYSIOLOGIC AGING

But evidence is accumulating that appropriate nutrition throughout life, especially when instituted when the propositus is *in utero*, has the potential for slowing down the rate of normal physiologic aging. The studies with rats referred to above at least sustain the hope that nutritional manipulations decelerate the rate of aging by some mechanism as yet unknown.

The very fact that observations half a century old have never been explained in mechanistic terms by biological scientists indicates not only the failure of aging to obtain a high priority among scientific causes, but more importantly the extreme complexity of the process. This complexity and the long intervals of time required to engage in studies of aging have led most scientists to pursue fields in which results and recognition are more easily and quickly attained.

AGING HYPOTHESES

Aging as a biological process is presently explained by a number of different theories. While these compete with each other for popularity, no one of them has become the front runner. In all probability, aging is a phenomenon of pluralistic origins. Nonetheless, to comprehend the phenomenon and to evaluate the impacts of environmental factors such as nutrition on it, one need have familiarity with certain of the major theories relative to aging.

Loss of Homeostasis

Scientists have achieved consensus in the opinion that aging is associated with a loss of homeostasis accompanied by a reduction in reserves. Consensus has not been attained, however, in opinions regarding what brings these changes about. No one theory seems to explain the process. Hence, without mechanisms to explain causality, no approaches to decelerating the aging process have achieved credibility when subjected to evaluation by the scientific method.

The Hayflick Phenomenon

One phenomenon *in vitro* related to, though far from explanatory of aging *in vivo,* is that named for Hayflick.[103] He demonstrated that human diploid cells, strain WI44, *in vitro* are able to maintain a constant doubling time for fifty doublings after which the doubling time increases exponentially and the culture is eventually lost. Hayflick and Moorhead[104] also showed that this *in vitro* capacity to double decreases with the age of the cells when cells of different ages are introduced into the same cultural media, ruling out the role of cell nutrition, pH changes, contamination by microorganisms or viruses or the accumulation of toxic levels of the end products of cell metabolism. Martin, *et al.,*[105] confirmed this by showing that human dermal cells from one hundred subjects ranging from those *in utero* to those ninety years of age decreased their doubling ability by two-tenths (0.2) doublings per year of donor age. Moreover, since the mass of the simplest and lightest possible molecule (composed of two hydrogen atoms), if needed in each of the 2^{50} cells would exceed the mass of a single cell, the loss of doubling capacity in no way can be attributed to the depletion with time of some essential factor found only in cells derived from the donor.

Interpretations of the Hayflick phenomenon pertinent to *in vivo* aging have suggested no relationship between mortality and the inability of certain cell populations to double indefinitely. Usually the phenomenon has been viewed as one intrinsic to the cell, specific to the species and related to the cell population's age. Some have suggested[106] exhaustion of proliferative capacity may be accompanied by exhaustion of other cellular functions whose failure would terminate organisms' homeostatic responses to changing environments.

The Nucleic Acids

Failure of homeostasis related directly to the passage of time suggests failure of cellular function related to enzymatic malformation which in turn can be related to defective RNA derived by transcription from DNA damaged by a variety of factors intrinsic to terrestial environment and proportional to the duration of exposure. Medvedev[107] has listed some of these: random errors in RNA from DNA; radiation; micro-emission of heat and radiant energy; blocking of active groups; micro-denaturation; incorporation of analogs and products in side reactions; and changes in the ratios of substrates during RNA and protein-synthesis.

To this list may be added free radicals which some have claimed do direct damage to nucleic acids[108] but to which most investigators attribute peroxidation of unsaturated lipids found in biologic membranes of cell surfaces, mitochondria, ribosomes and microsomes.[109-111]

In addition, autoimmunity developing in inverse proportion to agewise decrements in isoimmunity may impair protein synthesis.

Immunology in Aging

The science of immunology, while long identified with the prevention of various diseases and the pathogenesis of others and, in a general sense, with aging, has emerged within the last two decades as a powerful tool in investigating the etiology of aging as a process. Scientists utilizing this tool have found data from their experiments compatible with many phenomena known to be characteristic of biologic aging. Among these phenomena is that named for Hayflick *(v.s.)*. Of particular interest to those concerned with the prolongation of life in animals achieved by lifelong caloric undernutrition[21] is the fact that changes in immune responses characteristic of young animals may be prolonged and those characteristic of old animals be deferred by caloric undernutrition.[112,113] Immune responses in animals and in humans with diseases and conditions characterized by premature aging are characterized by deficient isoimmunity and accelerated autoimmunity. Animals and humans afflicted with neoplastic disease, statistically far more common among the aged, also demonstrate decrements in isoimmune responses and increments in autoimmunity.[114] In spite of the ability of scientists in the field of immunology to correlate their data with many of the phenomena associated with biologic aging, they have been unable to elucidate clearly the biochemical mechanisms responsible for these correlations. In a sense, therefore, the science of immunology adds but one more body of descriptive data to the compendium of descriptions of the phenomena of biologic aging.

Endocrinology and Aging

The female menopause and the male climacteric in humans and related phenomena in animal species long ago suggested to clinicians and scientists interested in aging that endrocrine deficiencies might be of significance in the etiology of this inexorable process. The failure of endocrine replacement therapy to provide more than palliative support in specific instances (e.g. surgical castration in young adults) has induced scientists interested in endocrinology and aging to turn their investigative sights toward more fundamental aspects of endocrine research. Results of these investigations suggest, as was the case with those in the field of immunology, that many correlations do exist relating endocrine changes with those associated with aging as a biologic process. Excellent summaries of these studies may be found in reviews by Adelman[114] and Cristofalo.[115] Here again the mechanisms responsible for the changes in endocrine functions have not been elucidated.

Theories of Cellular Aging

Two Categories: Scientists in general have turned to the genetic material, nucleic acids, in search for explanations of biologic aging. Broadly speaking the theories proposed may be broken down into two categories.

The first is based on the hypothesis that exogenous factors induce changes in the nucleic acids (deoxyribonucleic acid [DNA] and ribonucleic acid [RNA]) which in turn are reflected in the biosynthesis of enzymes which are afunctional. When the ratio of afunctional to functional enzymes inside a cell rises to a critical level, cell death, an ubiquitous fact of cellular aging, occurs.

The second is based on the hypothesis that in the hereditary material of each species there exist(s) a gene or genes which specifically program(s) the process of aging and determine(s) thereby, within limits relatively impervious to environmental factors, the life span of the species.

Exogenous Factors: Those exogenous factors which, according to the first hypothesis, contribute to aging include those listed by Medvedev (*v.s.*) and are thought by some[109-111] to include free radicals (*v.i.*). In the decade following the introduction of atomic weapons, considerable attention was focused on the similarities between aging and the pathologic phenomena associated with exposure to atomic radiation. In more recent decades, however, much evidence including observations on humans exposed to atomic blasts at Hiroshima and Nagasaki, have suggested that the contribution of atomic fission and, for that matter, of cosmic radiation to biologic aging, while potentially present, is percentage-wise of small quantifiable importance.

Of all exogenous factors shown to have an impact on aging as a biologic process, nutrition and particularly the Calorie undernutrition first reported by McCay and subsequently investigated extensively by Ross and colleagues (*v.s.*) has proven to be the most enduring but at the same time the least well explained.

Another environmental factor which has a demonstrable and statistically highly significant influence on lifespan and related phenomena in poikilothermic animals (e.g., certain fish, rotifers) is that of environmental temperature. Poikilothermic animals raised in cooler environments, although demonstrating satisfactory growth, suggesting no decrement in metabolic activity associated with reduced temperatures, have been shown to have older average ages at death. In one interesting set of investigations, environmental temperatures were maintained at either 20°C. or 15°C. for eight months for experimental and control groups, and then switched for the remaining life of the fish under investigation.[116] Lower temperatures during the latter half of life were associated with longer lifespans and the correlated retention of immune capacity and deferment of autoimmune phenomena. This study is especially pertinent to considerations of nutrition and aging, since most investigators have found nutrition to have its predominant effect on aging as a biologic process during the very early phases of life with relatively little impact during the latter phases of life.

Genetic Programming: In most respects, the theory of programmed aging provides an hypothesis compatible with the more experimental data and correlating better with descriptive information. The hypothesis also provides the infrastructure on which to develop additional hypotheses with which to explore with reasonable promise of positive results mechanisms underlying the observed impact of such environmental phenomena as dietary Calorie restriction and ambient temperature on aging as a biologic process.

The programmed aging theory presumes that one or more genes possibly located in specific chromosomes control the rate of biochemical phenomena which in turn influence the rate of biologic aging. These biochemical phenomena include the rate at which DNA unwinds to permit transcription of RNA which in turn leads to the assembling of amino acids into functonal or afunctional enzymes. They also include the amount of histone binding and of activation and inactivation of "active" sites on the DNA molecule. They include the accuracy with which RNA transcribes the information on DNA. They include in addition the rate of and quantity of healing of environmentally induced changes in DNA structure, as might be produced by so-called "aging hits."

The theory of programmed aging is compatible with two broad generalizations about aging as a biological process. The first of these is that each species has a life span which is characteristic of that species. The second is that environmental factors such as Calorie undernutrition or reduced ambient temperature may increase the average and even the maximum life expectancy but have never produced changes in life span of a magnitude suggesting a true change in that characteristic of the species. Since a true change in life span would involve, according to the theory of programmed aging, genetic engineering of an order now being attempted under only the most highly controlled experimental conditions,[117] the theory of programmed aging poses a challenge of reasonable dimensions, *viz.*, utilize every possible means to prolong life and defer death until the shortest possible time prior to the lifespan of a given species.

Such a challenge affords more than enough opportunities for practitioners of applied sciences, while leaving the more esoteric and potentially hazardous pursuits of genetic engineering to qualified basic scientists. Embedded in the challenge are such items as the prevention of accidents; the prevention of diseases; the successful treatment of accidents and diseases which have not been prevented; appropriate nutrition of mothers during pregnancy, of infants and young children, of adolescents and of mature adults with particular emphasis on avoiding Calorie overnutrition at appropriate phases to the life cycle; regularly scheduled physical exercise; adequate sleep; total abstinence from smoking; great discretion in the use of alcohol; elimination of occupational hazards; and avoidance to the greatest extent possible of potentially harmful environmental influences ranging from excessive exposure to ultraviolet light to long stays in environments with extremely high air quality indices.

The Lessons of History

Survival curves from ancient Rome, from the United States in 1900, from the United States in 1940, from the United States in 1980, from modern India, and from that hypothetical nation in which control of environmental factors including accidents and disease predisposes its citizens to death only a few hours or at most days before the life span of the species indicate the success of the dissemination of knowedge and of modern technology and suggest the marked differences that still exist between technically developed and technically less progressive societies.

The differences between the survival curves for ancient Rome and the United States at the turn of the century may be attributed largely to the marked advances in microbiology which occurred in the latter part of the 19th century. Differences between the United States in 1900 and in 1940 represent extensions of microbiologic knowledge to the realms of public health including such items as improved water supplies and better food sanitation practices. They also represent marked advances, many resulting from the experiences of World War I, in the practice of surgery and the growing concern for asepsis, particularly in hospital environments.

The marked advances of the next four decades represent the influence of several related factors. One of these was the introduction of antibiotics which led to an unprecedented ability of man to control the spread of infections. Another was the marked increase in the understanding of many hitherto mysterious diseases of which protein-calorie-malnutrition (Kwashiorkor) is most familiar to nutritionists. Still another factor was the development of improved methods of diagnosis which permitted earlier definitive treatments of curable diseases and disabilities. Finally, the differences between 1940 and 1980 in the United States can be viewed as the result of the tremendous increases in the quality and quantity of medical care available to the American public. These increases were the direct results of large sums of money made available for medical research and for medical care through such media as the National Institutes of Health, third-party health insurance, Medicaid and Medicare.

In monetary terms, it is indicative of popular concern to note that Federal funding of the National Cancer Institute in 1973 amounted to $2.00 per capita, whereas funding for the then aging research activities of the National Institutes of Health amounted to $0.03 per capita. The fact that aging is an inexorable process affecting everyone, whereas neoplastic disease affects less than 25% of the population is in itself an indicator of the priority inversion which frequently accompanies the American system of administering health-related concerns.

The differences in survival curves between modern day India and modern United States are attributable in large measure to the lack of resources in all technically underdeveloped societies of which India is a prime example. These deficiencies in absolute resources are aggravated by a relative lack of per capita resources because of the marked population growth which usually exceeds the percentage growth in gross national product. High infant mortality rates, poor nutrition of many millions of Indians throughout growth and development and an appalling low level of quality medical care throughout life reflect conditions which those Americans who have never visited India may find difficult fully to appreciate.

Nonetheless, in modern India as in ancient Rome and as in the United States at the time of the revolution, in 1900 and today, the life-span of man defined as the oldest age to which any member of the species has survived has remained the same. As one wag has put it,

Roman senators lived as long and performed as well as many of our senators of today. In Hunza, now a part of Pakistan but formerly a part of British India, biomedical scientists like Alexander Leaf (*v.s.*) are attracted by the legendary longevity of the Hunzakuts. While it is unlikely that the longevity of residents of Hunza, of the Transcaucasian Republics of the Soviet Union or of certain parts of Latin America is so great as often maintained, there is no question but that many residents of these areas are still alive in at least their tenth or eleventh decade. No well-documented evidence exists that mankind has survived beyond the lifespan of one hundred fourteen years reported in the Guinness Book of World Records.[100] In fact, Medvedev has estimated that, of the four billion persons alive today, only two will reach that age at which all systems will disintegrate simultaneously and the death certificates may legitimately attribute death to old age *per se.*[102]

Noncellular Aging

This discussion of aging has focussed so far on the processes in living cells. However, the aging process also manifests itself among those tissues which are essentially nondynamic. Collagen and elastin, for example, have such long half-lives as to preclude their being turned over at all. European investigators have used the maturation of collagen as an objective index of the biological age as opposed to the chronological age of both men and animals. The tendons from the tails of thirty-month-old rats showed greater contractility on heating to 65°C. than the tendons from five-month-old rats.[118] Similarily old collagen was shown to have prolonged relaxation time when compared to that from younger animals.[119] One European investigator found that dietary Calorie restriction produced tendons with biological age far younger than the animals' chronological age.[120] Investigators in the same laboratory also observed that collagen from the tail tendons of wild Norway rats had a lower biological age than fibers from the tail tendons of domesticated rats of the same age.[121] At a later date, it was demonstrated that intermittent feeding and fasting of domesticated rats led to an inhibition of the normally occurring increase in the stability of collagen usually seen in rats of the same strain, suggesting that altering the feeding patterns of domestic animals to correspond more closely to that of their wild counterparts resulted in a reduction in the biologic age of the collagen involved.[122]

These findings have been attributed by many investigators to the increased number of hydrogen and ester bonds forming cross-links among molecules within the collagen fiber.[123,124] Since collagen is not renewed in the lifetime of an animal, cross-links between the molecules would accumulate in increasing numbers, resulting in the prolonged relaxation time following thermally induced contraction at 65°C.

Since collagen constitutes about 40 per cent of the protein in the human body, and since it is an important component of connective tissue which enables all cells to maintain contact with the external environment, collagen aging may well explain some cell death through its contribution to oxygen and nutrient transport failure. Verzar[125] and Piez[126] have suggested that the molecular aging of collagen is itself genetically programmed, again emphasizing the extreme importance of greater understanding of molecular mechanisms involved in aging.

Other Theories of Aging

Histone Binding: VonHahn, observing that DNA from old animals was denatured at a higher temperature than DNA from the young, postulated stronger intramolecular bonding in old DNA.[127] He suspected that histone may be the substance which represses structural genes, preventing the DNA helix from unwinding and hence from transcribing RNA, thereby preventing the formation of functional enzymes. According to his theory, aging of DNA results from the stabilization of the double helix by firm binding of histone, as opposed to the temporary binding of histone to DNA which characterizes normal repression of RNA synthesis. Since transcription of the genetic information on to RNA requires the local unwinding of the double helix, the firmer binding of histone could interfere with the transcription mechanism preventing thereby the formation of RNA and enzymes and resulting ultimately in cell death.

Free Radicals: The free radical theory of aging has been proposed particularly by Harman.[109] Harman maintains that death, the end result of the superimposition and intertwining of basic aging processes and diseases states, may be successfully deferred by minimizing the effects of degradative changes associated with free radical reactions. These reactions have been named for the transient presence during metabolic reactions of highly reactive intermediates designated free radicals. The high reactivity of these intermediates enables their production of a variety of end products. These reactions are invariably irreversible. These more or less random, endogenous, irreversible reactions by free radicals are believed by Harman to produce a multiplicity of intra- and extracellular changes, all of which are compatible with the superimposition and intertwining of aging process(es) and disease states.

Harman perceives the differences in the relative rates of such reactions in members of a given species as being attributable to genetic and environmental (including nutritional) factors. In studies of a variety of strains of mice, Harman has shown increasing ages at death when the daily diet has been supplemented with chemicals capable of removing free radicals. The free radical inhibitors used have been antioxidents such as butylated hydroxytoluene (BHT) and 2-mercaptoethylamine hydrochloride. Such results may be due to the influence of a 2-mercaptoethylamine, a lathyrogenic agent, on connective tissue or the effect of BHT on lipid metabolism. Regardless of the mechanism of their action, Harman has observed no significant differences in the technical or maximum lifespans observed in the treated groups. Other investigators have attributed the effects of free radicals to their damage to biologic membrances which are characterized by high concentrations of unsaturated lipids.[128] The possibility of free radicals influencing directly and impressively the genetic programming of cells is regarded as minimal.

Lifespan Immutable Within Species

From this discussion it should be evident that aging is a process which manifests itself in many ways. Environmental factors, be they Calorie undernutrition, reduced ambient temperature, successful aging hits or the presence of free radicals, seem incapable of altering the lifespan of particular species. The lifespan is characteristic of species and seems, therefore, to be one of the few undisputed facts about aging as a biologic process.

-3-

What Is Nutrition?

DEFINITION

Nutrition has been defined by Professor Frederick J. Stare, Emeritus Professor of Nutrition at the Harvard University School of Public Health, as "the science of food and its relation to health." That terse nine-word statement describes an agglomerate of such great magnitude that amplification on four key words is essential.

Science

First, nutrition is a science. As with most sciences, it is a mixture of facts, figures, data from experiments, painstaking research and innumerable quantifiable parameters, but it is also an art without which much of the value of the data base would be lost to mankind. Ingredients of the science of nutrition range from meteorology and agronomy through animal husbandry to economics, politics, biochemistry, biophysics, and mathematics.

Food

The term food is familiar to everyone. However, as part of the definition of nutrition, food must be thought of in terms of its production, harvesting, storage, processing, warehousing, ditribution, merchandising, purchase, shelf life, preparation into meals, consumption, disposal of inedible portions and plate waste, and the recycling of the utensils or the disposition of the disposable items with which it is served for human consumption.

Food in modern day America involves the financing of seed, fertilizer, farm machinery, and land itself as well as the complexities of the futures' market. Production is dependent upon favorable climate and particularly on the availability of either rainfall or water for irrigation. Only slightly less capricious than those of the weather, the vagaries of politics, especially those concerned with subsidies, price supports, export and import controls, food stamps, food distribution and regulations imposed by the Departments of Agriculture and Health and Human Services, not to mention those of the Federal Trade Commission, the Interstate Commerce Commission and the various departments of the States, themselves determine for many Americans the quantity and quality of the food they consume.

Health

Health as it relates to nutrition must be viewed from two perspectives. First of all, adequate nurition quantitatively and qualitatively is absolutely essential to the maintenance of good health. Second, good health sustained through the prevention of diseases and disabilities and through the prompt and effective treatment of those diseases and disabilities which inevitably occur is absolutely essential for the maintenance of good nutritional status.

Dietary deficiencies of specific nutrients produce distinctive nutritional deficiency syndromes which have been described in detail by studies performed both within and without the United States. Less well understood are those so-called degenerative diseases such as atherosclerosis, diabetes, neoplasms, disorders of metabolism and inherited diseases which are based at least in part on some nutritional fault.

But even the best nutrition will not resolve the problems of the person who is suffering from an untreated illness or disability. The patient anemic from blood loss from a remedial carcinoma of the rectum, for example, will not be made well by any nutritional maneuvers but can be returned to a state of good health by a combination of therapy for the neoplasm and adequate nutrition before, during and after the therapy. Persons chronically ill with congestive heart failure cannot benefit by adequate nutrition no matter how well-planned until appropriate therapy restores the competency of the myocardium. Diabetes mellitus, particularly the insulin-dependent variety, cannot be managed by diet alone without treatment by competent professionals using insulin, weight control and exercise therapy. Gout, which once was managed by diet alone with modicum of success, can now be managed with great benefit to the patient by therapy with specific drugs.

Relation

In other words, good health is the basis for good nutrition, just as good nutrition is the basis of good health. Hence the fourth word in the definition — relation — becomes the keystone of nutrition's meaning to mankind. Before food can contribute to man's well-being, it must be masticated, requiring effective dentition. Next food must be digested, then absorbed and next transported to the sites where it may be metabolized or stored. Finally, the end products of metabolism must be excreted. All of these processes require a body maintained in an optimum state of health.

THE NUTRIENTS

Chemically Defined and Undefined

That healthy body, however, will be dependent not only on appropriate medical and dental care but also on the ingestion of a dietary containing appropriate nutrients. The nutrients essential for life are protein, fat and carbohdrate, all contributers to the Calorie content of the dietary, minerals including trace elements, vitamins, and water. Numerous studies including some in man have demonstrated clearly that life may be sustained by nutrient mixtures in which every component is definable chemically and soluble in water.[129] Such regimens, however, are extremely costly and deprive the ingestor of certain components of natural foods. Among these are those nutrients which are yet to be identified chemically, of which Schwartz' factor G is a good example.[130] Also included in natural, but to date excluded from chemically defined regimens, and far more popular in recent years, is dietary fiber, a general term encompassing crude fiber and a variety of other forms which will be described later (*v.i.*).

Essential and Nonessential

Whether consumed as natural foods or as chemically defined nutrient mixtures, the dietary for man or other species must include all those nutrients which can not be synthesized by that animal's own metabolism or by the intestinal microfloria normally synthesizing nutrients for absorption from the intestinal tract. Nutrients are customarily divided into essential and nonessential varieties. Essential nutrients are those which a specific animal is incapable of synthesizing in its own metabolic system from less complex elements. Nonessential nutrients are those which may be synthesized by the animal's metabolic system from less complex elements. Species differ in the number of essential nutrients required in their diets. A classic example of an essential nutrient in man and the guinea pig is vitamin C which neither of these two species can synthesize in their own metabolic systems. Vitamin C however can be synthesized by the rat, the mouse, and most other species of animals and therefore for them is nonessential whereas for man and the guinea pig it is an essential nutrient. In man, eight amino acids are regarded as essential, since they can not be synthesized within the human body. All other amino acids are nonessential for man with the qualification that under certain circumstances the synthetic rate may be insufficient to provide a needed quantity of a specific amino acid without supplementation from the outside.

Standards for Nutrient Intake

Standards for nutrition have been promulgated by various official bodies throughout the world. The standard for the United States is that set by the Food and Nutrition Board of the National Research Council — National Academy of Sciences and is referred to as the Recommended Dietary Allowances (RDA).[92a] Comparable recommended standards have been put forth by United Nations bodies (WHO-FAO),[132] and by official groups comparable to the Food and Nutrition Board in a variety of other countries. Such standards are designed for use in population groups and presume the availability of a variety of food stuffs. The recommended standards for each nutrient are set sufficiently high so that better than ninety-five per cent of total population in any society will receive adequate nutrition if the standard is met. Obviously such standards are not the minimum requirement and on the other hand do not purport to provide adequate nutrition for those with special nutritionally related problems. Nonetheless, they do provide guides to planners dealing with population groups.

The 1980 R.D.A. makes recommendations for all persons 51 years of age and older as well as for those in a variety of younger age groups and physiologic conditions (*viz.*, pregnancy and lactation). From the viewpoint of those interested in nutrition and aging, the recommended dietary allowances for those 51 years of age and older adjusted for sex and body weight are a satisfactory starting place. The marked variance of measurable parameters among older individuals requires, even more than among young, great individualization of diet to meet the specific nutrient requirements imposed by the variable histories of the older persons.

Physical Work

New recommendations regarding nutrition would be incomplete without mentioning what may be regarded as the "eighth nutrient group," physical work. There is consensus among nutrition investigators that the Calorie needs of man and animals are related to energy expenditure. A characteristic of aging is a gradual decline in both basal (the lesser decrement) and activity (the greater decrement) metabolism with advancing age from about age 25 onward. Obviously if Calorie intake is not decreased in proportion to the decrement in Calorie expenditure, unused Calories will be stored and the ingestor of those Calories will become obese.

For persons in the older age group physical work is a particular need, because the knowledge and other resources required to provide an intake of high nutrient density low in Calories are not always possessed by older persons. Foodstuffs of average nutrient density are more readily available and may be ingested without the consequences of obesity provided their extra Calories are expended in the performance of physical work.

But Calories and obesity are not the only concern. Work is essential to maintain the integrity of the cardiovascular system and particularly to maintain the collateral circulation around the major vessels in the heart, a major factor in preventing fatal myocardial infarctions. Experiences with exercise regimens among older people have indicated that general well-being is markedly improved subjectively and objectively by the participation of the elderly in regimens of exercise or other forms of work.[133] However much of this improvement may be deemed of psychological origin, many objective parameters also show improvement. Among these are pulse rate recoveries after exercise, tolerance for climbing such as the Harvard step test, evidences of improved collateral circulation, greater muscle strength, improved cardiac indices, improvement in maximal breathing capacity and improvement in maximal work performance.[134,135]

ENTERAL AND PARENTERAL ALIMENTATION

The amplifications on the definition of nutrition given above refer primarily to situations with people and animals with normal gastrointestinal tracts who are able to consume food by mouth. Among all populations, small segments exist who cannot for a variety of reasons tolerate food by mouth. These persons are usually seriously ill or disabled and must be fed by nasogastric tube, by gastrostomy, or by one of the many forms of parenteral nutrition. Proper mixtures of nutrients including Calories and water are essential to the maintenance of health and to the restoration of health in those who have been victims of disease or accidents. Tube and parenteral feeding regimens generally do not resemble in superficial appearances regimens composed of common foods unless, in the case of tube feedings, they are prepared by grinding common foods into a thin slurry. In terms of nutrient content, however, both tube and parenteral feedings, if adequate to sustain life and restore health, contain identical nutrients to those described above for regular dietary regimens. Parenteral feedings must be sterile, apyrogenic and nonallergenic. These requirements impose restraints on the nature of the components entering the regimens and in general result in far higher costs than regular diets or tube feeding regimens.

NONNUTRIENT REQUIREMENTS ESSENTIAL FOR PROPER NUTRITION

Also involved in nutrition are considerations of such disparate matters as housing, transportation, consumer protection, income maintenance, crime prevention and law, to mention only a few. Housing is essential for the storage of food, for the preparations of meals and as a place for their consumption. Transportation is required to carry shoppers to markets and shoppers and their purchases back to their places of residence. It is also essential to deliver patients to and return them from various sites of interface with the health industry. Consumer protection is required to assure elderly persons with limited resources maximum value for their scarce dollars. Income maintenance is needed to assure the elderly of the maximum possible financial resources to which they are entitled. Crime prevention is essential if the elderly are to be relieved from fear of walking on the streets whether for the purposes of shopping or merely for socialization. Legal assistance is necessary for the numerable problems related to probate, exchanges of property and maintenance of rights by those elderly who do not have their own lawyers.

THE NUTRITION AGGLOMERATE

In summary, nutrition is an agglomerate of all the biologic, basic and clinical sciences, economics and the political and social sciences. As such an agglomerate, its complexities in providing optimum benefits to the elderly are manifold. While only a nine letter word, nutrition implies involvement by all parts of every society. As an environmental factor directly under the control of each individual, it provides mankind with one of the few relatively easily controlled factors which may, with proper education on the part of the user, maintain and improve health and even decelerate aging as a biologic process.

-4-

What Is Health?

AN OBJECT OF NEGLECT BY ALL AGE COHORTS

Health, like beauty, is often in the eye of the beholder. This is especially important in considerations of the entire field of aging, whether dealing with aging as a lifelong biologic process or with those issues of concern to those who are already old.

For the majority of young persons, all of whom are aging, health is usually synonymous with the absence of illnesses serious enough to impair their mobility and the ways of life to which they have become accustomed. Indicated management of known chronic conditions in the early states of pathogenicity is often disregarded. Prudent behavior directed at health promotion and prevention of diseases and disabilities in future years may be totally ignored. When youth's attention is focussed on the innumerable health problems of today's aged, defensive denial mechanisms are engendered along with statements expressing repugnance at the very thought of living so long as to endure so disquieting a state of existence. But the young are not alone in their disdain for prevention and their scorn for concerns about their health. Those in middle age and even those approaching the borderline of senior citizenship not only ignore prevention and health promotion but actually feign contempt for those curative health services which may be indicated.

Neglected dentition, inappropriate or totally absent control of known metabolic disorders, continued smoking, excessive alcohol intake in the face of contraindications, self medication with various over-the-counter drugs, absence of an orderly lifestyle, deliberate shunning of mental hygiene issues, dietary indiscretions ranging from gluttony to sporadic resort to fad diets, professed fear of physicians and professed fatalism characterize a vast majority of Americans of all economic levels. Among the aged the problems characteristic of middle age are compounded not only by intrinsic difficulties such as economic deprivation, less perceptive intellect and limitations on mobility, but also by the fact that the rest of society has assumed a totally unprogressive posture toward promoting better health among those already old. Even physicians who may exhort young and middle aged patients to be more attentive to health related matters often will advise the elderly to be thankful for having lived so long and having selected parents with such elegant genetic constitutions.

GOOD HEALTH: A PERSONAL RESPONSIBILITY

These unfortunate perceptions of health reflect an ignorance of what health really is and how good health depends in the first instance on recognition by individuals of their personal responsibility for the maintenance of health, for the attainment of health in its absence, and for promotion of health and the prevention of disease and disabilities in future years.

CHANGE IN PERCEPTIONS REQUIRED

In the early years of its existence, the World Health Organization defined health in utopian terms: "A state of complete physical, mental and social well-being and not merely the absence of disease and infirmity".[1] The very fact that four decades later finds mankind groping as in a game of blind man's bluff toward realization of that utopian goal suggests that too little attention has been paid to promoting personal recognition of responsibility for health. Obviously, changing the recognition of personal responsibility from its almost negligible quantity today into an irresistible force is achievable only with great difficulty in a democratic society. What is required is a total change in attitude which in turn requires altering the perceptions by Americans of all ages of many hallowed values.

Among them is the notion that old age of necessity implies an era characterized by disease, disability, immobility, faulty perception, loneliness and poverty from which death is the only escape. Among them also is the fatalistic view that nothing can be done to prevent the inexorable consequences of aging and its associated diseases and disabilities. Among them is the misapprehension that physiologic and chronologic aging march *pari passu* throughout life. Disease and disability, the antithesis of health, are no respectors of age. The teenager who has suffered in microseconds a broken neck with irreparable cervical cord damage through a carelessly induced auto accident has suffered instant aging with all the consequences — physical, emotional, metabolic, economic, those inducing dependency and social — which might under other circumstances have characterized his eleventh decade.

In other words, recognition of the individual's responsibility for health and promotion of the concept that that recognition is a truly positive factor which may, if correctly channeled, bring this nation far closer with the utopia envisioned in the World Health Organization's definition, are measures not yet effectively implemented which need the attention and the imagination of all interested in improving life in America today.

NUTRITION: THE PREDOMINANT HEALTH FACTOR UNDER THE CONTROL OF INDIVIDUALS

Nutrition, *i.e.,* the entire agglomerate *(v.s.),* is directly related to health in ways unmatched by other environmental factors. In the United States, nutrition is an environmental factor directly under the control of individuals or, in the case of very young children and other dependent persons, of the guardians of those individuals. In nations where food is abundant, individuals have the ability to determine for themselves and their dependents the quantity and quality of foodstuffs ingested daily. Knowing what to buy, when to buy it, how to prepare it, how much to eat and how frequently to eat it, are some of the determinants enabling individuals to control their nutritional environment in such a way as to promote health, prevent disease and disability and defer physiologic aging until the latest possible time.

NUTRITION'S PROMISES TO BE REALIZED THROUGH EDUCATION

Obviously, for nutrition to deliver on these promises, education of all in all aspects of the nutrition-health-gerontology triad is essential. For those who are very young, the World Health Organization's definition of health as "a state of complete physical, mental and social well-being and not merely the absence of disease and infirmity" may with appropriate attention to lifelong nutrition come close to being reality. However, for those who are already old, who already have diseases and disabilities which were not prevented by appropriate attention to nutrition and other health related concerns, the objective becomes one of compromising with the W.H.O.'s definition. Since nutritional problems of most elderly are attributable to diseases and disabilities — physical, emotional, and/or attitudinal — the management of disease and disability becomes of primary importance in the prevention of malnutrition and hunger. Conversely good nutrition delivered at appropriate times is the key to the maintenance of optimum health and to the prevention of further diseases and disabilities. Education of all ages in the interrelationships of nutrition-health-aging triad is required if mankind is to take full advantage of his ability to use nutrition for improving his prospects for a long, healthful and productive life.

-5-

How Do Nutrition, Health, and Aging Interact?

MORE INFORMATION NEEDED

The discussions in the three preceeding chapters leave little doubt that interactions exist among the components of the nutrition-health-aging triad. The direct relationship between nutrition and certain deficiency diseases or diseases caused by nutrients taken in doses so large as to be toxic has been proven and the biochemical explanations for the disease states described. The impact of disease on nutritional status is no less well documented. Deficiencies in knowledge of interactions exist, however, when the nutrition-aging or the health-aging relationships are critically examined.

MULTIFACTORIAL PATHOGENESES DEMAND MORE FUNDAMENTAL RESEARCH

The problem is complicated still more by virtue of the fact that certain diseases, *e.g.* atherosclerosis and neoplasia, are more prevalent among the elderly and are related in manners yet poorly understood to the intake of certain nutrients. The multifactorial etiology of atherosclerosis, of neoplasia, and of aging as a process underscores the great difficulty of accumulating additional convincing data in man descriptive of the interactions of the components of the triad. This situation leaves without question the need for more fundamental research if mysteries of the nutrition-health-aging relationships are to be unraveled.

BETTER APPLICATIONS OF EXISTING KNOWLEDGE INDICATED

Nonetheless, sufficient information is now available enabling American society to catalyze the application of this knowledge to present problems. By application of existing knowledge to the problems of today, present society may uncover leads which will simplify and accelerate progress in the basic sciences.

The issues raised by lack of basic scientific knowledge are not esoteric ones rooted in academia. They have very deep roots in the political fabric of American society. Deficiencies in our management of the health and nutrition of older Americans have been highly publicized by the media and have become the grist for the mills of political campaigns. These deficiencies result not from absolute unavailability of health services or of food but rather from an appalling ignorance on the part of many elderly about how, when, where and why to take advantage of health services and nutrition services available to them.

Improvement in our ability to translate existing knowledge in health and nutrition into application which will benefit those who are already old will remove a major stumbling block to obtaining financial support for much needed basic research in the nutrition-health-aging triad interrelationships. If satisfied that their own needs are receiving needed attention, the eighty per cent of 32 million senior citizens who vote in America will don their altruistic togas and become strong supporters of investigations whose major beneficiaries will be younger cohorts and those yet to be born.

Part II

SPECIFIC NUTRIENTS AND THEIR RELATIONSHIP TO AGING

PROLOGUE

In Part II, the tempo changes from the orientation of generalists with overall interests in the NHA triad to the orientation of persons with professional-level concerns about nutrition and its relation to health and aging. This change is designed to provide nutritional biochemists and their graduate students, physicians and their residents and fellows, dietitians and their interns and trainees, nutritionists and all students of applied nutrition basic information and extensive references about health-related and aging-related aspects of specific nutrients essential to human health.

The dissection of foods — the customary vehicles for nutrients — into the nutrients discussed in this section is a by-product of academic necessity which has both fortunate and unfortunate aspects. On the fortunate side, nutrients in biologic systems can be examined scientifically best by raising or lowering single nutrient concentrations in given meal patterns otherwise constant and adequate by modern standards in all but the nutrient under investigation. On the unfortunate side, such examinations overlook the possibility that there are among nutrients numerous interrelations whose value may be minimized or whose hazard may be maximized by unilateral changes in an otherwise constant dietary.

Apart from scientific considerations, most experimental regimens for human beings are monotonous and often unpalatable. As the cost of traditional metabolic investigations has risen logarithmically, investigators have resorted more and more to utilization of liquid diets which are readily prepared. have precise nutrient composition, are relatively inexpensive in terms of components and, most importantly, may be prepared with minimal labor costs.

These considerations raise two issues: (1) is the information derived from such studies comparable to that which might be derived from studies using more conventional foods?; and (2) do the subjects who volunteer for such studies together with other nonfood-related conditions of such experiments induce results which may not be representative of results to be found in a randomly selected age-stratified population sample investigated under less rigid conditions?

The debate over these issues has gone on for decades and will continue as long as disputants on the issues continue to press their opposing views. From a practical standpoint, the debate is senseless. Only available data from studies among aging and elderly subjects are utilizable, and much of present knowledge has yet to be applied. The chances of getting more and better data will improve only with the development of more acceptable, effective and cost-effective methodology and with the application to clinical investigations of basic biochemical information on aging as a process, information which has been frustratingly slow in its promulgation. However, information among the aged (*i.e.*, persons 86 years of age or older) is so sparse that even the most simple clinical and laboratory parameters are worth acquiring. In brief, the data presented in this section in many instances is unique, having been collected at a time when the studies producing such data were feasible. Much can be learned by their study and much can be achieved by applications derived from that study. The void in data among the truly aged is great and deserves high priority in a scientific environment where painful choices must be made.

The information in Part II provides all — scientists, clinicians, practitioners of health industry professions, students and interested lay persons — with data and interpretations of that data which will be scientifically and medically useful but which also may aid in clarifying the confusion caused by the flood of nutrition, health and aging presentations through various media. While these chapters have been written to provide material meaningful to scientists, they have also been prepared with sufficient explanatory information to make their contents intelligible to readers with curiosity about and appreciation for human biology. Capable readers will readily locate the material most useful to them.

-6-

Protein

MINIMUM PROTEIN REQUIREMENT FOR THE AGED STILL CONTROVERSIAL

In its relation to aging and the requirements of the aged, no nutrient has received so much attention and been the object of so much controversy as protein. The ease with which the intake and the excretion of nitrogen, sixteen per cent of protein by weight, could be measured by the Kjeldahl method at times when measurement of the overall metabolism of other nutrients was technically extremely difficult led to a plethora of investigations of nitrogen balance as an indicator of protein requirements. Various investigators using the nitrogen balance technique have found increased,[136-139] decreased,[140-142] and similar[143,144] minimal protein requirements for the aged when compared to the young. Considering the relatively enormous variance of the measurement of any parameter in the aged as opposed to similar measurements in the young, such differences are not surprising in view of the small numbers of subjects studied in each of the investigations. Details of these early investigations have been summarized elsewhere.[145-148]

AMINO ACID REQUIREMENTS

In line with scientific trends toward greater detail in the investigation of nutrient requirements, considerable emphasis has been placed since the middle 1950's on requirements for specific amino acids, the building blocks of protein. Most investigations have concerned the minimum requirements of essential amino acids using techniques not vastly different from those employed by Rose in his early investigations of the minimum essential amino acids requirements of young men.

Rose's Studies with Rats

Rose's now classic studies began in rats in 1931. By the middle of the decade, with the identification of threonine, McCoy, Meyer and Rose were able to achieve satisfactory growth in rats fed diets containing only pure L-amino acids but no protein.[149] During the next decade Rose's laboratory successfully eliminated from the diet mixture all but the essential amino acids and published their best estimates of the amount of each required for growth for rats.[150] The same investigators showed that non-amino acid nitrogen sources such as diammonium citrate could stimulate growth when diets contained only minimal levels of essential amino acids, clearly suggesting that all other amino acids could be synthesized, in the presence of adequate nitrogen sources, within the bodies of the animals.[151]

Studies in Young Humans

Rose's studies in young men produced estimates of the minimal levels of essential amino acids needed to maintain nitrogen equilibrium when the subjects were fed a highly purified diet containing pure amino acids as almost the sole source of nitrogen.[152,153] Leverton[154] using techniques similar to those of Rose has estimated the amino acid requirements of young women. Holt and Snyderman,[155] using nitrogen balance and growth as criteria, have estimated the amino acid requirements of infants.

Amino Acids Essential for Man

The essential amino acids, as defined by Rose, were those which could not be synthesized fast enough from nitrogen sources normally available in the diet to meet the needs of the body. The amino acids which have to be supplied by food itself and therefore are essential for man include isoleucine, leucine, lysine, methionine (cystine, cysteine), phenylalanine (tyrosine), threonine, tryptophan, and valine.* In rats and other species satisfactory growth repair and maintenance may require additional essential amino acids, but those given above suffice for man.

*Both cystine and cysteine are essential, but both may be derived from methionine. Similarly, tyrosine is essential but may be derived from phenylalanine. However, the reverse is not possible, *i.e.*, cystine or cysteine can not be converted into methionine nor can tyrosine be converted to phenylalanine.

Nonessential Amino Acids

The nonessential amino acids are those which can be synthesized by a given animal but need not be supplied by that animal's diet. These nonessential amino acids actually are no less important than the essentials in growth, repair and maintenance. When an essential amino acid is missing from the diet, or is present in inadequate amounts, that particular diet is inappropriate for growth or maintenance even though it may contain an excess quantity of amino acids. The nonessential acids need not be present in the diet, since they can be produced in an organism from the intermediary products of carbohydrate and fat metabolism and from such nitrogen sources as urea by the process of transamination.

Los Angeles and Tuskegee Studies in the Aged

Studies by Mertz, *et al.*,[156] and Albanese, *et al.*,[157] on traditional intakes of older persons suggested that the elderly self-select diets deficient in methionine and lysine. More quantitative data were obtained by Tuttle *et al.*,[158] who studied men aged 52 to 58 utilizing L-amino acid mixtures based on the composition of 18.75 grams of egg protein containing also, in addition to the eight essential amino acids, the L-forms of histidine, cystine and tyrosine. Glycine was used to bring the nitrogen content of the regimen up to that of natural food (7.0 grams per day). All the old men receiving this regimen were in negative nitrogen balance. When three additional subjects were fed egg protein in an amount equivalent in terms of essential L-amino acids to the amino acid mixture, they too were in negative nitrogen balance. These studies suggested that older men may have a higher requirement for one or more of the essential amino acids or that glycine may be less well utilized by the aged than by the young in the synthesis of nonessential amino acids.

In spite of the statistical conclusiveness of the data collected by Tuttle *et al.*, Watts, *et al.*,[159] a trainee of the Tuttle group, using comparable techniques and Negro male subjects ranging from 65 to 84 years of age, observed positive balances at the 200, 280 and 360 milligram tryptophan levels of the FAO pattern.

When these same old men were fed essential amino acids in the milk pattern rather than in the FAO reference pattern, Watts, *et al.*, reported methionine requirements ranging from 0.29 to 0.60 grams of methionine as opposed to the 2.4 and 3.0 gram requirements reported by Tuttle, *et al.*[160]

Tuttle, *et al.*,[161] investigated the essential amino acid requirements of old men in relation to the total nitrogen content of their diet. They observed that the essential amino acid requirement increased as the total nitrogen content of the diet was increased by additions of diammonium-citrate and glycine. They suggested that there is a dependence of essential amino acid requirement on total nitrogen intake in older men, since reports of a similar dependence have not been made in respect to younger men and women.[162]

Tuttle, *et al.*,[163] using men ranging from 50 to 70 years of age, studied the effect of the kind of nonessential nitrogen in the diet on the requirement for dietary essential amino acids. When a nonessential amino acid mixture replaced glycine as the source of supplemental nitrogen, greater nitrogen retention occurred in 5 out of 6 subjects. In spite of the increased retention of nitrogen when nonessential amino acid mixtures replaced glycine, 2.4 grams of essential amino acids daily were required to achieve nitrogen equilibrium in all subjects, even though one had achieved nitrogen equilibrium on 1.2 grams of the essential amino acid nitrogen daily. These studies demonstrated clearly the marked variability in amino acid requirements among the aged. In addition, they suggested that the nonessential as well as the essential amino acid composition of diet may influence the essential amino acid requirement. They also bring up the interesting issue of whether there may be a failure of certain nonessential amino acid synthetic pathways with advancing age.

Studies by the Los Angeles investigators[160,164,165] indicated a far higher requirement for methionine than reported by other investigators[153,166] in young men and women and also by Watts, *et al.*, *(v.s.)* in older men. The possibility exists that the increased requirement would be accounted for by a decreased efficiency of the conversion of methionine to cystine. The same investigators also reported higher lysine requirements than had been proposed for young subjects in general. The data of the Los Angeles investigators suggest that old men require more than twice the quantity of methionine and lysine needed for nitrogen equilibrium in young adults. As noted above, Watts, *et al.*,[159] were unable to confirm findings of the Los Angeles investigators in studies performed in Tuskegee, Alabama.

CAMBRIDGE STUDIES OF THE PROTEIN AND AMINO ACID REQUIREMENTS OF THE AGED

Nitrogen Balance Studies

Interest in the protein requirements of elderly adults has been renewed by a series of provocative studies performed at the Clinical Research Center of the Massachusetts Institute of Technology in Cambridge. In the first of these studies, Tontisirin[167] observed that a nitrogen intake equivalent to 0.5 gm. egg protein per kilogram per day is sufficient to maintain positive nitrogen balance in healthy elderly persons, just as the same level had been found to be adequate for maintaining positive nitrogen balance in young adults.

Plasma Amino Acids *vis a vis* Amino Acid Intake

The remainder of this study concerned the relationships among plasma tryptophan concentrations, tryptophan intakes and tryptophan requirements. After fourteen elderly subjects, four men and ten women 73 ± 5 years of age, had received 10 milligrams tryptophan per kilogram per day (four subjects) or 5 milligrams tryptophan per kilogram per day (ten subjects), tryptophan intake was gradually reduced through consecutive four day intervals, during which the diet was maintained isonitrogenous, until a level of tryptophan intake of 0.5 milligrams per kilogram per day was reached. Fasting and postprandial plasma tryptophan levels were determined at the end of each diet interval. The plasma tryptophan concentration decreased as tryptophan intake was reduced to the 2 milligram per kilogram per day level, thereafter remaining constant in spite of further reductions in the tryptophan intake. The authors interpreted this data as indicating that the mean minimum tryptophan requirement of healthy old subjects approximates 2 milligrams per kilogram body weight per day, or less than the value of 3 milligrams per kilogram per day previously reported for young men studied by the same method.[168]

In a second study using identical techniques but examining the threonine requirement of young men and elderly women, Tontisirin *et al.*,[169] found a minimum requirement for threonine of 6.8 ± 1.7 milligrams per kilogram per day in young men and 7.6 ± 2.2 milligrams per kilogram per day in one male and twelve female subjects aged 62 to 82 years of age. A lack of statistically significant differences in this data was interpreted as indicating that the threonine requirement per unit of body weight does not change with advancing age.

In spite of these data, the MIT investigators concluded their 1974 contribution with the suggestion that the data were not of practical significance and that the low "break point" on the curve of plasma amino acid response to stepwise decreases in intake of an essential acid might underestimate the actual needs for that amino acid.

In another discussion of the same data, Young, *et al.*,[170] have argued that such data in reality mean that the requirement per unit of total body protein increases with age, because lean body mass is reduced and the portion of the body fat increased in the older subject. They report that the preliminary data on a valine response curve in the elderly also suggest that the valine requirement may be higher per unit of cell mass in the elderly than in young adults, although no differences on a milligram per kilogram body weight basis were observed.

Young, *et al.*,[170] also have argued that the optimal pattern of essential amino acid requirements may change during old age. They have noted that other investigators[163] *(v.s.)* have maintained that the source and the amount of nonessential nitrogen in the diet influence utilization of dietary nitrogen and may influence the requirement for essential amino acids.

Factorial Approach to Estimating Requirements

Young, *et al.* [170,171] have used other methods in evaluating the protein and amino acid requirements of the elderly. Among these is the factorial approach in which the losses of "obligatory" nitrogen via urine and feces are measured and combined with other nitrogen losses through the skin and other quantitatively minor routes. When these losses are measured after the subject has been on a nitrogen-free diet for several days, the combined losses are regarded as equivalent to minimum dietary protein requirement of good quality protein. When obligatory urinary nitrogen excretion was measured in healthy elderly women, Young, *et al.*,[170,171] found values similar to those for young women when these obligatory urinary nitrogen losses were expressed in terms of milligrams per kilogram per day or grams nitrogen per day. However, if expressed in terms of milligrams per kilogram of body cell mass per day (body cell mass having been measured in elderly women using whole body ^{40}K measurements), milligrams per basal Calorie, and grams per gram of urinary creatinine, the derived values for elderly women were appreciably higher than those for young women. They also observed that the obligatory fecal nitrogen loss from elderly women was comparable to that reported for young women. Total obligatory nitrogen losses were also found to be similar.

Using all their collected data and applying the factorial approach, Young, *et al.*,[170,171] have concluded that 0.42 grams of protein per kilogram per day would be a safe, practical allowance for healthy elderly women.

Role of Disease Among Older Persons

Young, *et al.*,[170,171] have also reported studies of minimum protein needs of elderly women using the nitrogen balance approach which, in the hands of others, has produced inconclusive or contradictory results. Their preliminary findings support the views of others[143,144] that the minimum protein needs of healthy older adults are no greater than those of healthy young adults. They conclude that the recommendations of the Food and Nutrition Board (National Academy of Sciences — National Research Council) in its 8th revision of Recommended Dietary Allowances (RDA) in 1974[92] are adequate for most healthy, elderly persons. However, Young, *et al.*,[170,171] and Young and Scrimshaw[172] stress the influences of infection, altered gastro-intestinal function and metabolic changes prevalent among the aged as reasons for increasing the amount of protein in the diet.

Whole Body Nitrogen Turnover Studies

Perhaps more significant than other parts of their investigations, Young, *et al.*,[170,171] have reviewed whole body nitrogen turnover in the young and the elderly and have reported data collected by their application of the Picou and Taylor-Roberts model in four elderly women. This method involves administration of a tracer dose of ^{15}N-glycine continuously or at frequent intervals during a thirty to sixty hour experimental period. ^{15}N enrichment of urinary urea gradually increases to achieve a plateau from whose level it is possible to estimate the disposal rate of nitrogen through the metabolic pool and the rates of total body protein synthesis and breakdown. The data of Young, *et al.*,[170,171] suggest that protein synthesis expressed per unit of body weight gradually falls with age so that healthy elderly people have only 60 to 70 per cent of the protein synthetic capability observed in young adults. The decrement of total body protein synthesis in the elderly paralleled the decrement in their total body cell mass. Consequently, when protein synthesis per day was expressed as grams per kilogram of body weight, the figures for the elderly were 63% of those of young adults. However, when expressed as grams per kilogram of body cell mass, they were 102%. When expressed as grams per gram of creatinine excretion per day, they were 140%. When expressed per Calorie of basal metabolic rate, they were 100%.

The MIT investigators interpret these observations in the light of their hypothesis that, as muscle mass is reduced with age, creatinine excretion is decreased, and there is a greater contribution by visceral tissues to whole body protein metabolism.

N^2-methylhistidine Excretion Studies

They extended their observations on this aspect of the issue by measuring urinary N^2-methylhistidine (3-methylhistidine) excretion in young adults and elderly persons. This amino acid, present in actin of all muscles and in myosin of "white" muscle fibers, is quantitatively excreted in the urine, not being reutilized for purposes of protein synthesis. It therefore can be used as a measure of the rate and extent of the muscle protein breakdown. Investigations in six elderly women and two young men indicated that the daily output of 3-methylhistidine is much lower in old women than in young men.

When expressed per gram of urinary creatinine, the output of 3-

methylhistidine is considerably lower in elderly women, suggesting to the authors that the rate of muscle protein breakdown per unit of muscle mass declines with advancing age.

Using certain assumptions derived from an analysis of the 3-methylhistidine concentration in the mixed protein of human calf muscle, Young, *et al.* [170,171] estimate that the excretion of 277 micromoles of 3-methylhistidine is equivalent to the daily breakdown of 150 grams of muscle protein, suggesting, therefore, an equivalent amount of muscle protein synthesis in young men. By these assumptions, therefore, muscle protein accounts for more than two-thirds of the estimated rate of total body protein synthesis in young men. In contrast, the excretion of 3-methylhistidine in elderly women equals about 50 grams of muscle protein breakdown or less than fifty per cent of whole body protein synthesis. The authors maintained that such data support the thesis that protein metabolism in muscles accounts for less total body protein turnover in the elderly than in the young. From these phases of their investigations, the MIT investigators concluded that the greater contribution to total body nitrogen metabolism made by the liver and other viscera might, indeed, reduce the need for exogenous sources of nitrogen and essential amino acids.

ROLE OF ANABOLIC HORMONES

Anabolic hormones, particularly male hormones, have long been regarded as possible means of inducing nitrogen retention. The inter-relationships between the protein content of diets and androgen administration was examined by Watkin, *et al.*[173] When combined with a high protein diet, the androgen induced somewhat greater retention in eight elderly men. However, the increment achieved by androgen administration, while the subjects were consuming a low protein regimen, was less than the increment achieved by a high protein diet alone. An analysis of variance performed on data from the four men fed high and the four men fed low Calorie diets[174] revealed no Calorie influence but a marked effect of the level of protein. A modified "t" test analysis was performed to examine the role of protein level on the response of androgen administration. This analysis suggested a significant effect of hormone therapy on nitrogen balance at both levels of protein intake. However, the influence of the dietary protein level itself was of far greater statistical significance. No hormone-protein interaction was revealed from their data. The authors concluded that high protein intake is a greater stimulus to nitrogen retention than either added Calories or androgenic hormone.

RESPONSES OF OLDER PERSONS TO ABRUPT CHANGES IN PROTEIN AND AMINO ACID INTAKE

Since old age is often correlated with diminished ability to respond to stress, Watkin, *et al.*,[175,176] compared the metabolic responses of four elderly and three middle aged men to abrupt changes in protein intake. Dietary intake was changed from medium (7.0 grams nitrogen per day) to low (4.3 grams nitrogen per day) to high (13.3 grams nitrogen per day) protein content. After shifting from the medium to the low protein diet, the elderly men attained a minimal level of nitrogen loss four days sooner than did the middle aged men. When the protein intake was increased from the low to the high level, the elderly retained more nitrogen than the middle aged men both during the first five days and for thirty days after the change. No statistically significant differences in cumulative nitrogen balances between young and old were found after any shift in dietary protein level.

Couch, *et al.*,[176,177,178] made similar observations in the 70 year old man subjected to complete nitrogen withdrawal while consuming a 2800 Calorie diet containing all essential nutrients except amino acids. The subject reduced his urinary nitrogen to 2.5 grams a day, a level comparable to that observed in younger subjects, long before the end of the 12 day nitrogen free period. When L-amino acids in a casein pattern were added to the chemically defined water soluble regimen, the subject responded with strongly positive nitrogen balances.

These studies suggest convincingly that the aged respond normally to protein withdrawal and that their protein synthesis accommodates rapidly to the presence of appropriate amino acids in the substrate supplied by the diet.

SUMMARY OF PRESENT KNOWLEDGE OF PROTEIN NUTRITION AND AGING

All available evidence suggests that the protein needs of healthy elderly persons are adequately fulfilled by the 0.8 gm. protein per kg. per day of the 1980 Recommended Dietary Allowances (RDA) of the Food and Nutrition Board, National Research Council, National Academy of Sciences, Washington, D.C.[92a]

Recent claims[170,171] that specific diseases, trauma and stress, always prevalent among the elderly, increase protein needs merely restate principles enunciated by Shaffer, Coleman and DuBois[179,180,181] beginning in the first decade of this century.

Reduced renal function caused by nephron death from physiologic aging[182,183] and/or disease may require reduced protein intake and special concern for increasing the biological value of the lesser quantity of protein ingested[184]

Minimum requirements of elderly subjects for specific amino acids vary from person to person. The capacity to produce nonessential amino acids is also highly variable. These characteristics may be either disease related or the result of variable rates, presumably genetically determined, of pure physiological aging.

Investigations among carefully selected, healthy, aged (86 years of age) human subjects using modern technology have yet to be performed and are required to resolve specific scientific issues.

From a pragmatic standpoint, the protein nutrition of elderly persons should be tailored to meet their specific individual needs. These needs may reflect the older persons' exposure to disease, to trauma, to life styles or to previous eras of nutritional deprivation or nutritional excesses. The greater variance of any quantifiable biologic parameter among older persons combined with the fact that "old age" encompasses a time interval of half a century, strongly suggests that nutritional guidance should not be generic but rather individualized to meet the requirement of specific persons.

–7–

Fat

CLASSIFICATION OF DIETARY FAT

Glycerol

A three carbon alcohol, glycerol ($C_3H_8O_3$), which also has three hydroxyl groups (a trihydric alcohol), is the invariable component of all glycerides.

The Glycerides

The glycerides are esters formed by the chemical union of generally unbranched, even numbered monocarboxylic acids — the fatty acids — with glycerol. Such esters may contain one fatty acid (monoglycerides), two fatty acids (diglycerides) or three fatty acids (triglycerides). Naturally occurring fats are almost always triglycerides, all of which usually contain two or three different fatty acids.

The Fatty Acids

The fatty acids, joined by the glycerol molecule to form triglycerides in food, are characterized by their chain length, *i.e.*, the number of carbon atoms each contains, and by their degree of unsaturation, *i.e.*, the number of double (or unsaturated) bonds between adjacent carbon atoms in the chain.

Although very short chain fatty acids do exist (*e.g.*, acetic and butyric acids) and have unusual (for fatty acids) characteristics (*e.g.*, solubility in water), most fatty acids found in nature are long-chain (*e.g.*, palmitic with 16 carbon atoms and stearic with 18 carbon atoms) and are insoluble in water. Medium chain fatty acids (6-12 carbons) have received considerable attention in both animal and human nutrition in the past two decades by virtue of their availability in the form of medium chain triglycerides (MCT),[185,186] especially useful in the treatment of patients with malabsorption syndromes characterized by inability to absorb long chain triglycerides (LCT) containing from 12-18 carbons. However, triglyceride mixtures containing significant quantities of medium chain fatty acids are not found in nature but are prepared by fractionating coconut and other palm kernel oils and may be obtained through commercial processors, *e.g.*, Mead Johnson and Company, Evansville, Indiana, and Unilever Research Laboratorium, Vlardingen, Netherlands.

The fully saturated fatty acids have no double bonds and are represented by capric (10 carbons, found in coconut oil and butter), lauric (12 carbons, also found in coconut oil), myristic (14 carbons, nutmeg butter and coconut oil), palmitic (16 carbons, many animal and vegetable fats), stearic (18 carbons, also in many animal and vegetable fats), and arachidic (20 carbons, found in peanut oil).

The common unsaturated fatty acids contain from one to four double bonds and are represented by oleic acid (18 carbons, one double bond, found in olive oil, depot fat and milk), linoleic acid (18 carbons, two double bonds, found in increasing amounts in cottonseed, soybean, corn, sunflower and safflower oils), linolenic (18 carbons, three double bonds, found in linseed oil and soybean oil), and arachidonic (20 carbons, four double bonds, found never in vegetables but in relatively small pecentages of total fatty acids in depot fat and milk of animals, including man).

The polyunsaturatd fatty acids have never been demonstrated to be synthesized in rats or man and hence are frequently referred to as essential fatty acids (EFA).[187] In fact, they have also been referred to as "vitamin F".[188] However, the quantities required are very small, making it difficult to demonstrate deficiency states even in the rat, let alone in man whose diet worldwide usually contains sufficient EFA to prevent signs of deficiency.

Other Dietary Lipids

The Steroids: Steroids are grouped with the lipids largely by virtue of their mutual solubility in fat solvents but also because of certain metabolic relationships. Included in the steroid group are precursors of certain vitamins, especially the provitamins D, ergosterol in plants and 7-dehydrocholesterol in animals; many types of hormones; bile acids; certain naturally occurring drugs and poisons; and, from the standpoint of a dietary component, the sterol or steroid alcohol, cholesterol. All steroids have in common the four-ring cyclopentanoperhydrophenanthrene nucleus.

From the point of view of dietary lipids, only three steroids will be mentioned here: cholesterol, 7-dehydrocholesterol, and ergosterol.

Cholesterol is found in virtually all tissues of the human body. In blood plasma and other tissues outside the nervous system, it is found in greater quantities esterified with fatty acids. In blood plasma it is carried by lipoproteins. Cholesterol is synthesized from 2-carbon fragments such as acetic acid in the body. The synthetic rate is such that plasma cholesterol levels may remain elevated or in the normal range in the absence of any dietary cholesterol, a point which will be elaborated on below. Foods high in preformed cholesterol include, in descending rank order of milligrams per 100 gms of edible portion, brain, egg yolk, chicken liver, sweetbreads, mammalian liver, butter, shrimp, Parmesan cheese, cream cheese, turkey dark meat, and veal.[189] Cholesterol has attained notoriety in clinical medicine because of the direct correlation between plasma cholesterol levels and the prevalence of cholesterol-containing atheromatous plaques in arteries leading to a high incidence of myocardial infarcts and cerebrovascular and peripherovascular accidents (*v.i.*).

The provitamin D_3, 7-dehydrocholesterol, is found in tissues of animals in whom it is synthesized in the intestinal mucosa from cholesterol. However, to acquire vitamin D activity, it must be transported to the skin where, with exposure to ultraviolet rays, it is transformed into active vitamin D_3.

The provitamin D_2, ergosterol, is found in plants. In its nonactivated form, it has no nutritional value, since it is not absorbed in significant amounts from the intestine. However, when exposed to ultraviolet rays, ergosterol becomes activated into calciferol (vitamin D_2) which is readily absorbed.

Preformed vitamin D_2 is very rarely found in nature. Preformed vitamin D_3 is widely distributed in foods of animal origin, particularly in items such as egg yolks, milk, and fish liver. Pragmatically, however, natural foods contain so little preformed vitamin D that they can not be relied upon, in the absence of artificial enrichment, to supply a amount of vitamin D adequate for minimal human needs.

The Phospholipids: From a dietary point of view, the only phospholipid worth mentioning is lecithin, since it has been mentioned as a dietary component whose absence may lead to higher incidence rates of rheumatic heart disease[190] and since it has been a popular item in many health food stores. The most common source of dietary lecithin is egg yolk. Another source is brain. Some is of vegetable origin.

Chemically, lecithin is composed of glycerol, two fatty acids, phosphoric acid and the quarternary ammonium base, choline, an essential dietary ingredient for rats, chicks, turkeys, etc., but not for man.

ROLES OF DIETARY FAT

Calories

Fats provide on an average mixed diet 9 Calories per gram, or more than twice the number per gram supplied by carbohydrates and proteins, both of which provide only 4 Calories per gram. Hence, fats represent concentrated sources of energy. This characteristic assumes great importance in those situations demanding large numbers of Calories in small volumes and light weights of food, whether they are consumed by mouth or administered parenterally. It also is an important consideration in the design of diets for weight control, a complex topic which will be dealt with later (*v.i.*).

Specific Dynamic Action (SDA)

The specific dynamic action (SDA), sometimes called the specific dynamic effect (SDE), is the increase in heat production following the ingestion of food. According to Rubner,[191] ingestion of 100 Calories (25 grams) of protein results in the production of 130 Calories of heat; 100 Calories (25 grams) of carbohydrate, 113 Calories; and 100 Calories (11.1 grams) of fat, 105 Calories. Although Rubner's figures are universally regarded as too high, the relative size of the SDE when protein, carbohydrate and fat are fed individually is correct. Thus, fat would appear to be the most efficient source of Calories, since it results in the least loss or the least excess expenditure of Calories as a result of its ingestion. Furthermore, classic studies by Forbes and Swift[192] and Forbes, *et al.*[193-195] demonstrate that partial replacement of carbohydrate by fat in a mixed diet containing protein diminishes the energy lost via SDE. Their studies in growing animals revealed greater gains in live weight, higher protein digestibility, and greater retentions of nitrogen and energy as fat contents of diets were increased from 2 to 5 to 10 to 30 per cent. In adult animals fed 2, 5, 10, and 30 per cent fat at two Calorie levels, 45 and 65 daily, their studies demonstrated that the Calories wasted via the SDE of the extra 20 Calories decreased from 36 to 20 per cent as the fat content of the diet was increased from 2 to 30 per cent. The net effect equaled an additional 3 Calories daily for the rats on the isocaloric but higher fat diet.

The practical importance of the SDE in human nutrition has probably been overemphasized. Nonetheless, in theoretical terms, diets containing reasonable levels of fat apparently spare energy which might be wasted on diets with lower fat levels. Studies of the SDE in aged adult humans or aged animals have not been reported.

Taste

Fat is renown for its ability to increase the palatability of food. In part, this may be due to its lubricating effect. In large measure, however, the increased palatability stems from the taste imparted to the food by fats and particularly by those charred by intense heat. Fat increases the satiety of a diet by decreasing the sense of hunger between meals, since its peak absorption is delayed until about $3^1/_2$ hours after its ingestion.

Vehicle for Fat-Soluble Vitamins

Dietary fat serves as a vehicle carrying fat-soluble vitamins, *i.e.*, A, D, E, and K. As dietary fats are emulsified by bile acids, so are the fat-soluble vitamins they carry. In clinical conditions characterized by steatorrhea, *i.e.*, excessive quantities of fat in stools, symptoms and signs of deficiencies of fat soluble vitamins may occur.

Essential Fatty Acids (EFA)

Essential fatty acids, simply defined, are those which either cannot be synthesized at all or cannot be synthesized in sufficient quantities by animals that require them for growth, maintenance, and the proper function of a variety of physiologic processes. Most investigations of EFA have been conducted in growing rats.[196-198] Studies in man have included those in children[199] and in a particular East Indian condition, phrynoderma, or "toadskin".[200,201]

Since EFA are polyunsaturated fatty acids, the issue of their role in the pathogenesis of hypercholesterolemia and of atherosclerosis naturally has received considerable attention.[202,203] This aspect, however, is usually considered apart from the essential quality of fatty acids and will be dealt with later (*v.i.*).

In 1964, Van Dorp, *et al.*[204] and Bergstrom, *et al.*[205] demonstrated that prostaglandins, all derivatives of C20-cyclopentonoic (prostanoic) acid, could be synthesized from polyunsaturated fatty acids. Van Dorp, *et al.*,[206] observed that the biologically active prostaglandins are formed only from the fatty acids with considerable EFA activity. They proposed that EFA were essential solely by virtue of their role as precursors of prostaglandins. However, this theory has not been substantiated in rats, since oral or intravenous administration of prostaglandins has failed to reverse EFA deficiency.[207] Nonetheless, since prostaglandins influence blood pressure, water and electrolyte excretion, the female and male reproductive systems, the pulmonary tree, the upper respiratory system, the gastrointestinal tract,[208] the secretions of pituitary hormones,[209] and the enhancement of erythropoiesis,[210] it seems only logical that they and their precursors, EFA, may play roles in biological aging and the diseases associated with old age.

Role of Dietary Cholesterol

Dietary cholesterol is absorbed in direct proportion to the quantity of fat and the chain length of dietary fatty acids.[211] The increased absorption of cholesterol in proportion to fat intake has been attributed to the increased flow of bile occasioned by fat and the increased number of fatty acids with which cholesterol is esterified in the intestinal mucosa.[212] Cholesterol also is absorbed in proportion to the quantity in the diet, although the efficiency of absorption diminishes with increasing dose levels. Various authors disagree on the maximum quantity of exogenous cholesterol absorbable daily.[213,214,215] The range, from 0.3 gm to 2.0 gm daily, aproximates the intake range summarized by Keys for western societies.[216]

In spite of the numerous purposes cholesterol serves in the animal body, it is not an essential nutrient, since all needs for cholesterol may be fulfilled by its endogenous synthesis. The cholesterol molecule is synthesized from acetyl groups, the combining form of acetic acid.

The complete synthesis of cholesterol from acetyl-CoA and acetoacetyl-CoA is a fifteen step process.[217] One of these steps, the conversion of β-hydroxy-β-methylglutaryl-CoA (HMG-CoA) to mevalonic acid (MVA), is worthy of special mention, since it has been suggested as the point in cholesterol synthesis at which negative feedback from dietary cholesterol may reduce *in vivo* synthesis of cholesterol.[218] This negative feedback operates in animals in the liver but not in extrahepatic tissues. The same is true for man. Impairment of hepatic cholesterol synthesis has been demonstrated in persons with hypercholesterolemia.[219,220] Others have regarded hepatic negative feedback control in man as questionable.[221,222]

The HMG-CoA to MVA step has received attention more recently by virtue of some surprising results of studies by Mann and Spoerry designed to test the hypothesis that surfactants in food would increase cholesterol absorption and lead to hypercholesterolemia.[223] These studies, conducted among Massai males aged 16 to 23 who drank daily over eight liters of fermented milk containing about 1100 mg of cholesterol, revealed universal weight gains but, to the authors' surprise, reductions rather than increases in serum cholesterol levels of the Massai whether or not the milk contained the surfactant, Tween 80. The authors suggest that the fermented milk contains a substance inhibiting cholesterol synthesis. In addition, they suggest that the inhibitor may work by diminishing the activity of HMG-CoA hydroxylase, an enzyme regulating conversion of HMG-CoA to MVA. This work opens a new approach to the control of hypercholesterolemia in man.

Role of Lecithin

As noted previously (*v.s.*), the only dietary phospholipid with a real or potential role in human nutrition is lecithin. Soy lecithin has been used extensively in the preparation of fat emulsions for intravenous alimentation where it serves as an effective emulsifying agent.[224] Lecithin also is a source of choline, an essential dietary ingredient for rats, chicks, turkeys, etc., but not for man. In consideration of its role in the prevention of fatty livers in animals, choline has been used in certain therapeutic regimens for the treatment of fatty livers in humans.[225] However, such supplementation has little value if a diet adequate in protein is eaten regularly by the person with the fatty liver,[226] presumably because the methionine containing proteins provide the labile methyl groups with which the body synthesizes choline.[227]

While some dietary lecithin may be absorbed directly by the gut,[228-230] most is hydrolyzed, the components absorbed, and resynthesized in the intestinal mucosa. Since the components of lecithin (*v.s.*) are abundantly present in human diets, the practice of consuming preformed lecithin has little scientific justification. The reports of Coburn[190] emphasizing the possible role of egg lecithin deficiency in the pathogenesis of rheumatic fever and rheumatic heart disease are interesting, but have yet to be confirmed in definitive investigations and conceivably could be attributable to other dietary or environmental factors.

QUANTITY OF FAT IN HUMAN DIETS

Historical Perspective

The January, 1977 Staff Report of the United States Senate Committee on Nutrition and Human Needs entitled *Dietary Goals for the United States*[231] summarized a U.S. Department of Agriculture report[232] which showed a rise of over 25 per cent in the food Calories derived from fat in the six decades between 1910 and 1970. This was associated with a five per cent decrease in total Calorie intake, a two per cent decrease in protein Calories and a decrement of 23 per cent in carbohydrate Calories. The same Staff Report,[231] summarizing U.S. Department of Agriculture published[233] and unpublished data, indicates that the fat Calories in the average American diet increased from about 32 per cent during the 1909-1913 baseline period to 46 per cent in 1975. In the interval between 1900 and 1973, the amount of nutrient fat per capita per day increased from about 125 gms. to 156 gms.,[234] equal to an increase of over 11 kilograms per person per year.

During the last seven years reported, meat provided the greatest source of the increase in fat. Using data acquired from the American

Meat Institute, Morgan[235] reported a rise in per capita beef consumption from 38.7 kg. to 51.4 kg. between 1960 and 1971 with an additional increase to 58.4 kg. between 1971 and 1976. Not only did beef consumption rise, but the amount of fat in every kilogram of beef rose as a result of the introduction in the 1950's of feedlots where beef cattle were stuffed with more and more corn made cheap and plentiful by the introduction of hybrid seed varieties, chemical fertilizers and energy intensive methods of planting, cultivating, and harvesting.[236]

Comparable trends have been observed in other industrialized countries and have led to suggestions[237] comparable to that in the report of the U.S. Senate Select Committee on Nutrition and Human Needs which recommends a reduction of fat Calories to no more than 30 per cent of energy intake.[231]

An end to this spiraling increase in fat Calories is in sight. Unprecedented demands for American grain used to fatten animals, crop failures associated with bad weather, premature slaughtering of cattle in view of low beef prices in relation to costs of feed, and educational efforts to impress on the public the long range dangers associated with a diet high in fat Calories have combined to cause some reduction in fat intake. The Nutrition Program authorized by Title IIIc of the Older Americans Act, as Amended, recommends a nutrient standard method of menu planning and monitoring which requires meals in the menu cycles containing less than 40 per cent fat Calories.[238]

Geographic Perspective

The fat Calorie content of the American diet has increased dramatically since the first decade of the twentieth century. This increase has paralleled the rise in productivity of American agriculture, the rise in the American gross national product, and the rise in per capita income. Citizens of few countries in the world spend so small a percentage of per capita income on food as do Americans. Hence, Americans have been able to afford the substantially higher costs associated with diets high in fat Calories.

Comparisons of certain health-related parameters among Americans and citizens of countries consuming diets with lower percentages of fat Calories leave little doubt that high percentages of fat Calories contribute to the unacceptable measures of morbidity and mortality found among Americans.[239-241]

Confirmation of these gross geographic epidemiologic findings has come through studies specifically focusing on genetically related population groups residing in the United States on the one hand and in the countries from which the American groups migrated on the other. Classic among these are the studies of persons of Irish descent living in Boston and their relatives residing in the Republic of Ireland.[242]

Even more extensive are the studies of Japanese residing in the United States (both in Hawaii and in the contiguous 48) and Japanese residing in Japan.[243] In this connection, additional data on the impact of changes in diet in post World War II Japan on certain parameters among the Japanese themselves have given additional support to the concept that diets high in fat Calories are associated with higher prevalence rates for obesity and hypercholesterolemia and higher incidence rates for myocardial infarction.[244]

As suggested by findings reported by Leaf,[12] the dietary fat Calorie content needs to be related to the activity level of the particular population groups under study. Studies in Finland,[245] for example, have shown that strenuous physical work will keep plasma lipid levels in the normal range in spite of high fat diets. Mann's studies with the Massai[223] suggest not only the role of physical work but also the role of dietary substances suppressing endogenous cholesterol synthesis in controlling hypercholesterolemia in persons on diets high in fat Calories.

In regard to geographic considerations among those who are already old, data on the impact of fat Calories is sparse. Studies like Leaf's among Soviet citizens in the Trans-Caucasian Republics show little concern for excluding fat from diets but, on the other hand, indicate that diets high in yogurt and life styles replete with abundant strenuous work are associated with healthy, very active, long lives. The diets of other presumably long-lived population groups in Ecuador and Hunza[13] do suggest an association with diets low in fat Calories.

Interpretations of geographic considerations are complicated by the fact that in technically underdeveloped societies, among whom low fat, high carbohydrate, low protein diets are common, the numbers of people reaching old age by American standards are few, many dying from infectious diseases and accidents prior to reaching what Americans regard as old age.

In addition, birth and death records among technically underdeveloped societies are notoriously inaccurate, making precision in interpretation impossible. Finally, the cultural reverence for old age among societies where the total numbers of aged are small creates a protective screen about those who are old, making comparisons with conditions among the old in technically developed societies highly unrealistic.[246]

Economic Perspective

The high fat content of currently traditional American diets not only has unfavorable connotations in terms of health and happiness but also reflects an almost profligate use of economic resources. During the fattening of animals in feed lots prior to their slaughter, thousands of tons of commodities which could be consumed directly by man are transformed into fat. Relatively little is transformed into protein. The transformation of commodities into fat is associated with a very low feed efficiency ratio,[247] even lower than the low feed efficiency ratios traditionally found in the routine production of lamb, beef, or pork.[248] Hence, the over-fattening of animals used for meat production wastes resources in two ways: first, by virtue of the low feed efficiency of fat production and, second, by virtue of the fact that trimmable fat which can be readily removed from cuts of meat is included in the price of the cut. Many American consumers not only remove trimmable fat but also drain melted fat from the cut after cooking. The economic waste of these practices is obvious. For the elderly, the higher prices inspired by them are particularly onerous. Unfavorable weather in recent memory resulting in poor crop yields and higher animal feed costs promises to aggravate this already oppressive burden.

Sociological Perspective

Many present day elderly Americans passed through and out of middle age at a time when "keeping up with the Joneses" was as essential in food consumed as it was in dress or household furnishings. Not only was meat an essential staple but prime and choice cuts well marbled with saturated fat also were the order of the day. In addition, social pressures promoted by the mass media encouraged the use of butter instead of vegetable oils or margarine and downgraded nonfat dry milk solids to the status of animal feed. These forces, operating throughout American society created startling fallout. For example, diets planned for consumption by the armed forces were designed to contain as high as 50 per cent fat Calories. This planning did not result from any scientifically proven need but rather from pressures generated among citizens who firmly believed their sons and daughters deserved, while in the services, exactly the type of food they were accustomed to have placed before them at home.[249] In view of the age of most military conscriptees or recruits, the ready availability of high fat Calorie diets in the services reconfirmed, and fixed indelibly, food preferences inimicable to the health of the troops in later life, whether military or civilian. These military personnel became more liable to the diseases and disabilities associated with preferences for high fat Calorie regimens reinforced by their military dietary experiences.

Mayer[250] has referred to the need for a new American mentality to cope with the craving American society has displayed for high fat Calorie foods. The key to developing such a new mentality lies in creating new sociologic values which place premiums on the type of nutrition sanctioned by modern science,[231] rather than that evolved from market economy pressures promoted via the mass media.

In market economies, market analysts constantly assess demand for specific products and work closely with media personnel in manipulating not only the magnitude but also the qualitative aspects of this demand. Often, as pointed out by McLuhan,[251] the medium is the message, *i.e.*, persons within societal groups demand certain products and qualities in products because those products and qualities are promoted by mass media. Profit considerations, not considerations of health, usually dictate the messages rendered by the media. To add to the complexities of the problem, negative health values are actually used in promotions, *e.g.*, "product X is least likely to lead to disease Y."

The resolution of this conundrum is not easy but obviously must come from increasing the understanding by the public about the content of appropriate nutrition and from increasing the sophistication and skepticism of the public about the content of mass media messages promoting various food products. This resolution implies a massive effort by change agents in the hope of influencing public action in the direction of behavior more consonant with optimum health and vitality throughout life, including the latter two-fifths of the life span now categorized as old age.

More than ever before, elderly Americans are in position to become the vanguard of citizens whose actions resolve the conundrum, not only for themselves, but for other segments of society as well. First, they now represent an appreciable segment of the total market in the United States.[252] There are over 32 million who are 60 years of age or over, representing about 14.5 per cent of the population. Second, while one-quarter or about 8,000,000 of these live under less than ideal economic constraints,[253] three-quarters live reasonably comfortably. The disadvantaged quarter have available various income maintenance mechanisms and needs-meeting programs[253a] which assure them the means to participate by exercising consumer preferences in influencing the messages put forth by the consortium of market analysts and promoters via the mass media. Third, the elderly are organized as never before through voluntary associations who voice their needs and interests effectively to both the private and public sector.

Finally, through a network of community-based aging agencies,[254] aided by Federal and State technical assistance, the elderly are learning the application of good nutrition practices and developing sufficient knowledge and sophistication to instruct younger members of society.[254a]

Leadership of the elderly in reducing the fat Calorie content of American diets is spreading beyond their own numbers and is slowly but surely beginning to influence the content of media messages, of the fiscally-oriented messages market analysts deliver to their top management and of the political messages received by legislative and executive branches of government. The promulgation of *Dietary Goals for the United States,*[231] the first Federal action specifically directed at changing the American dietary in the direction of lower fat Calories, less salt and fewer refined carbohydrates, is only one measure of the success of consumer education and action at the political level. The amazingly large demand for this document in the first months following its release is further testimony of interest — professional, public and industrial —, interest which generated attention and some interesting action among the market analysts, mass media promoters and government officials.

While the first two of these reacted promptly and predictably to the ground swell of public interest in the *Dietary Goals for the United States,*[231] Federal government officials were more cautious, procrastinating until February, 1980, before issuing for public consumption in a booklet entitled *Nutrition and Your Health: Dietary Guidelines for Americans*[254b] information supporting the concepts incorporated in the Dietary Goals. In regard to dietary lipids, these Guidelines, although phrased to allow for modification under political pressure, stressed the role of high blood cholesterol as a major risk factor for myocardial infarction.

The Guidelines then stated: "Eating extra saturated fat and cholesterol will increase the blood cholesterol in most people." As this statement was being promulgated, the National Heart, Lung and Blood Institute, a component of the National Institutes of Health of the Department of Health, Education and Welfare (now Department of Health and Human Services), was about halfway through the sixth year of its sponsorship and direction of a ten-year double-blind clinical trial[254c] designed to test the lipid hypothesis, *i.e.,* lowering the concentration of serum cholesterol (in this instance, by use of the bile-sequestering agent cholestyramine) in human beings will reduce the incidence of myocardial infarction and certain other manifestations of atherosclerosis. Although the association of elevated serum cholesterol concentrations with atherosclerotic lesions has been known since the first decade of the twentieth century, no study in humans has demonstrated that reducing serum cholesterol concentrations will reduce morbidity and mortality in man from atherosclerosis.

While acknowledging the controversial nature of the Dietary Goals,[321] the USDA-USDHEW 1980 Guidelines[254b] described as "sensible" that the U.S. population *as a whole* (italics by the promulgators) reduce their consumption of total fat, saturated fat and cholesterol.

In May, 1980, the other side of the acknowledged controversy was officially promulgated in *Toward Healthful Diets,*[254d] a 32-page publication of the Food and Nutrition Board prepared by a six-person task force and approved by the Governing Board of the National Research Council. In regard to lipids, the task force noted that hypercholesterolemia is one of eight risk factors statistically associated with an increased incidence of atherosclerosis. However, the task force reminded readers of their statement that risk factors ". . . cannot, without independent evidence, be considered to be causative agents of the disease."

The task force reviewed data collected world-wide in regard to the results of lowering serum cholesterol concentrations by diet and by drugs. They concluded that "... it has not been proven that lowering these levels (of high serum cholesterol and low-density lipoproteins [LDL]) by dietary intervention will consistently affect the rate of new coronary events." They recommended adjusting fat intake to the Calorie requirements of the individual, noting that many subsets of the U.S. population (*viz.*, infants, adolescent boys, pregnant teenage girls and adults performing heavy manual labor) have no need to reduce the fat content of their diets below 40 per cent of fat Calories. They recommended against an increase in the polyunsaturated : saturated (P:S) ratio.

With respect to dietary cholesterol *per se*, the task force noted that cholesterol is poorly absorbed from the gastro-intestinal tract at high levels of intake and that feedback mechanisms exist in the human body which adjust endogenous cholesterol synthesis to meet body requirements. They noted also that neither the Framingham Study[317] nor the Tecumseh Study[315,316] had demonstrated any significant correlation between cholesterol intakes and serum cholesterol concentrations among free-living persons. They reported that the Canadian Department of National Health and Welfare[254e] similarly had reached the conclusion that healthy persons deserved no specific recommendations in regard to dietary cholesterol.

The release of the Food and Nutrition Board's guidelines led immediately to a battle largely waged in the media[254f] in which the proponents of the so-called prudent course confronted those who demanded more scientific evidence before recommending as a public health measure radical changes in the American diet. As is often the case in emotionally charged issues, the battle was waged over personalities and fiscal considerations but not — simply because none existed — over scientific data.

For the elderly, publication of the two sets of guidelines,[254b,254d] although a source of media-created confusion as to optimum dietary lipid intake, placed lipid nutrition in the headlines and/or radio and television in an unprecedented manner. From these discussions, elderly persons who have a comprehension of the scientific method and some knowledge of the data base from which the conflicting opinions arise should be able to gain some useful insight into the issues challenging policy makers in the nutrition field. They should recognize that the recommendations on both sides of the dietary lipid issue have little relevance to them. They must recognize too that the lipid hypothesis with respect to the pathogenesis of coronary atherosclerosis is now for the first time being tested and that the results of that research will not be available until the middle of the decade. Finally, elderly persons must recognize that no information is presently available regarding the influence of lipid nutrition on the health of persons who are truly aged, *i.e.*, those 86 years of age and older who have survived more than three-quarters of the technical life span of man. Serious, long and expensive longitudinal studies will be needed to provide data which may yield guidance for future generations.

Ready Reserves of Dietary Human Fat

Frequently unrecognized is an enormous reserve of fat available as an energy source for the American population. It is that fat already present in the adipose tissue of millions of Americans. This fat is available not via cannibalistic consumption as occurred among survivors of the tragic Andean plane crash of October, 1972,[255] but rather via normal metabolic processes induced to an appropriate quantitative level of activity by combinations of reductions of dietary Calorie intake and increments of Calorie expenditures by physical work.

If one assumes: (1) an American population aged 18 and over composed of 71.46 million males and 78.54 million females;[252] (2) a mean ideal weight for white and nonwhite adult males of 70 kg. and mean ideal weights for white adult females of 58 kg. and for nonwhite adult females of 57 kg.;[256] (3) obesity defined as 120 per cent of ideal weight;[257,258] and (4) prevalence rates of obesity of 15 per cent among all white adult males (n = 63.51 million), 10 per cent among all nonwhite adult males (n = 7.953 million), 20 per cent among all white adult females (n = 69.25 million) and 30 per cent for all nonwhite adult females (n = 9,291 million),[256] a minimum of 336,940,420 kg. of excess fat is available among the obese alone for purposes of providing energy. This is a conservative estimate, sinçe mean weights of measured population groups always exceed median weights,[256] suggesting that many obese Americans weigh more than 120 per cent of ideal weight.

In terms of energy, these kilograms of excess fat amount to over three trillion Calories, 1.30 trillion Calories for obese adult males and 1.73 trillion Calories for obese adult females. If an allowance of 2400 Calories per day is granted to men and 1800 Calories per day to women,[92a] the excess fat in the obese men alone would provide enough Calories for 52.5 days for all obese adult men and for 57.8 days for all obese women, assuming no other Calorie intake.

These approximations strongly suggest the rationale of limiting dietary fat Calories intake as well as total dietary Calories, since the high concentration of Calories in fat provides the most efficient and taste appealing way of producing Calorie imbalance and thereby obesity in man. Recognition of this huge reserve and deliberate planning to utilize it as an energy resource for man are steps which could improve the physical, emotional and fiscal health of Americans.

Although obesity is less common among the elderly,[259] it does exist and should be treated as it should be in members of younger age groups. However, in view of data recently assembled by Andres,[259a] great care should be exercised in determining what degree of obesity deserves vigorous treatment. Most importantly, if obesity can be avoided or treated successfully in youth or middle age, fewer adults will reach old age disabled by the various stigmata associated with excessive corpulence.[260-263]

HEALTH AND DIETARY FAT

Quantitative Aspects

Obesity: Imbalance between Calorie intake and Calorie expenditure, if favoring the former, inevitably will lead to overweight which, if sufficiently in excess of ideal standards, may be categorized as obesity. The high Calorie density of fat, nine Calories per gram, makes fat the nutrient which has the greatest potential for contributing to human obesity. This potential is enhanced by the excellent flavor which fat imparts to foods of which it is a component, making such foods more irresistible to persons attempting to limit their Calorie consumption. Dietary regimens comprising 40 per cent or more of fat Calories have the greatest potential for contributing to high prevalence rates for obesity. While it is true that total Calorie intake from whatever source must be balanced against Calorie expenditure if any person's body weight is to remain constant, the high Calorie density and the seductive flavor of fat give it the properties which enable it to contribute more than carbohydrate or protein to the high prevalence of obesity in the United States.

Obesity has long been associated with high prevalence rates for cardiovascular-renal diseases, diabetes, biliary tract and other liver diseases, arthritis, and hernias.[257,260-265] Among the elderly, obesity is common in the age group 60-70 but becomes increasingly rare in later decades. Cross sectional studies [266] show declines in average body weight with age after 60. This often has been interpreted as indicating higher mortality among the obese resulting in diminished average weight among lighter survivors. Recent longitudinal studies in Baltimore [267] in which specific individuals were followed over intervals of eight years suggest that average weight decrements occur within individuals starting with the decade between ages 55 and 64. Cross sectional studies of dietary intake of participants in the Baltimore study [268] and in others,[269] have shown decrements in total Calorie intake during the interval of weight loss and, significantly, also decrements in intake of dietary fat.

In interpreting the more recent data, it is important to recognize that the Baltimore longitudinal data were derived from studies in highly motivated, well-educated, relatively prosperous persons who were or had been engaged in professional or managerial occupations.[270] These comprise a population characterized by a low prevalence of obesity and who are receptive to health education messages pointing to the hazards of obesity and of consumption of dietary regimens high in fat Calories. The data should not be interpreted as indicating that obesity is a benign condition which will go away with advancing age or that it has no relevance to effective longevity.

Not only are prevalence rates for diseases far higher among obese, but incidence rates for accidents also are higher. Since many of the victims of such diseases or accidents require treatment entailing confinement to bed, the nursing care involved in their treatment is made inordinately more difficult merely by virtue of their excessive weight. Hence, not only does obesity contribute to the need for treatment in bed, but also obesity diminishes the chances for top quality care and thereby decreases the salvage rates well below those characteristic of normal weight persons suffering comparable pathology.

However, theory and statistical associations render no scientific proof in the sense of validating that cause (in this case, obesity) yields effect (the diseases associated with obesity.[257,260-265]) In fact, Andres [259a] has reported lower mortality rates for persons in the 110-130 per cent of ideal weight (defined as the center of the range in the medium frame desirable weight table of the Metropolitan Life Insurance Company) [259b] categories than for those in the 80-110 per cent categories. His reports have been confirmed by reanalyses of data collected during the Framingham Heart Study.[259c] Both groups have ruled out the role of persons with disease-induced cachexia by observing that no decrements in weight occurred in participants in longitudinal studies prior to the diagnosis of an illness which would terminate their lives in one year or less. Andres offered two interpretations of these findings.[259a] First, some persons may be harmed by overweight while others may be helped provided it is not morbid obesity (130 per cent of standard weight or more). More research will be needed to characterize accurately those who will be harmed and those who will be helped. Second, the Metropolitan Life Insurance Company's desirable weight tables give values that are too low. In this second interpretation, Andres enjoys the concurrence of the Framingham investigators.[259c]

Obviously, prevention of obesity or overwieght by judicious limitation of fat Calorie intake throughout life would be an ideal resolution of a serious problem. But what can be done or should be done for an elderly person who has survived even though obese? This is an issue charged with emotion. Unfortunately, little data exists which might enable serious investigators to substitute knowledge for passion. Efforts to change dietary habits and to induce weight reduction among the overweight and obese elderly are often ridiculed by those who believe the elderly deserve tolerance of their ingrained habits or who are convinced that elderly persons cannot be changed regardless of the intensity of the efforts directed at them.

Evidence is abundant that elderly persons can, will, and do change their behavior when instructed how and encouraged to do so.[271] Whether such changes should be instigated is at present a matter more in the philosophical than in the scientific realm. Since presently available objective data are inadequate to draw firm conclusions as to the value of dietary intervention in diminishing the prevalence of obesity in the younger aging, a philosophical stand, rooted in logic and the need-to-know the results of carefully planned intervention, is the only stand presently acceptable. Such a stand expressed for the older person was eloquently stated by the late Justice of the Supreme Court of the United States, Oliver Wendell Holmes:[272] "Some people you know as they approach 70 begin to read the Bible and prepare to die; others prepare to live until they are 90. Now if the ones who prepare to live to 90 die at 70, they won't know the difference. But if the ones who prepare to die at 70 live until they are 90, their last 20 years will be hell." Justice Holmes died at 93.

Such philosophy, applied to the fat Calorie content of the diet of the obese and overweight elderly individual, suggests the need to reduce fat Calorie intake and, of course, keep the total Calorie intake below estimated Calorie expenditures. In view of data acquired in the Baltimore longitudinal studies, such reductions induced early in old age may merely accelerate a trend which, without intervention, might occur at a later time. Such acceleration, when considered in the light of obesity's association with morbidity[257,260-265] and now its uncertain status *vis a vis* mortality,[259a,259c] in theory might lead to more years of effective longevity or, on the contrary, to a more rapid demise.

Philosophical approaches, no matter how logical to the nonstatistically oriented, are generally unacceptable to the scientific community until substantiated by well-designed and meticulously conducted investigations producing quantifiable, objective data subject to conclusive statistical analysis. Because of the time, personnel, and equipment involved in implementing and conducting such investigations in adequate numbers of people, such studies are becoming increasingly rare.[273] As a result, the lay public is receiving, via mass media and publishing houses, substantial quantities of advice based on no evidence or on scientific concepts distorted to meet the needs of the promoter. Obesity is a favorite condition toward which such advice is directed.

A recent example of such advice is contained in *Dr. Atkins' Diet Revolution: The High Calorie Way to Stay Thin Forever.*[274] The best-seller status of this publication not only revealed the public hunger for slenderizing without deprivation[275] but also engendered a forceful critique from the Council on Foods and Nutrition of the American Medical Association.[276] The critique noted that low carbohydrate and therefore high fat diets were not new, having been prescribed by William Harvey[277] and attested to favorably by a patient, William Banting, in 1863.[278] Over the years, many such diets have received public acclaim only to fall into obscurity. Meanwhile, in spite of periodic resurrections of diets promising universal and painless weight reduction, the prevalence of obesity has continued to rise.

In their critique, the Council on Foods and Nutrition presented evidence that the rationale used by Atkins was without scientific merit; that no controlled clinical studies to validate the claims had ever been conducted; that the diet was potentially hazardous to patients with atherosclerosis; that such a regimen produces anorexia and some transient weight loss but has little potential for widespread acceptance; and that "... no reliable mechanism exists to help the public evaluate and put into proper perspective the great volume of nutritional information and misinformation with which it is constantly being bombarded."

The critique contained over 40 references to scientific work which severely indicted the concept promoted by Atkins. Why then has the Atkins' diet been one of the more enduring of a long series of comparable regimens? In part, its popularity may stem from the fact that detection of ketone bodies in the urine by a simple dip-stick or tape test enables the dieter to check regularly his adherence to the regimen. In part, also, is the fact that, indisputably, the diet succeeds in inducing short-term losses of weight in many who try it. Since the first law of thermodynamics has not been circumvented, it must be assumed that the low carbohydrate, high fat regimen results in diminished Calorie intake.

Recently, Lewis, *et al.*[279] compared in 10 obese young men the responses to two cholesterol-free liquid formula diets, both containing 10 Calories per kg. body weight per day and 20 per cent of total Calories derived from protein. One diet contained 70 per cent carbohydrate Calories and 10 per cent fat Calories; the other, 70 per cent fat Calories and 10 per cent carbohydrate Calories. A weight maintenance diet containing 30 Calories per kg. per day, 20 per cent protein Calories, and 40 per cent both fat and carbohydrate Calories was used as a control diet before and after use of the experimental diets.

Weight loss on the high fat was greater than that noted on the high carbohydrate regimen. However, when the control diet was resumed after 14 days on the experimental diets, marked retentions of water and sodium and rapid weight gain occurred only after the high fat regimen, with the result that no significant difference in weight decrement between diets was observed. The authors attributed the difference to aqueous loss during consumption of the high fat diet. The high fat diet also led to a seven-fold increase in ketonemia, greater decrements in fasting glucose and insulin concentrations, lesser decrements in fasting glucagon concentrations, a 50 per cent fall in the insulin:glucagon molar ratio, and greater falls in serum triglyceride ($p < 0.01$) and cholesterol concentrations (not significant), attributable entirely to decrements in very low density lipoproteins. Hyperuricemia developed during consumption of the high fat diet. Free fatty acids increased similarly on both diets, suggesting in the light of other data, a shift of hepatic free fatty acid metabolism away from triglyceride synthesis and toward ketone body production.

Lewis, *et al.* conclude that the equal efficacy in lasting weight loss of the two diets, the greater hyperketonemia and the hyperuricemia observed with the high fat diet and the striking decrement in the insulin: glucagon ratio on the high fat diet suggest that high carbohydrate diets are preferable weight loss regimens.

While their experiment was conducted in young men for only a short period of time, the results attained in a meticulously conducted metabolic study suggest that elderly persons seeking to lose weight should avoid high fat regimens and should seek weight loss via diets low in fat accompanied by appropriate physical activity.

The gullibility of a public ever seeking easy solutions to difficult problems has been demonstrated once more by the heyday of the "Last Chance Diet"[279a] just before being branded a potential hazard to health by the U. S. Food and Drug Administration[279b] and the Center for Disease Control.[279c] This regimen comprises predigested proteins derived from hides and tendon to which flavoring agents are added to disguise the otherwise offensive taste and odor. Taken in liquid form, these proteins apparently satiate appetite enabling the consumer to tolerate the low Calorie regimen. Consumer ketosis indicating fat catabolism is also observed. While psychologically effective, this regimen containing only protein of low biological value leads in faithful adherents to potassium losses from muscle and myocardium which in several persons have led to cardiac arrythmias and death. The cost of such regimens exceeded $5.00 per pint, a high price to pay for an undistinguished and potentially dangerous substitute for willpower and common sense.

Emaciation and cachexia: While obesity and overweight have received major billings near the top of the rank order in terms of their prevalence as health problems in the United States *(v.s.),* underweight and particularly those degrees of underweight which may be characterized as emaciation and cachexia, while ranked far lower in rank order of priority based on their prevalence, are no less menacing to the affected individual. Moreover, they pose therapeutic problems of magnitudes and complexity far greater than do those associated with the treatment of overweight and obesity.

Among the elderly, especially those in the older age groups, *i.e.*, those 76 years of age and older, emaciation and cachexia may have many roots, all of which may be interrelated. Imperative, therefore, in planning the management of such problems is a thorough diagnostic evaluation. The details and the complexities of such an evaluation have been described.[280] They encompass careful considerations of potential anatomic, physiologic and biochemical pathology. Among the potential components of such pathology are neoplastic disease; untreated diabetes mellitus; adrenocortical insufficiency; hyper- and hypothyroidism; untreated myocardial failure; renal insufficiency; anemias of a variety of pathogeneses; residisua of cerebro- and peripherovascular accidents; inherited and acquired neurologic disease; arthritides; disabilities from accidents; visual, auditory, gustatory and olfactory pathology; pulmonary diseases; complications of prior surgery; oral and dental pathology and/or poorly functioning prostheses; and functional disturbances of the gastrointestinal tract.

Obviously, the accumulations of lifetimes of exposure to pathogenic organisms; environmental hazards; deleterious personal habits such as smoking and drug and alcohol abuse; dietary indiscretions; accidents; and inappropriate medical and dental care increase the complexities inherent in diagnoses when only straightforward biomedical pathologies are involved. When psychiatric disorders and socioeconomic problems, common among the elderly, are added to this list, another order of magnitude is added to the complexities of diagnosing and managing emaciation and cachexia among the elderly. In addition, the problems mentioned above initiate vicious cycles in which the original disorders are aggravated by malnutrition when the latter develops through ignorance on the part of or neglect by others of elderly persons.

The prevention of emaciation and cachexia among the elderly is a matter of education of those still young or middle aged or of the elderly who still manifest ideal weight. The education consists largely of indoctrinating the pupils with the concepts of the nutrition-health-aging triad which have been enunciated above *(v.s.)*.

However, when elderly persons are already emaciated and cachectic, their rehabilitation involves the judicious use of fat Calories in conjunction with other nutrients. The previously described high Calorie density of fat and the excellent flavor it imparts to food are properties which enable fat to serve admirably in the management of emaciation and cachexia. Creating accumulations of Calories in excess of expenditures is an essential step, equal in importance to attacking any underlying pathology which may be present. Whether incorporated into tube feedings, into orally administered diet supplements, or into regular meals, fat provides a maximum number of Calories in the smallest possible volume. When combined judiciously with other nutrients and Calorie sources, it affords the best and quickest route to Calorie accumulation. When parenteral feeding is indicated, fat in emulsified form provides the same desirable high caloric density per unit volume.

Important also in such rehabilitation is attention to the regularity with which the therapeutic regimen is consumed. Even the most scientifically and artistically designed regimens will do no good unless they are consumed consistently.

Also essential in such rehabilitation is incorporation of the "eighth nutrient group", *i.e.*, physical exercise, into the process. At its inception, such exercise may consist only of very simple passive and active movements in bed.[281] As soon as possible, however, the exercise regimen should include sitting, standing, walking, and even more vigorous activities. Such physical activity is essential to achieve the maximum anabolic effect of the fat-nutrient dietary mixture.[282] In addition, such exercise improves the microcirculation in the heart and skeletal muscles.[283] It is associated with dramatic increases in life satisfaction and morale.[284] It effectively counteracts the various undesirable results of consuming diets high in fat Calories.[285]

As the emaciated person gains weight, consideration need be given to adding more carbohydrate foods and reducing the quantity of fat served. Weaning the formerly emaciated person away from the high fat Calorie regimen and onto a more conventional dietary regimen is the final stage of the nutritional rehabilitation process.

Cardiovascular diseases: Apart from their potential for inducing obesity, which in itself has strong associations with cardiovascular pathology, dietary regimens high in fat Calories have been associated with high prevalence rates for hypercholesterolemia which, in turn, have been associated with high incidence rates for myocardial infarctions.[285-291] However, agreement on the influence of dietary fat Calories on serum cholesterol levels is by no means universal.

In their classic study of human starvation,[292] Keys, *et al.* summarize data on acute starvation from 1913 through 1943 by observing that "during short fasts there is no consistent change in lipids other than cholesterol" whose serum concentration generally increased. While methodologic problems made interpretation of semi-starvation during World War I and World War II difficult, Keys, *et al.* interpret the literature as indicating that "semi-starvation produces little if any change in the blood lipid levels except for a decrease in cholesterol . . . in contrast to the suggestive slight increase in this component during acute starvation."

In the "Minnesota Experiment" conducted from November, 1944, through December, 1945, Keys, *et al.* compared plasma cholesterol levels of 23 male subjects in their early twenties at the end of a 12 week period on a control diet and at the end of a 24 week period on a semi-starvation regimen. The control diet averaged 3180 Calories of which 37.1 per cent was derived from fat. The semi-starvation regimen averaged 1704 Calories of which 18.2 per cent was derived from fat. The mean level of cholesterol per 100 ml. of plasma was 169.3 mg ± 24.0 (SD) at the end of the control phase and 150.7 mg. ± 21.7 at the end of the semi-starvation phase. All but five of the 23 subjects showed a decrease in plasma cholesterol concentration. While the absolute change was not large, the consistency of the change was such as to make it statistically highly significant. The authors concluded that the preponderance of evidence indicates that semi-starvation regimens, almost always low in fat Calories, are associated with decreased concentrations of serum or plasma cholesterol.

Since the subjects lost an average of 6.80 kg. of fat during 24 weeks on the semi-starvation regimen, they added to the 34.4 gm of dietary fat (comprising the 18.2 per cent fat Calories) 40.5 gm fat daily from their own fat stores. Hence, the fat actually metabolized daily was 74.9 gm, or 39.6 per cent fat Calories, more than the 37.1 per cent fat Calories during the control phase when body weights of the 23 subjects were constant. It is possible, therefore, that factors other than the reduced fat Calories in the semi-starvation diet were involved in the reductions in plasma cholesterol.

Keys, *et al.* report plasma cholesterol concentrations after six weeks of rehabilitation in only five of the 23 subjects. The one on a diet of 1984 Calories had an increase from 157 to 218 mg. per ml of plasma; the one on a diet of 2329 Calories, from 127 to 171; the one on a diet of 2928 Calories, from 171 to 202; and two on a diet of 3035 Calories, from 188 to 191 and 128 to 193, respectively. All five, at the end of six weeks of rehabilitation, had plasma cholesterol concentrations higher than at the end of the control phase.

The "Minnesota Experiment" was among the first modern studies in man whose data relating diet to serum cholesterol concentrations can be accepted as valid. It also supplies data on a range of parameters, *e.g.*, changes in body fat mentioned above. Nonetheless, since dietary changes included reductions in total, protein and carbohydrate Calories as well as fat Calories, little can be said in regard to the effect of fat Calorie reduction *per se.*

More recent studies have left the influence of fat Calories on serum cholesterol in a somewhat less confused but still uncertain status. Studies of extremely low fat Calorie diets such as the rice diet[40,41,293] produced unquestionable reductions in serum cholesterol. Epidemiologic investigations of population groups consuming diets with various percentages of fat Calories have strongly suggested the direct relationship of dietary fat Calories to serum cholesterol concentrations.[294-298] Yudkin,[249] however, has cast doubt on the meaning of this relationship in comparable societies by noting the four-fold range of morbidity from coronary artery disease in Norway, Denmark, the United Kingdom, Canada, and the United States where fat intakes are essentially the same.

Clinical investigations in which dietary fat Calories were controlled have suggested that reduced fat Calories are more effective than lipotropic agents,[300] cholesterol restriction,[301] sitosterol ingestion,[302] or ethyl linoleate ingestion.[303] Many studies employing the diet suggested by the American Heart Association (AHA)[304] have been reported as showing reduction in serum cholesterol levels.[305-307] However, the AHA diet, in addition to containing 35 per cent fat Calories or less, also contains daily less than 300 mg. cholesterol, less than 10 per cent of Calories in the form of saturated fats, and emphasizes fruits, vegetables, and lean meat, fish or poultry.

In two varieties of monkey, the Rhesus[308] and the Cebus,[309] high fat diets have produced xanthomatosis and atherosclerosis.

Moore, Young, and Maynard,[310] studying women aged 16 to 66, found no relation between dietary fat or fat Calories and changes in lipids in the blood. However, their studies involved diets high in fat Calories and were conceived to study weight loss on low Calorie regimens. Apart from questions of adherence to the regimens, fluctuations in the blood lipid levels were wide. Schroeder[311] reported no significant changes in plasma cholesterol on diets containing less than 20 per cent fat Calories in patients who later responded to a combination of linolenic acid, calcium disodium ethylenediamine-tetraacetate and pyridoxine. Conner, Stone and Hodges[312] reported that the effect of dietary cholesterol was independent of that of dietary fat, noting that a cholesterol free diet resulted in reduced serum cholesterol in spite of a high saturated fat intake. Conner and Conner[313] reported a higher correlation between dietary cholesterol and mortality from atherosclerosis than for total or animal fat Calories.

Cox, *et al.*[314] reported that dietary fat alone produced no significant hypercholesterolemia in Rhesus monkeys.

In an investigation of the relationships of dietary Calorie sources to cholesterol and triglyceride levels in 957 men and 1082 women participating in the Tecumseh study, Nichols, *et al.*[315] found that the mean daily consumption of fat Calories (and other measured components as well) was virtually identical among all tertiles of cholesterol and triglyceride concentrations. Men consumed quantitatively more fat than women. Similar findings among Tecumseh participants have been reported by the same authors using the food frequency method of evaluating individual diets.[316] Other dietary surveys conducted among participants in the Framingham,[317] the Israel Ischemic Heart Disease,[318] and the Evans County, Georgia[319] studies have revealed no significant relationships between fat Calorie and other nutrient intakes and serum cholesterol levels.

The difficulty in obtaining a clear-cut answer to the question of whether quantitative reductions in dietary fat Calories are consistently associated with reductions in serum cholesterol concentrations is probably accounted for by the multifactorial etiology of hypercholesterolemia and of atherosclerosis. Hence, many investigations have been designed to explore influences other than fat Calories *(v.i.)*. The failure of the Tecumseh, Framingham, and similar studies to confirm positive influences of dietary fat Calories on serum lipid levels anticipated as a result of epidemiologic studies comparing population groups[242,243,294,320] in no way refutes the validity of the comparative studies. In the studies referred to,[315-319] fat Calorie intakes are at the upper end of the worldwide distribution of fat Calorie intakes. In many, obesity, also highly correlated with lipid concentrations, is prevalent.[316,321] Hyperglycemia,[322] season of the year,[319,323,324] age of the subjects,[325] their level of physical activity,[319,326] their dietary cholesterol intake,[312,313] possibly their fiber intake,[327-330] their intake (especially in men) of alcohol,[315,331-333] and the prevalence of hyperlipoproteinemias,[334,335] are all factors correlated with serum cholesterol concentrations. In population studies among relatively affluent, free-living societies, these factors may obscure the associations among specific nutrients and serum lipids which would be anticipated from comparisons of societies of widely differing economic conditions or from highly controlled investigations on metabolic study units.

For these reasons, proof by established scientific methods of the value of fat Calorie restriction in the control of cholesterol concentrations or of cardiovascular diseases technically is not available. This lack of proof has been responsible for such cautiously worded recommendations as those of the American Medical Association's Council on Foods and Nutrition[336] who espoused in 1962 the philosophy that manipulations of dietary fat should be regarded as experimental procedures only, as far as the prevention and treatment of atherosclerosis is concerned.

More recently, Ahrens[337] in 1976 has pointed to the unimpressive results obtained in major diet and drug trials.[45,338-347] He believes the lipid hypothesis has been inadequately tested and urges a two phase approach to testing the theory. First, he would establish that a combined diet/drug regimen is acceptable to, harmless to, and adhered to for years by adult male patients with hyperlipidemia. Second, he would proceed to use the acceptable, harmless, easy-to-adhere-to regimen in a study of its effectiveness in reducing the incidence of new coronary artery disease events. Until such data are available, Ahrens recommends that no broad scale recommendations on diets and drugs be made to the general public. As a major reason for his caution, Ahrens notes the need to have a convinced body of medical opinion supporting such public health measures if they are to be effective. He feels the medical profession is not convinced of the feasibility or the effectiveness of lipid lowering in preventing coronary heart disease. He submits that "no amount of public persuasion to change the American lifestyle will succeed until internists themselves become convinced on the basis of solid evidence." Nonetheless, he concludes by recommending that internists screen their patients for hyperlipidemia and, for patients who are found to have that and other risk factors, institute in stepwise fashion the measures which studies to date of the lipid hypothesis have proven most efficacious.

In spite of the lack of convincing proof, the U.S. Senate Select Committee on Nutrition and Human Needs in 1977 promulgated the *Dietary Goals for the United States*[265] in which the recommendation for diets containing 30 or less per cent fat Calories is included. The Select Committee, in effect, cut the Gordian knot.

For the elderly, many of whom are chronically ill with cardiovascular diseases, the issue of what if any dietary change to introduce has been, and will continue to be, present despite the Select Committee's bold and decisive action. Meaningful evidence that changes in diet after age 55 will alter the morbidity and mortality rates is lacking.[348,349,349a] Nonetheless, if for no reason other than the fact that consuming a diet low in fat Calories may lead indirectly to other improvements in the diet of the elderly *(e.g.,* increases in the intake of vitamins and minerals from protective foods through isocaloric substitutions for the empty Calories of fat), conformity by the elderly with the *Dietary Goals for the United States* is indicated. Furthermore, by setting examples for those who are not yet old, the elderly have an opportunity to participate in health promotion among younger age groups where restriction of dietary fat Calories has a far greater chance of affecting morbidity and mortality from cardiovascular disease for those who will be old in the future. Finally, since no data from longitudinal studies on the effect of reducing fat Calories in diets of free-living elderly have been published, there is no absolute scientific proof that benefits may not accrue, especially if reductions in fat Calories are combined with other recommendations in the *Dietary Goals for the United States.*

An exception to the evidence that plasma lipid concentrations are poor predictors of risk from coronary artery disease has resurfaced after lying dormant for over a quarter-century.[349b] High density lipoproteins, also referred to as α-lipoproteins and α-cholesterol, have been found to be better predictors of coronary artery disease than other plasma lipids.[349c-f] Particularly significant to those caring for persons already old is the fact that high density lipoproteins retain their predictive quality beyond age 55. The correlations are inverse, *i.e.,* the higher the concentrations of high density lipoproteins, the lower the incidence of coronary heart disease. Glueck, *et al.*[349g] have reported that elevated high density lipoprotein concentrations characterized long-lived families.

The relation of these observations to nutrition has yet to be examined in detail. One study among men of Japanese ancestry in Hawaii[349h] suggested that moderate alcohol consumption — up to 60 ml. per day, mainly from beer — was correlated positively ($r = 0.28$) with high density lipoprotein levels and hence with lower rates of incidence for coronary heart disease.

The mechanisms underlying the inverse correlations between high density lipoprotein concentrations to coronary artery disease (and obesity)[349c] are not understood. However, various investigators have suggested that the high density lipoproteins are scavengers removing cholesterol from deposits[349i] and disturbing the uptake of excess cholesterol by cells.[349j,349k]

Evidence that low fat Calorie regimens are harmful has not been presented. On the other hand, a substantial literature exists[40,350-355] indicating that diets high in carbohydrate Calories improve the clinical and biochemical status of diabetics, many of whom are elderly and all of whom, like the elderly, are at higher risk from cardiovascular diseases. One study in normal young men aged 18 to 22 showed marked deterioration of oral glucose tolerance tests when their diets were changed from a control diet with 43 per cent fat Calories to one containing 65 per cent fat Calories. The same subjects showed marked improvement when the glucose or sucrose content was increased to 80 per cent of total Calories.[356] Another study in which mild to severe diabetics were switched from an American Diabetic Association diet containing 34 per cent fat Calories to one containing 75 per cent carbohydrate Calories, 9 per cent fat Calories and 9.5 gm daily more crude fiber than the control diet, reported discontinuation of insulin or sulfonylureas in nine out of thirteen, reduction of insulin requirements in one, and no change in three with relatively high exogenous insulin requirements.[357] The group of 13 showed highly significant reductions in mean serum cholesterol and a 15 per cent reduction in mean fasting serum triglyceride concentrations.

Additional comments on dietary fat in diets of patients with diabetes mellitus appear immediately below.

Diabetes Mellitus: The nutritional aspects of the prophylaxis and treatment of obesity, atherosclerosis and diabetes mellitus share many common threads. Several of these have received attention in the sections on "Obesity" and "Cardiovascular Disease" above *(v.s.)*. Among them also are many of the same risk factors.[358] Hence, interventions directed at one condition may benefit the others. Among these interventions, changes in traditional patterns of nutrition loom large but by no means stand alone.

Among the elderly, diabetes mellitus is a common disorder, but how common is a matter of some dispute.[359,360] The controversy arises from the fact that studies applying various tolerance tests[361-364] have suggested that man's ability to metabolize carbohydrate is reduced with advancing age. By some, this is regarded as a function of the ever increasing incidence of true diabetes as age advances.[360] Andres,[365-367] and Andres and Tobin,[364] however, propose that this is a nonpathologic manifestation of aging in a general population. Andres and Tobin[364] have derived an oral glucose tolerance test nomogram[367] by which performance on tolerances tests may be judged in the light of the subjects' ages. They urge that this standard be used instead of an arbitrary number applying to all ages, and that the results of tolerance tests should be correlated with the results of long-term longitudinal follow-up studies. Andres[367] maintains that until it is clear (a) what level of tolerance test performance connotes increased risk, (b) that prophylaxis is possible and, (c) that treatment is helpful, a conservative attitude toward classifying middle-aged or elderly subjects as diabetics on the basis of poor tolerance test performance alone is indicated.

This controversy again reflects the difficulty faced by public health oriented medical scientists in making recommendations in regard to large population groups. If Andres is right, many middle-aged and elderly persons are saddled unnecessarily with the psychological, economic, and logistic burdens of diabetes mellitus. On the other hand, if he is wrong, as suggested by the relatively unsophisticated reappraisal[360] 22 years later of participants in the 1946-1947 Oxford, Massachusetts study, many true diabetics will be erroneously reassured and thereby fail to seek opportunities for prophylactic and corrective measures.

As pointed out in the section on "Cardiovascular Disease" above, the preinsulin and early insulin eras' concern for limiting the carbohydrate content of the diabetics' dietary regimens has slowly but surely given way to liberalization of the per cent carbohydrate Calories in the regimen and has been replaced by concerns over the total Calorie content of the regimen and, particularly, over its fat Calorie content. These concepts have been reflected in statements by an expert committee of the American Diabetes Association[368] and by others.[369,370]

West,[371,372] in analyzing and summarizing the problems and potentials of nutrition in the prevention and treatment of diabetes mellitus, has emphasized the differences in nutritional needs among the two major and other minor categories of diabetics. The two major types are (a) maturity-onset obese diabetics and (b) insulin-dependent nonobese diabetics. Other special types of diabetics may have more varied requirements. They include lean persons with mild diabetes who do not require insulin, insulin-dependent diabetics who are fat, and hyperlipemic diabetics whose blood lipid levels are especially sensitive to dietary carbohydrate. Another group not mentioned by West comprises those insulin-dependent diabetics whose β-cells still produce endogenous insulin at variable rates and who, therefore, must constantly be on the alert against hypoglycemia.

Among the elderly, maturity-onset obese diabetics have much to gain by adherence to regimens designed to decrease total Calorie intake, increase total Calorie expenditure through physical activity, or preferably both, with a view toward reduction of adiposity toward and to ideal weight. Not only does weight reduction reduce hyperglycemia, but also it reduces the insulin resistance associated with obesity, thereby improving islet beta-cell function. For these diabetics, limitation of diet Calories from whatever source is the primary therapeutic objective. Regular eating habits including the elimination of snacking between meals and at bedtime are helpful in achieving the desired goal. Elimination of all biochemical evidences of diabetes is unusual only because weight is rarely reduced to and maintained in the ideal range.[372] As noted in the discussions in the section of "Obesity" above, limitation of dietary fat with its high caloric density improves the chances of attaining and maintaining ideal weight.

Insulin-dependent, nonobese diabetics in the older age category have more complex schedules, physical activity regimens, dietary needs, and precautions to observe. First, they should receive their insulin at the same time or times daily. Second, their physical activity should be regularized as to time and amount daily or special provisions made to reduce insulin dosages or consume extra food. Third, they should consume daily meals and between-meal snacks so that their food consumption is distributed to conform as closely as possible to the time-action pattern of administered insulin. This helps prevent postprandial hyperglycemia and is an organized way of protecting against hypoglycemia. Finally, they should be trained in how to contend effectively with absent or delayed meals, unplanned physical exertion, and acute illnesses, and in how to recognize and respond to the early signs of impending hypoglycemia. Liberalization of carbohydrate and limitation of fat Calories to less than 30 per cent make meal planning within the Calorie range required to maintain weight simpler and afford, when the timing, division, quantities and qualities of the carbohydrates are appropriately planned, the greatest possible protection against hypoglycemia.

The more special types of diabetics require appropriate modifications of the regimens suggested above to meet their special requirements. Even diabetics with type IV hyperlipoproteinemia respond well to low fat, higher carbohydrate diets when complex carbohydrates are featured and sugars and total Calories are carefully controlled in regimen planning.

The major problem, especially for elderly diabetics, lies in convincing patients, nutritionists, and physicians that liberalizing carbohydrate and diminishing fat intake are not harmful to diabetics. Education is the only solution and admittedly takes time. As an aid in the education process, Committees of the American Diabetes Association and the American Dietetic Association, in cooperation with the

National Institute of Arthritis, Metabolism and Digestive Diseases, and the National Heart, Lung and Blood Institute, have prepared a new booklet entitled "Exchange Lists for Meal Planning".[373] When used in conjuction with the Food and Drug Administration's publication entitled "Using Nutrition Labels with Food Exchange Lists",[374] the patient, the nutritionist, and the physician have a means of implementing a modern diabetic dietary regimen. How these tools are used depends entirely on the success of the education process.

Neoplastic Diseases: Neoplastic diseases not only are prevalent but also are feared more by the elderly than are other diseases of old age. This latter characteristic of neoplasms arises from the obvious fact that, unlike diabetes, hypertension, or even myocardial infarctions, they produce in the middle and advanced stages of their natural histories dramatic changes in the physical and emotional health of their victims. Whereas diabetics, hypertensives and victims of myocardial infarctions usually look relatively normal, the victims of active neoplastic processes do not. Often the malignancies themselves are manifest on inspection. More often the victims are cachectic. Frequently they are anemic from neoplasia-induced hemorrhages, from cachexia-induced nutritional deficiencies, and/or from the suppression of erythropoiesis by the neoplastic process. Visible hemorrhage is not uncommon. Furthermore, most forms of therapy — surgical, radiologic, endocrine, or chemotherapeutic — result in some form of mutilation of body image. Most therapy, even in the modern era, is often uncomfortable, unpleasant, and disquieting. Finally, the elderly more than younger age cohorts associate the diagnosis of neoplastic disease as a harbinger of death, however unrealistic that may be.

This fear leads many to ignore obvious signs and symptoms, as if denying their presence would eliminate their cause. This, in turn, defers detection of neoplasms until they are well beyond their initial phases and their existence is undeniable. Consequently, among the elderly the neoplastic disease problem is primarily one of diagnosis and treatment, not one of prevention. In addition, the carcinogenic factors inducing the neoplastic process may have been operating for years, (*e.g.*, cigarette smoking or exposure to asbestos) so that prevention is not usually a realistic primary objective of a public health program in this age category.

Nonetheless, as has been noted so often in all matters concerning the health of the elderly, little data exists on the prospective value of preventive measures at any age, suggesting that prevention, while a secondary objective, should by no means be ignored.

Nutritional aspects of neoplastic disease received considerable attention in the decade and a half following World War II. Much was learned about host-tumor relationships and how nutrition related to them. Modest beginnings were made in the improvement of nutritional care of those afflicted. Some of this information has been presented and summarized.[375-381] In general, it suggested that the effectiveness of nutritional rehabilitation in patients with neoplastic diseases was inversely proportional to the activity of the disease processes. Since hyperalimentation raised the caloric expenditure (total daily metabolism, not just basal) and enhanced further the disease activity in patients with rapidly progressing neoplasms, available information suggested that aggressive nutritional rehabilitation would be counterproductive until other therapeutic measures had been given an opportunity to reduce the activity of the disease.

In the last half of the decade of the fifties, a 15 per cent cottonseed oil emulsion stabilized with soybean phosphatide and Pluronic F68 in four per cent glucose solution was studied extensively in patients with and without neoplastic disease.[382-384] Patients with neoplastic disease responded to the intravenous administration of about 900 Calories daily with weight gains, Calorie accumulations, and the retention of protoplasmic constituents in inverse proportion to the activity of their neoplasms. The patients with nonneoplastic conditions responded even more favorably (even including one who twice experienced bizarre reactions termed the "overloading syndrome"). The fat Calories in the oral plus the parenteral alimentation amounted to about 49 per cent of total Calories ingested or administered daily.

These studies confirmed the utility of the high density of Calories in fat in the rehabilitation of anorectic and cachectic persons with and without neoplastic disease. By providing 1.5 Calories per milliliter instead of 0.2 Calories per milliliter of parenteral fluid available with isotonic glucose, the 15 per cent fat emulsion was a promising and simply administered (via peripheral veins) vehicle for supplying the extra Calories needed for nutritional rehabilitation.

Despite its promise, the fat emulsion's use was severely restricted and ultimately prohibited in the United States primarily because of infrequent but extremely bizarre reactions when it was used daily over periods exceeding two weeks in duration.[385] Its place was taken by mixtures of protein hydrolysates and hypertonic glucose whose osmolarity was such that they could be administered only via catheters inserted into large caliber central veins. While these made major contributions to the total care of patients with advanced, active neoplastic disease, their utility was limited to sophisticated hospital environments by virtue of the requirement that the hyperosmolar solutions be administered by catheter into the large-bore central veins.

During this interval, a very significant step in the nutritional rehabilitation of patients with active neoplastic diseases was the demonstration that, during the course of treatment, hyperalimentation by the parenteral route could protect patients from the combined assaults of the neoplastic processes and the therapeutic regimens.[386,386a-386d]

Such parenteral hyperalimentation was achieved in the United States using mixtures of protein hydrolysates, hypertonic glucose, vitamins, minerals, and trace elements. In Europe, however, fat emulsions for clinical use were available and provided essential Calories in isotonic formulations.

In 1975, one of these European emulsions (Intralipid®, distributed in the United States by Cutter Medical, Berkeley, CA 94710) was approved by the Food and Drug Administration (FDA) both as a source of essential fatty acids and of Calories. The Intralipid® approved for use in the United States is composed of ten per cent soy bean oil, 1.2 per cent egg yolk phospholipids, 2.25 per cent glycerin and pyrogen-free water. It has been used primarily in the management of burns, trauma, and the complications of gastrointestinal surgery but has also been tried in the management of some patients with neoplastic disease.[386e-g] Twenty per cent fat Intralipid® was approved for use in the United States early in 1981.

In mid-1979, the FDA approved both as a source of essential fatty acids and of Calories another ten per cent fat emulsion (Liposyn®, produced and distributed by Abbott Laboratories Hospital Products Division, North Chicago, IL 60064). The Liposyn® approved for use in the United States is composed of ten per cent safflower oil, 1.2 per cent egg phosphatides, 2.5 per cent glycerine, and pyrogen free water. Although approved for general use for only a short time, Liposyn® has been tested under a variety of experimental and investigative conditions.[386h] A 20 per cent fat Liposyn® emulsion was approved by the FDA for general use late in 1981.

Baxter Laboratories have developed a 10 per cent fat emulsion marketed under the Travenol® label containing soy bean oil which was approved by the FDA in early 1982. A 20 per cent Travenol® emulsion will be approved after the completion of clinical trials late in 1982.

In those anorectic and cachectic patients for whom nonparenteral alimentation is feasible, fat-containing recipes and supplements and liquid formulas for administration *per os* or by nasogastric tube provide the maximum Calories in compact volumes. Fat emulsions for administration by mouth or tube containing as much as 40 per cent fat by volume (*e.g.*, Lipomul Oral®, produced and distributed by the Upjohn Company, Kalamazoo, MI 49001) have multiple applications. In patients displaying malabsorption of long chain triglycerides as a result of surgical removal of portions of, radiation to, or chemotherapy affecting the small bowel, medium chain triglycerides provide fat Calories in a more efficiently absorbable form.[387-389]

While fat plays an important role in the rehabilitation of anorectic and cachectic persons with neoplastic diseases, it is its essentially negative role in the pathogenesis of neoplastic disease which has attracted attention.[390,391] The background data engendering this renewed interest are essentially epidemiological, some from prospective but most from retrospective studies. These include comparisons of mortality and incidence rates in various countries; geographic incidence rate differences within countries; changes in rates among persons of similar genetic constitution who have migrated from one country or region to another; and time trends and varying rates among certain religious, racial, and socioeconomic groups.[392,393]

Examples are found in the increasing national death rates from cancer of the colon in both men and women as the national average per capita intake of dietary fat rises in 41 countries from less than 25 gm to more than 155 grams.[391] Studies comparing the incidence of colonic cancer in the United States and Japan, which in the past had far lower rates, have shown striking decreases in the differences as Japanese have increased their consumption of dietary fat and cholesterol.[394,395] Additional studies have shown increasing incidence and mortality rates among Japanese immigrants to the United States such that after three generations the rates are equal to those of the rest of the American population.[396,397] The largest changes in the diets of these migrants have occurred in the marked increases in consumptions of fat and cholesterol. In the United States itself, vegetarians have been found to have lower incidence rates for colon cancer than nonvegetarians,[398] whose intake of dietary fat is appreciably higher.

Breast cancer's geographic distribution and mortality rates in 41 countries are also highly correlated to the intake of dietary fat.[391] Experiences in regard to Japan and Japanese immigrants to the United States are similar to those for cancer of the colon. Breast cancer is relatively uncommon in Puerto Rico where the diet is also relatively low in fat and cholesterol.[399,400] A diet high in fat alters the hormonal milieu.[401] Prolactin production, for example, has been significantly reduced in American women when they were placed for four weeks on a vegetarian diet.[392] Studies in female rats have shown that the incidence of breast cancer induced by carcinogens is increased when animals are placed on high fat diets,[391,402] whether the fat is saturated or unsaturated. In the rat, the increase is related to the increased prolactin production with a resulting increase in the prolactin:estrogen ratio associated with consumption of the high fat diet.[402]

Similar data from other studies have suggested associations between obesity and neoplasias of the endometrium and kidney in women.[404] "Over-nutrition," which almost certainly includes intake of diets high in fat has also been implicated in the pathogenesis of cancer of the prostrate, pancreas, ovary, fallopian tube, and broad ligament.[405]

The meaning of these findings to proponents of the "prudent diet" is clear: apply to the cancer problem the same rationale which lipid hypothesis supporters have applied to the problem of atherosclerosis, *viz.*, adopt now a diet low in fat, saturated fat and cholesterol.[392,405,406]

The question arises as it did with cardiovascular diseases with respect to the elderly: should, as a matter of public health policy, the elderly be encouraged to adopt the prudent diet as one measure to protect them from neoplastic disease? Obviously, the scientific data needed to supply the answer are not available. Again, a philosophical answer is all that can be expressed, and that in the minds of most authorities is "yes." As Hegsted has put it,[406] "all of these diseases — heart disease, cancer, diabetes, obesity, etc. — clearly have a complex etiology. Diet is one of the factors, however, and diet *can* be modified. . . We know what the risks of current practices are and they are high. I believe there are no identifiable nutritional risks associated with these kinds of dietary modification, and the probable benefits are high."

The cancer problem has certain aspects which differentiate it from the problem of cardiovascular disease and which imply that the value of adopting a prudent diet as a hedge against neoplastic disease is definitely worthwhile. Unlike atheromatosis, neoplastic disease is usually not something which has existed since youth or middle age. The lesions have specific times of appearance. Hence, regardless of age, the die may not yet be cast, suggesting that prevention in the true sense may occur in response to appropriate precautions. Second, progression of neoplastic disease is slower in the old than in the young. It is conceivable, therefore, that elimination of the pathogenicity of a high fat intake by adopting a prudent diet might slow even further the rate of progression of the disease or perhaps even arrest it *in situ*.

In concluding this discussion on cancer, it should be noted that the association between death rates from carcinoma of the colon and atherosclerotic heart disease noted by Wynder[405] may have some plausible scientific rationale. Benditt,[407] after describing his hypothesis that the proliferating smooth muscle cells of an atheroscleratic plaque all stem from a single mutated smooth muscle cell,[408,409] points to risk factors shared by both carcinogenesis and atherogenesis (cigarette smoking, hypercholesterolemia, high blood pressure) and presents the concept that atheromata are in fact benign neoplasms in the sense that they do not spread by invasion and metastases. Ross and Glomset[410] have reported a chemical factor found in platelet aggregates at sites of endothelial loss in blood vessels which promotes the replication of smooth muscle cells in the arterial walls. Benditt envisions mutant cells which no longer require this factor to divide, thereby assuming neoplastic qualities which lead to formation of atherosclerotic plaques. In related developments, Daoud, *et al.*[411,412] have shown that certain factors in serum enhance the breakage of DNA and promote the migration and proliferation of arterial wall smooth muscle cells. These same factors activate serum lipoproteins which by themselves have no effect on cell proliferation. These factors as well as the concentrations of lipoproteins can be modified by changes in diet. Daoud, *et al.*,[413] in a double blind study, have shown that factors derived from the sera from patients with angiographically demonstrated atherosclerotic heart disease cause medial smooth muscle cells of swine to proliferate at rates higher than those caused by the sera of persons identified by angiography as having no demonstrable atherosclerotic heart disease. Coh, Gabbay, and Eglicki,[414] also studying patients with and without angiographically defined coronary artery disease, showed that serum cholesterol concentrations had a continuous association with the severity of the disease process rather than being related to any critical serum level.

If all of this information is integrated, the logic of a philosophically based reduction in fat intake for the elderly seems overwhelming, especially since no known hazards are created by such recommendation, and since such reduction would lower accepted risk factors for four diseases or conditions of multifactorial pathogenesis — cancer, atherosclerosis, diabetes, and obesity — for which the probability of obtaining conclusive scientific evidence in support of a relationship prior to promulgating a major public health recommendation is virtually nil.

Renal Disease: Fat's applications to the treatment of renal disease are derived primarily from its role as a concentrated source of Calories. Calories are presumed to spare protein, *i.e.*, provide energy from food thereby diminishing to a minimum the transformation of protein to glucose through the process of gluconeogenesis. The protein-sparing action of Calories becomes important in renal disease only when renal function is very seriously diminished, *e.g.*, glomerular filtration rates less than ten per cent of normal. Since glomerular filtration rates diminish linearly with age,[183] ten per cent is suggested rather than more commonly recommended lower values.

Very seriously compromised renal function implies the need for a comprehensive search for etiology of the condition. If no correctable pathology is found, patients may benefit by diets low in total protein, which should be of the highest biological value, and adequate in Calories. Since azotemia itself depresses appetite and since many patients accustomed to high protein regimens find low protein menus unappetizing, Calorie deficiency may vitiate the value of the low-protein diet by increasing gluconeogenesis to support Calorie requirements. This sequence of events may be modified by judicious use of fats which provide not only concentrated Calories but also desirable gustatory qualities to the foods of which they are a part. In debilitated patients, fat emulsions for oral administration provide concentrated Calories in an easily ingested and assimilated form.

In even further advanced renal disease (glomerular filtration rates approaching unity or below), peritoneal or hemodialysis may be initiated as life saving procedures. Under these circumstances, the high Calorie density of fat may again be useful in rehabilitating patients whose renal insufficiency has been of long standing and has led to poor nutritional status. In the unusual event that an elderly person should receive a kidney transplant, similar use could be made of fat.

Acute renal failure caused by ingestion of toxins, including overdosages of prescribed and over-the-counter drugs, may require low-protein, high Calorie regimens in addition to other indicated therapeutic measures until renal function has been restored. Here again fat plays a useful role.

Since excessive fat intakes are ketogenic and are felt by some to increase metabolism,[415-417] low protein, high Calorie regimens should contain sufficient carbohydrate to prevent development of ketosis. The importance of this may be even greater in view of the association of glucose intolerance with renal insufficiency. Improvement in glucose tolerance with hemodialysis has led to the hypothesis that a dializable insulin antagonist is active in renal failure.[418] Elevated glucagon concentrations are also characteristic of patients with uremia and may be reduced to normal by successful renal transplants but not by hemodialysis.[419] Since glucagon responses to experimental *(e.g.,* intravenous glucose) stimuli are intact in uremic patients, it would appear that homeostatic mechanisms that control plasma glucagon are set at higher than normal levels.[420] Since glucagon administered in pharmacologic doses intravenously increases urinary nitrogen excretion[421] and since the molar ratio of insulin to glucagon (plasma insulin $\times$ 22.3 $\div$ plasma glucagon) is inversely proportional to protein catabolism[422] and directly proportional to changes in lean body mass,[419] dietary maneuvers designed to keep glucagon levels as low as possible would seem advisable.

On the other hand, hyperlipemia and especially hypertriglyceridemia commonly accompany uremia, presumably because of a lipoprotein lipase inhibitor.[423] Since the inhibitor is poorly dialyzable, only intensive hemodialysis brings about a satisfactory triglyceride reduction.[424] Patients whose uremic states were treated with peritoneal dialysis, which involves a significant glucose load, were found to have significantly higher triglyceride levels than the same patients treated by hemodialysis.[425] The same authors, however, on the bases of comparing their patients' oral dietary intakes over a seven day period with that of nonuremic patients and that of average Canadians,[424,426] concluded that neither total Calorie intake nor the distribution of carbohydrate, fat or protein apear to be important in the production of uremic hyperlipemia.

It is apparent that much more investigation will be required to clarify the exact role fat may play in the management of renal diseases. Some recent reviews provide excellent background reading upon which to weigh future developments.[427-429]

Parenteral and tube feeding: Several references have been made to specific uses of fat emulsions in the nutriton of persons unable to obtain adequate Calories by the usual oral route. While emulsions containing 40 per cent fat for oral and nasogastric tube administration are commercially available, emulsions for parenteral use were not generally available in the United States. Some of the difficulties encountered in their use included anemia and a bizarre syndrome characterized by jaundice, hepatomegaly, splenomegaly, fever, sore throat and loading of the reticuloendothelial system with fat.[430] The signs and symptoms subsided rapidly when the infusions of the emulsion were halted. Reactions of this and other types were encountered frequently enough to depreciate the value of fat emulsions as components of routine parenteral alimentation. Studies of an experimental nature in the United States and clinical applications in Europe have led recently to the approval of Intralipid®, Lyposyn®, and Travenol® emulsions for use in the United States *(v.s.)*. Emulsions for oral or tube administration continue to provide a convenient means of increasing Calorie intake. Medium chain triglycerides have specific value in resolving some malabsorption problems *(v.s.)*.

The absence of fat from presently administered parenteral hyperalimentation regimens (80 per cent glucose, 20 per cent casein amino acid hydrolysates, minerals and vitamins) has been reported to be associated with a marked fall in linoleic acid in all plasma lipid fractions.[431] Although no clinical signs of essential fatty acid deficiency were observed, the authors concluded that essential fatty acid deficiency develops rapidly when fat-free diets containing glucose are given either intravenously or by nasogastric tube as 24-hour continuous infusions. While these studies were short in duration, the potential hazard of essential fatty acid deficiency may exist in patients receiving fat free regimens over longer periods of time. Added linoleic acid seems indicated.

Qualitative Aspects

Saturation and Chain Length of Fatty Acids: In the sections dealing with quantitative aspects of fat in the dietary regimen, much of the work involving the role of the saturation of fat in the pathogenesis of cardiovascular disease has already been reviewed. At this point, specific attention need be focused on the influence of the degree of unsaturation, *i.e.*, the presence or absence of double bonds, of ingested fat and its relation to cardiovascular diseases.

Kinsell, *et al.*[432,433] reported in 1952 and 1953 that formula diets high in vegetable oils produced in humans reductions in serum cholesterol concentrations, while formulas containing isocaloric amounts of animal fat led to cholesterol concentrations similar to those in persons on a normal, mixed diet. These findings have been confirmed by a host of studies[45,273,339-344,434-441] showing that serum cholesterol concentrations could be reduced by adding vegetable oils containing linoleic (C_{18}:2) and linolenic (C_{18}:3) fatty acids or even more highly unsaturated fish oils[442] to dietary regimens in place of fats containing saturated myristic (C_{14}) and palmitic (C_{16}) fatty acids.[443,444] Saturated stearic acid (C_{18}) has little or no influence on serum cholesterol concentrations[443,444] nor do medium chain triglycerides[445,446]. Monounsaturated oleic acid (C_{18}:1) has no effect on serum cholesterol concentrations in the *cis*isomeric configuration[447] but acts like saturated myristic and palmitic acids in the *trans*isomeric configuration.[448]

As Ahrens has pointed out in his commentary on the lipid hypothesis,[337] the question is not how lipid lowering should be undertaken but rather whether it should be contemplated at all. The cost of undertaking the field trials in a sufficient number of subjects has to date deferred implementation of such investigations.[449,450] Meanwhile, circumstantial evidence accumulates suggesting that dietary changes do improve mortality but, as was pointed out in the discussion of quantitative aspects of fat in the diet *(v.s.)*, these are countered by other studies implying little or no effect or suggesting possible undesirable results.

The question is nowhere more moot than among considerations of the appropriate course to recommend to those who are already old. Data on hand *(v.s.)* suggest that little can be accomplished for those who have given no heed to dietary considerations in the past. However, most of these arguments are based on epidemiologic studies or on intervention trials among those who already have been seriously afflicted and, therefore, are already poor risks. What Ahrens is suggesting for younger adults[337] in terms of a phased, long term approach to this problem has never been suggested and even has been actively opposed[49] for implementation among the elderly. The fact that persons who have reached sixty years of age in good health and still performing well are known already to be candidates for a reasonably long life should make a group of this kind acceptable candidates for a phased, well-controlled intervention trial.

The fact that the Select Committee on Nutrition and Human Needs of the U.S. Senate has cut the Gordian knot[231] by recommending general adoption of a prudent diet may add some stimulus to such studies, since public knowledge of and interest in such dietary measures will be heightened. However, as Ahrens has suggested,[337] the ability of the public in general and especially those who are already old to put such measures into meaningful effect is conditional on the assistance from the health industry which can not in any way be assured without the intellectual interest of the medical profession in observing and documenting the results of such interventions.[451]

Influence of Dietary Cholesterol: Many references have already been made to this topic because of the interactions of dietary fats and carbohydrates with dietary cholesterol in determining the serum cholesterol concentrations in man. This is an appropriate opportunity, therefore, to summarize the consensus of thinking in regard to dietary cholesterol. First, cholesterol is in no way a dietary essential for man. Man can synthesize endogenously all needed cholesterol. Second, dietary cholesterol is a problem because so many foods desirable from the viewpoints of availability, price, taste, and habit are high in cholesterol. Hence, the task of tearing the American public away from these desirable foods will be difficult. Third, evidence indicates that dietary cholesterol does relate linearly to serum cholesterol. Biofeedback suppression of endogenous cholesterol synthesis by dietary cholesterol is imperfect; hence, each mg of cholesterol ingested adds to the serum cholesterol concentration. Fourth, analyses of data such as that collected in the Framingham study suggest that serum cholesterol concentration is proportional to risk of coronary artery disease over its entire range, and, therefore, no arbitrary level can be set as the upper limit of normal. Fifth, potential benefit from lowering serum cholesterol concentrations decreases with age, suggesting that efforts to lower serum cholesterol should begin early in life. Sixth, since endogenous synthesis is the major contributor to the serum-tissue pool of cholesterol, efforts directed at blocking endogenous synthesis may ultimately be more productive than dietary restrictions in reducing serum cholesterol concentrations. Finally, the serum cholesterol concentration is determined by multifactorial inputs, as are the diseases with which it is associated. This makes interpretation of data imprecise and, when considered in conjunction with interindividual variability, suggests that no older person should be discouraged from reasonable efforts to lower serum cholesterol, assuming he or she is motivated to try.

FOOD PREPARATION PRACTICES

In the fast-food era, more and more fats and oils are entering the human diet, not as selected dietary items, but as vehicles for the rapid heating of foods. Fish, shellfish, and potatoes are popular and commonly eaten items cooked in fats or oils for the sake of convenience.

In the direction of more tasteful eating, the cookbooks at home and the recipe files of the best restaurants contain instructions figuratively dripping with fats and oils. Meats sold in the market are graded and priced in proportion to their fat content.

The only rational explanation for the continuing emphasis on fat in the American dietary is that the American people like meals prepared with fat and hence encourage the producers of food and the providers of meal service to provide them what they desire. While media may be partially to blame for promoting such a dietary, the media spend even more time promoting the ideal of a lithe, slender, active, productive population. The media devote time and space daily to promoting foods and exercises designed to counteract the results of excessive consumption of fat-containing foods and foods prepared in fats and oils. Obviously, the American public needs the results of some clear thinking to assist in the resolution of this absurd but very real problem.

The nation's elderly who have survived in spite of the system may be the most effective change agents in setting new standards for themselves but more importantly for the younger age cohorts who have the most to gain. Getting the elderly involved in eliminating much fat from food preparation practices is a project with ingredients of interest to them all and one which could snowball through them into a far broader application of the nutrition-health-aging triad concept to all age groups.

SUMMARY OF PRESENT KNOWLEDGE OF FAT IN NUTRITION AND AGING

The high Calorie density of fat endows it with opportunities to serve mankind both constructively and destructively. In providing essential fatty acids, as a vehicle for the fat soluble vitamins, and as a means of rehabilitation of victims of caloric undernutrition, fat serves a constructive role. Fat adds markedly to the taste and texture of many foods. It has become a symbol of the good life, of prosperity and affluence, but it is also a symbol of a high energy consuming, low efficiency economy. Most destructive of all, it is associated with diseases and disabilities through its facility in producing obesity and its presumed role in the pathogenesis of cardiovascular and neoplastic diseases. While statistical data proving an absolute association of excess dietary fat and disease are not available, sufficient epidemiologic and clinical studies have been done to suggest the value of reasonable reductions in total Calories daily to a level of 30 per cent or less. Such a reduction achieves at the same time a reduction in dietary Calories, cholesterol and saturated fat and, therefore, in a single move reduces the impact of three potential risk factors.

Reduction of fat Calorie intake per se is no panacea. It should, in the vast majority of Americans, be accompanied by a reduction in total Calorie intake and an increase in Calorie expenditure through increased physical activity. Such changes must be accompanied by an increase in knowledge about all aspects of nutrition, since diminishing Calorie intake increases the need for wise selection of foods to guard against inadvertent vitamin, mineral and trace element dietary deficiencies through selection of foods with low nutrient as well as low Calorie density.

For some elderly, pursuit of the above recommendations may entail few changes in dietary habits, since many, for economic as well as for health-related reasons, may already be on a relatively low fat intake. But many of the younger elderly are still obese, still at high risk for cardiovascular and neoplastic disease. For them, reducing fat intake may improve their own outlook for the future. If those who provide them with leadership in regard to health matters would also collect data on the results achieved by such dietary changes, the medical and scientific community could resolve in the process questions for which no acceptable answers now exist.

-8-

Carbohydrate

CLASSIFICATION OF DIETARY CARBOHYDRATES

Monosaccharides

The monosaccharides of importance in human alimentation are the hexoses, *i.e.*, those having six carbon atoms. The monosaccharides most important in human nutrition are glucose, fructose and galactose.

The Oligosaccharides

Oligosaccharides contain from two to ten monosaccharides. The ones most commonly associated with human nutrition are sucrose (glucose and fructose), lactose (glucose and galactose), and maltose (glucose and glucose).

The Polysaccharides

Polysaccharides contain more than ten monosaccharides. The ones of importance in human nutrition are starch, the storage form of carbohydrate in plants, and glycogen, the storage form of carbohydrates in animals. Cellulose, the structural form of carbohydrate, is indigestible by man but is an important source of food for ruminants.

ROLES OF DIETARY CARBOHYDRATE

Maintenance of Blood Glucose Concentration

A principal role of carbohydrates in human nutrition is the maintenance of the blood glucose concentration within the extremes of 50 to

200 mg per cent. An elaborate homeostatic mechanism comprising insulin, glucagon, epinephrine, adrenal cortical hormones and thyroxine together with glycogenesis and glycogenolysis has evolved for this purpose.

Blood glucose in an acceptable range is the fuel of choice for most organs but is absolutely essential for proper function of the brain. When excess carbohydrate enters the body by the ingestion of sugars or starches, what can not be readily utilized in the production of energy is stored as glycogen (glycogenesis) in liver, muscle, brain, and other tissues or converted to and stored as fat. Glycogen in liver may be called upon to supply glucose (glycogenolysis) when maintenance of blood glucose concentration is required. The glucose in muscle glycogen in not available through the same rapid glycogenolytic processes found in liver. Hence, glycogen reserves are limited and serve primarily for the maintenance of blood glucose concentrations, not as long-term reserves of energy, that role being played by fat.

Carbohydrates in many societies are the principal source of Calories. What is not immediately utilized or converted into glycogen is stored in the adipose tissue of the body as fat. Once changed into fat, carbohydrate can not be reconverted to carbohydrate. Hence, when glycogen stores are exhausted, they are replaced and/or blood glucose concentration is maintained by glucose derived to a minor extent from the glycerol of fat being metabolized for energy and, to a greater extent, from protein through a process called gluconeogenesis. Such utilization of protein is undesirable, since it results in diminution of lean body mass and requires the excretion of the unoxidizable residues of protein metabolism, principally urea, ammonia, creatinine, and uric acid, by the kidney.

The potential for losses of protein through gluconeogenesis has been indicated in studies using the fasting, phlorhizinized dog as the experimental animal. Phlorhizin is a glycoside causing glucosuria by blocking reabsorption by the renal tubule of glucose in glomerular filtrate. Such animals, when fasting, derive virtually all of the blood glucose essential for bodily function via gluconeogenesis, since the animal's glucose pool is depleted by constant glucose losses as blood passes through the kidneys and since glycogen stores in the liver are quickly exhausted and not replenished during fasting. Such studies indicate that every 3.65 gm of glucose appearing in the urine is accompanied by one gm of nitrogen derived from the breakdown of protein. Since protein is 16 per cent nitrogen (protein = N x 1/0.16 or N x 6.25), every gram of glucose produced by gluconeogenesis requires the degradation of 1.71 gm protein (6.25/3.65 = 1.71) and the excretion of its nitrogenous end products.[452] While this interpretation of the glucose/nitrogen ratio in the phlorhizinized dog is greatly oversimplified and no longer regarded as a precise index of the degree of gluconeogenesis from proteins, it does point out the importance of minimizing gluconeogenesis by incorporating carbohydrate into dietary regimens at sufficiently regular intervals to maintain reasonable stores of liver glycogen.

This is particularly important in the very old and the very ill whose lean body masses have already been reduced by the inexorable process of cell death or by the influences of disease. The importance of such management has been stressed in discussions in Chapter 7 on the management of acute illnesses. Here attention should be called to its importance in the management of chronic conditions as well, especially those where anorexia is present.

In discussions of diabetes mellitus in Chapter 7, stress was placed on the role of carbohydrate in the modern management of that disease. Here, in addition, the work of Cohn and various colleagues[453-458] suggests that frequent carbohydrate ingestion using isocaloric, isonitrogenous diets has resulted in lower serum cholesterol concentrations and greater nitrogen retention than when similar quantities were ingested three times daily. This work suggests appropriate prophylaxis against gluconeogenesis in old, debilitated and anorexic patients.

Calorie Source

Carbohydrates digestible by man not only provide glucose for immediate use throughout the body but also may be converted to fat for storage as an energy supply when sources of glucose are not readily available. Excessive consumption of carbohydrate can therefore lead to obesity. However, since carbohydrate supplies only four Calories per gram, it is a less concentrated source of Calories than is fat. Among elderly living on limited incomes, foods high in carbohydrates, because of their relatively low cost, are a principal source of Calories. Unfortunately, many of the dietary regimens that result from these high carbohydrate foods are low in proteins, vitamins, minerals, and trace elements compared to the concentrations of the same nutrients found in foods of animal origin. This has led to concern that high carbohydrate diets were merely vehicles of "empty Calories" to certain categories of older persons.[459-461]

A 1972 reevaluation[462] of survivors of the 1948 Michigan State University study[461] showed that carbohydrate intake had decreased from 191 gm per day in 1948 to 143 gm per day in 1972. Although total Calorie intake had fallen by 376 Calories, protein intake had risen appreciably and had been accompanied by some reduction in fat as well as carbohydrate.

While changes may have occurred in carbohydrate content of diets among elderly women in Michigan, 1973 studies among 343 middle Tennessee elderly women[463] revealed that those receiving two-thirds or more of the 1974 Recommended Dietary Allowances (RDA)[92] numbered 81.5 per cent for protein, 69.5 per cent for vitamin C, and 65.9 per cent for calcium but only 44.3 per cent for iron, 42.8 per cent for vitamin A, 38.5 per cent for thiamin, and 36.8 per cent for riboflavin. In this sample, vegetables were the most widely used foods.

Data on nutrient intake collected by the 24-hour recall method on a large national probability sample of older women during the Health and Nutrition Examination Survey (HANES) conducted from 1971 to 1974 by the National Center for Health Statistics[464] showed Calories, protein, calcium and iron intakes to be less than the full RDA but more than two-thirds the RDA, whereas intakes of vitamins A, C, B_1, and B_2 were far in excess of the RDA. The differences in the two studies may suggest a regional problem in middle Tennessee. The HANES study data fail to confirm the "empty Calorie" legend about foods for the elderly. Some of this may be the result of fortification with vitamins of many carbohydrate foods such as breads and cereals since the earlier observations made in the 1940's.

Vehicle for Sweetness

The intense public outcry in early 1977 against the Food and Drug Administration's proposed ban on saccharin as a sweetner can leave little doubt of "the power of the American sweet tooth".[465] The craving for sweets is a result of cultural conditioning. Children may be conditioned to crave or not to crave sweets, a characteristic that carries over into adult life. Americans consume more sugar per capita than persons of almost any country. The outcry among the elderly at the time of the saccharin ban suggests that they, too, retain the intense craving for sweetness.

Carbohydrates in many forms, but particularly sucrose, contribute to the flavor of many foods. In this sense, the sweet carbohydrates have characteristics similar to fat and, like fat, are often consumed in excess for that reason. Consumption of carbohydrates will be quantified in a later section.

Components of Major Dietary Fibers

For many years fiber was studied primarily by scientists concerned with wood, grasses, animal feeds, and ruminant nutrition. In the early 1970's, fiber burst into considerations of human nutrition and health, particularly those considerations concerned with function and diseases of the colon and those concerned with lipid metabolism and diabetes. Clearly, fiber is of concern to those dealing with the nutrition and health of the elderly. As a result of massive publicity, fiber has become a houschold word. Unfortunately, few who bandy about the term understand what fiber really is.

Fiber is a catch-all term generally used to describe carbohydrate components and lignins found largely in plant cell walls. They are thought to be neither digested nor absorbed in the upper gastrointestinal tract.[466] Fiber includes the following carbohydrates: celluloses, hemicelluloses, pectins, plant gums, mucilages and storage polysaccharides. Lignins which are not carbohydrates are also included in most definitions. Algal polysaccharides, though obviously carbohydrates, are usually classified separately because they are derived from algae and seaweed. The algal polysaccharides include such commonly found ingredients of processed food as alginic acid, agar and carrageenin. Nonnutritive synthetic fibers include cellophane and highly refined cellulose from wood pulp, all carbohydrates but not consumed by man as part of his normal diet.[467]

Any discussion of carbohydrates would be incomplete without noting that fibers which are indigestible in the upper gastrointestinal tract of man ultimately provide man with much of his food supply, though by an indirect route. This route is man's consumption of the milk and meat of herbivorous animals, particularly ruminants such as cattle, sheep, goats and deer (pre-acid fermentaton types), and hares, rabbits, rodents, and horses (post-acid fermentation types).[468]

In ruminants, fibers such as cellulose and hemicellulose are fermented in the rumen by rumen bacteria and protozoa to various volatile fatty acids which are absorbed in a portion of the stomach called the omasum and are, therefore, available to the ruminant, as is glucose in man, to satisfy metabolic needs. Most protein in the ruminants diet is derived from the bodies of rumen microorganisms which are absorbed in the ruminant's intestine after being killed in the hydrochloric acid secreting portion of the stomach, the abomasum.

Animals of the postacid fermentation type achieve the same bacterial fermentation and absorption of volatile fatty acids in a portion of the cecum. However, the microbial cells which provide protein to ruminants can not be utilized before being voided. Hence, some of these animals practice coprophagy.

Birds usually eat only animals, fish, plant seeds, or other easily digested material, but even those like ducks and geese who do ingest grass and aquatic plants do not obtain any nutrients from the fiber ingested.

Hence, fiber, although not digestible by man, provides the raw material from which man derives his dairy products and his meat. The herbivores who consume the fiber may be looked upon as living factories converting fibers indigestible by man into foods edible and metabolizable by mankind. As such, the herbivores add immeasurably to the world's food supply, and, through them, the carbohydrates in fiber serve as a vast reservoir of food potentially available to mankind.

QUANTITY OF CARBOHYDRATE IN THE AMERICAN DIET

As pointed out in the discussion of the quantity of fat in the American diet, the quantity of carbohydrate has decreased reciprocally as consumptions of fat and protein have risen. According to U.S. Department of Agriculture estimates for 1974,[232] carbohydrate Calories for that year accounted for only 46 per cent of the total, 24 per cent of which was derived from refined sugar and only 22 per cent from complex carbohydrates. These estimates contrast sharply with the 58 per cent total carbohydrate Calories containing no more than 15 per cent refined sugar recommended in *Dietary Goals for the United States.*[231]

The annual consumption of refined sugar has increased from 76.4 pounds per capita in the 1909-1913 interval to 101.5 pounds per capita in 1971.[469] While direct consumer use declined from 52.1 pounds per capita in the 1909-1913 interval to 24.7 pounds per capita in 1971, the quantity per capita of refined sugar in processed foods and beverages has increased three and one-half fold. In beverages alone the increase has been almost seven fold to a per capita level of almost 23 pounds annually.

Changes in carbohydrate consumption from geographic, economic, and sociologic viewpoints have been reviewed in Chapter 7.

HEALTH AND DIETARY CARBOHYDRATE

Carbohydrate Intolerance

This subject has been discussed in detail in Chapter 7. While liberalization of carbohydrate intake of diabetics is gaining greater acceptance, and while higher percentages of carbohydrate Calories at the expense of fat Calories are being recommended, it is well to recall that such changes call for increases in complex carbohydrates, not refined sugars.

Hypoglycemia

Hypoglycemia — low concentration of blood glucose — may be produced in the fasting state by excessive strenuous physical activity, by functioning adenomas of the islets of Langerhans of the pancreas, by extensive parenchymal disease of the liver, by deficiencies of hormones which normally counteract insulin, and by the presence in the body of certain large tumors (apart from those secreting insulin).

In the fed or postprandial state, hypoglycemia is caused by a lack of synchronism between rises and falls of blood glucose and insulin concentrations following ingestion of food (reactive hypoglycemia).

Such lack of synchronism in elderly persons may be found in those who have had gastrectomies or surgical procedures which cause food to bypass the pylorus. In these persons, food reaches absorptive sites in the small intestine more rapidly, resulting in sharp rises in blood glucose concentrations which in turn evoke greater than normal secretion of insulin. Glucose is utilized quickly with blood glucose concentrations falling sharply, the insulin being unbuffered by the delivery of more glucose to absorptive sites from stomach contents. Hypoglycemia of this type is part of the symptomatology of the "dumping syndrome" which occurs in many patients following surgical treatment of duodenal ulcer.

Hypoglycemia in elderly persons may also occur with normal rates of glucose absorption when release of insulin is sluggish as in early maturity-onset diabetes mellitus. The high blood glucose concentrations evoke high insulin concentrations which may result in a relative hyperinsulinism if the glucose utilization rate exceeds the rate of glucose replacement from intestinal contents.

In young persons, so-called functional hypoglycemia of unknown etiology is occasionally found especially in tense, hyperkinetic and compulsive personality types. In the elderly, however, such a diagnosis should be scrupulously avoided until other causes of hypoglycemia have been systematically eliminated.

In persons of all ages, but more commonly in older adults, the most common form of hypoglycemia is that caused by exogenous hypoglycemic agents used out of phase with ingestion and absorption of food which contains or may be readily metabolized into glucose. While such hypoglycemia may be induced factitiously in anyone, the most common victims are patients with diabetes mellitus whose dietary pattern, level of physical activity, or endogenous insulin secretion may change, thereby making them more susceptible to hypoglycemia from their own prescribed medications.

In the fasting state, a drug which produces hypoglycemia independent of insulin action is alcohol. In adults, alcohol induces hypoglycemia after relatively long fasts. It acts by interfering with gluconeogenesis in the liver. Alcohol is particularly dangerous in insulin-dependent diabetics who may continue to take insulin while imbibing heavily and abandoning appropriate dietary practices.

The management of hypoglycemia comprises first correcting the low blood glucose concentration by prompt administration by mouth or parenterally, if the patient is unconscious, of glucose or a food containing glucose or quickly metabolizable to glucose. Once the patient is stabilized, the cause of the hypoglycemia should be diagnosed and appropriate corrective therapy instituted. Very often, hypoglycemia can be managed successfully by redistributing components of dietary intake, *e.g.*, increasing the frequency of meals and snacks during the day.

In diabetics, redistribution of insulin dosages in concert with dietary intake redistribution may be required. Very importantly, insulin-dependent diabetics should be trained to recognize the very early symptoms of hypoglycemia and warned never to go anywhere without a supply of glucose or glucose-containing oligosaccharide *(e.g.*, sucrose) immediately available for ingestion when the first early symptom appears. Since hypoglycemia may be associated with loss of consciousness with or without convulsions, avoiding hypoglycemia is a matter of top priority. Injuries from falls and convulsive seizures can seriously incapacitate persons in all age groups but are particularly life threatening to the elderly *(v.s.)*.

Obesity

While the high Calorie densities of fat and alcohol make them prime villains in the dietary pathogenesis of obesity, the potential role of carbohydrate as a co-conspirator can not be overlooked. Since carbohydrates do not have the satiety value of either fat or protein, foods high in carbohydrate may be eaten in larger quantities with the resultant intake of Calories being equal to or greater than would have been consumed if foods containing other Calorie sources had been ingested. Since carbohydrate-containing foods are usually cheaper than foods with higher concentrations of protein and fat, they are consumed by persons in the lower income brackets, including many elderly. Since the nutrient density of carbohydrate containing foods is low, large amounts must be eaten to acquire adequate amounts of protein and certain minerals and vitamins. In present-day America, highly refined carbohydrates — particularly those in processed foods and in beverages — pose the greatest problem in considerations of carbohydrate's contribution to obesity. Such refined carbohydrates represent true "empty Calories," providing nothing other than Calories to the person consuming them. Elimination to the greatest extent possible of refined carbohydrates from the American dietary would remove a substantial number of useless Calories and could thereby contribute effectively to maintenance of ideal weight.

Elimination of refined carbohydrates from processed foods and from beverages does not *ipso facto* serve as justification for the addition of so-called artificial sweeteners to the foods and beverages involved. Quite apart from their potential carcinogenicity, artificial sweeteners are high in sodium. In addition, their use by infants and children creates a "sweet tooth" or craving for sweets which is satisfied not only by the low Calorie beverages but also by candy and other confections and by the addition of sucrose to such items as breakfast cereals or even fresh fruit. Ideally, the carbohydrate moiety of a diet should comprise complex starches and sugars occurring naturally in the foods eaten without attempts to use either refined carbohydrates or artificial sweeteners merely to impart a saccharine quality to the foods or beverages consumed.

Cachexia

In persons who are emaciated and cachectic, the refined carbohydrates do play a constructive role. First, parenteral hyperalimentation and hydration involve the use of hypertonic or isotonic glucose solutions. Second, since most Americans have a "sweet tooth," foods and beverages sweetened with refined sugar are often more acceptable than foods composed of complex carbohydrates. The ease with which Calories may be ingested when refined carbohydrates are combined with fats and oils make such combinations ideal for rehabilitation of emaciated and cachectic persons. Third, under these circumstances, the "empty Calorie" charge can be overlooked, since Calories in any form are needed and since the health industry personnel supervising such rehabilitation would include in the formulas utilized appropriate quantities of proteins, minerals, vitamins, trace elements and water.

Dental Caries

A striking decrease in the incidence of dental caries during World War II in the United Kingdom, Scandinavia, Finland, and Japan has been attributed to the enforced reduction in consumption of readily fermentable carbohydrates and especially to the amount available for eating between meals.[77] Other studies conducted among Eskimos,[470] in urban and rural areas in Ghana,[471] among members of Antarctic expeditions,[472] among institutionalized patients,[473,474] and among students fed sucrose or sucrose free sweets,[475] leave little doubt but that sucrose is the leading plaque former and therefore caries producer in man. Plaque is the film containing bacteria and polysaccharides which accumulates on teeth, especially in the absence of good oral hygiene. The bacteria in the plaque produce organic acids from the fermentable carbohydrates which lower the pH sufficiently to demineralize some tooth enamel. The bacteria also synthesize from the fermentable carbohydrates polysaccharides which serve as an energy reserve enabling the microorganisms to continue to produce acid even in the absence of environmental carbohydrate.[476]

The physical properties of the food containing fermentable carbohydrates determine its efficacy as a caries inducer. For example, sugar in solution produces little or no increase in caries, whereas caramels and toffees are highly cariogenic.[474] In addition, the frequency of exposure of teeth to fermentable carbohydrate, such as occurs in nibbling or between-meal snacking, is directly proportional to the incidence of dental caries.[477] Desirable foods for use as snacks between meals include all raw, fresh frozen or waterpack fruits or vegetables or their juices prepared without the addition of sugar. When taken in the absence of added sugar, dairy products, meats and nuts are also acceptable. To be avoided are sugared gums; candies of all kinds; sugar-containing beverages, jellies, gelatins, ice creams or sherbets; and most cough drops, throat lozenges and sugared pharmaceuticals.

Important in the prevention of dental caries is the practice of regularly scheduled brushing and flossing of teeth. Ideally, this should be done after every exposure to carbohydrate-containing foods. Obviously, this is not practical. A desirable compromise comprises brushing and flossing teeth after meals and at bedtime. Such care removes plaque from the teeth and thereby prevents acid formation which in turn leads to caries.

While the teeth of children are more susceptible to caries than are the teeth of older adults, those adults who have retained their teeth through proper oral hygiene and regular, periodic dental care should practice every measure possible to assure retention of their natural teeth throughout life. Selection of appropriate between meal snacks and systematic brushing and flossing of teeth following meals combined with regular professional dental care provide the best protection against dental caries.

Cardiovascular Health

Carbohydrate first received attention in the cardiovascular field as a result of epidemiologic studies by Yudkin.[478] He showed highly significant correlations between sucrose consumption and the incidence of ischemic heart disease. Although he acknowledges a high correlation between sucrose and fat intake, Yudkin believes the correlation of ischemic heart disease with sugar intake is significant ($p < 0.001$), whereas that with fat is not ($p > 0.1$). Additional studies by Cohen[479] in Yemenite Jews who migrated to Israel showed they had a marked increase in the incidence of coronary artery disease related to a considerable increase in their intake of dietary sugar. Such conclusions have been criticized because many other factors in the environment also reveal associations with coronary artery disease.[480]

The issue of carbohydrate's relation to cardiovascular disease has been highlighted by the promulgation of *Dietary Goals for the United States* by the Select Committee on Nutrition and Human Needs of the U.S. Senate.[231] These goals include one to the effect that carbohydrate should comprise 58 per cent of total Calories as contrasted to the present estimated 46 per cent. However, they also include another goal to the effect that the consumption of refined or processed sugars (cane and beet sugar, corn sugar, syrups, molasses, and honey) should be reduced from the present estimated 18 per cent of Calories to 10 per cent and that complex carbohydrates (fruits and vegetables, grain products) and "naturally occurring" sugars (those which are indigenous to the food) should be increased from 28 to 48 per cent of Calories. Among the reasons cited for these goals are the low incidence of cardiovascular disease among populations consuming diets high in complex carbohydrates[481] and the higher incidences of cardiovascular disease among those consuming large quantities of refined and processed sugars. Authories generally agree that carbohydrates should be substituted for fat; however, there is little agreement with Yudkin's condemnation of refined sugar.

As noted earlier in Chapter 7, *Dietary Goals for the United States*[231,265] was an attempt by certain members of the U.S. Senate to cut the Gordian knot and bring constructive action to a field immobilized by controversy. In regard to carbohydrate, paticularly that goal proposing a reduction in intake of refined sugars, the *Dietary Goals* have been attacked by the medical[482] and scientific communities.[483] For the latter, Harper decries the simplistic view (except in the case of dental caries) that sugar has already been indicted as contributing to cardiovascular and other diseases. He pleads for more information prior to promulgation of recommendations to the public at large and joins the American Medical Association[484] in recommending that each disease and each patient receive individual consideration, attention and therapy. In a reply to an invitation addressed to health professionals from the Center for Science in the Public Interest to join the Center in petitioning the President of the United States to adopt the *Dietary Goals,* Harper[485] states the issue and expresses succinctly the viewpoint of health professionals and scientists toward the *Dietary Goals.* He urges "... using a sound scientific approach to problems rather than techniques reminiscent of those of some of the less ethical Madison Avenue advertising agencies."

Quite obviously, consensus on the *Dietary Goals* among health professionals, politicians, consumer activists and consumers themselves will be long in coming. For the elderly as well as all others, a rational approach to this conundrum is suggested by Harper himself.[483] Citing advice given in the 1974 *Recommended Dietary Allowances, Eighth Edition,*[92] Harper notes that persons consuming diets low in total Calories (the elderly, the physically and emotionally ill, the injured, those recovering from surgery and those on weight reduction diets) should avoid "dilution" of nutrients with such pure Calorie vehicles as refined carbohydrates, fats and alcohol. Certainly, elderly persons whose reduced activity, illnesses and disabilities, and medications may result in markedly reduced Caloric intake not only should avoid "dilution" with empty Calories but also should consume carefully planned regimens of high nutrient density, including foods containing complex carbohydrates.[486]

The work of Fredrickson and many colleagues[334,335,487] has popularized another aspect of the relationship of dietary carbohydrate to lipid metabolism which in certain persons has implications for cardiovascular disease. Persons with types IIb, III, IV and V hyperlipoproteinemias are advised to limit carbohydrate (and alcohol) consumption to reduce concentrations of circulating endogenous triglycerides in the form of VLDL. This advice applies only to persons with particular forms of familial hyperlipoproteinemias and should not be applied to the public at large. Stamler, in fact, has reported[488] no significant triglyceride increases in persons who shift to diets in the 55-60 per cent carbohydrate Calorie range.

Renal Diseases

Carbohydrate's role in the management of renal disease lies in the ability of small quantities of ingested carbohydrate to reduce gluconeogenesis from body protein, thereby minimizing the products of nitrogen metabolism which must be excreted by the diseased kidney if their concentrations in body fluids are to remain in the acceptable ranges. In the management of far advanced chronic renal disease or of acute renal failure, carbohydrate used in conjunction with fat and with protein of high biologic value serves to prevent ketosis which may be encountered if sufficient carbohydrate is omitted from the dietary regimen. See Chapter 7, page 87 for a more extensive discusson of diet in renal diseases.

Role in Physical, Sensory and Intellectual Peformance

Carbohydrate serves as the principal fuel or energy source for muscles throughout the body, including the heart. While muscles can function on energy supplied by fat and by glucose supplied by protein through gluconeogenesis as well as that furnished by the glycerol component of metabolized glycerides, carbohydrate is a more efficient energy source and is used preferentially when available.

Unlike muscle, the nervous system is almost totally dependent on carbohydrate for its normal functions. Sensory and intellectual processes are seriously impaired by hypoglycemia. Bizarre motor behavior may be observed during hypoglycemia, sometimes culminating in grand mal seizures. These can be particularly dangerous because they may occur while the victims are standing, resulting in severe injury to the head and other parts of the body when the victims fall to the ground. The most frequent victims of hypoglycemic episodes are diabetics treated with insulin. All insulin-treated diabetics should be taught to recognize the most minimal and earliest symptoms and signs of hypoglycemia. They should also be conditioned never to go anywhere without a readily accessible supply of easily ingested and readily assimilated carbohydrate on their persons. Small paper bags filled with sucrose, served in restaurants and on airlines for sweetening coffee and other beverages, are one convenient form of available carbohydrate which diabetics can carry wherever they go. The only acceptable rule to follow is, if in doubt, take some carbohydrate and do it fast.

One pair of sensory organs — the eyes — are particularly susceptible to changes in glucose concentrations in the blood. The crystalline lens changes its refractive index when blood sugar remains higher than the normal range leading to a reversible form of myopia.[489] Similarly, low blood sugar concentrations may be associated with failure of near vision compounded by oculomotor disturbances and intellectual malfunction of the central nervous system. In either case — hyper- or hypoglycemia — correction of the abnormal blood glucose concentration by appropriate therapy is mandatory.

Dangers of High-Carbohydrate, Low-Protein Dietary Regimens

Kwashiorkor, the so-called sugar-baby disease, described in detail by Cecily Williams[490] and first given by her the name used by the natives of the Gold Coast (now Ghana)[491] (a name later adopted by Brock and Autret[492] following their Food and Agriculture Organization (FAO)-sponsored survey of ten African countries and territories) has for over four decades been the classic example of a syndrome associated with ingestion of quantities of carbohydrate far in excess of the amount justified by the protein present in the diet. The victims of this syndrome are usually infants and young children whose superficial physical appearance suggests that they are thriving on the high-carbohydrate, low-protein regimens proffered them by well-meaning adults who have little insight into the problems of carbohydrate-protein imbalance. Infants and children with kwashiorkor appear to be well nourished by virtue of their retaining larger quantities of water in the subcutaneous tissue. Associated with this are the characteristic reddish cast to the usually black hair of dark-skinned children, low concentrations of serum albumin and a variety of other abnormalities in blood chemistries, hematology, body composition and intellectual performance data.[493] If diagnosed in time, such infants and children may be returned to excellent physical health by proper therapy including appropriate quantities of protein or protein mixtures of high biological value and adequate nonprotein Calories.[494]

In view of the popular belief that many older persons eat low-protein, high-carbohydrate diets by reason of personal choice, habitual practice, economic necessity or insufficient nurition education, the question of the prevalence of adult kwashiorkor among the elderly is frequently raised. Fortunately, this condition among elderly Americans is rarely found. Data from the Ten State Survey[495] and from the

HANES evaluations[496] and even from hospital records describing elderly persons admitted with a variety of diseases rarely describe pure versions of the typical kwashiorkor-like syndrome. Elderly adults with chronic debilitating diseases and disabilities, alcoholism, and drug-induced anorexia who have neglected themselves or have been neglected by others may manifest the edema, hypoproteinemia, skin and hair changes associated with the syndrome. Usually, however, adults on low protein diets also consume diets low in total Calories; hence, a marasmus-like syndrome is far more common than that caused by an excess intake of carbohydrate in the absence of adequate protein.

In the United States, even inexpensive foods such as bread, pastas, beans and rice contain far more protein than is found in the high-carbohydrate foods (sugar, cornstarch, cassava, maize, etc.) which comprise much of the diets of infants and children who develop kwashiorkor in technically underdeveloped countries. In addition, the availability of relatively low cost animal protein foods (*e.g.*, nonfat dry milk solids) which complement the amino acid mixtures found in the cheaper vegetable proteins is widespread. While food faddism among some elderly may lead to a true kwashiorkor-like syndrome, excesses in carbohydrate intake in the absence of protein are rarely found among elderly adults.

SUMMARY OF THE ROLE OF CARBOHYDRATE IN NUTRITION AND AGING

Carbohydrate is the fuel of choice for energy in all organ systems and is absolutely essential for appropriate function of the central nervous system. Ingested carbohydrate may be hydrolyzed to glucose and absorbed and used directly as an energy source. Excess glucose may be stored for short intervals as liver and muscle glycogen or in adipose tissue but for long-term storage is converted by a one-way reaction into fat which cannot be converted in any significant quantities back to carbohydrate. Protein, however, through the process of gluconeogenesis, can be converted to carbohydrate with accompanying losses of lean body mass and increases in the renal excretory load of unoxidizable residues of protein metabolism.

Carbohydrate is the principal vehicle for sweetness in human food. An acquired taste for sweets developed during childhood is usually carried over into the mature and older years of life. Carbohydrates and particularly sucrose rank with fats and salt as major components imparting desired flavors to many food products.

While fiber is technically a carbohydrate and while its role in supplying unabsorbable bulk to the dietary is often desirable, its major role in world nutrition is the provision of food for ruminants who in turn provide meat and dairy products for human consumption.

Carbohydrate intolerance increases with advancing age in adults and must always be distinguished from true diabetes mellitus. Hypoglycemia may be found among elderly persons from a variety of causes; however, hypoglycemia from exogenous insulin with or without physical exertion, unbalanced by appropriate carbohydrate intake is the most common.

Carbohydrates contribute to obesity if eaten in great excess of Caloric needs over periods of time measured in days.[497,498] They present particular hazards when consumed as pure (or empty) Calories, unassociated with other nutrients, unless care is taken to balance or cover the empty Calories with adequate quantities of protective nutrients.

In the management of illnesses associated with cachexia, parenterally administered solutions containing glucose are widely used. In addition, the widespread acceptability of most carbohydrates when taken in small, frequently ingested quantities makes them useful in nutritional rehabilitation when undertaken via *per os* feeding.

Dental caries have long been associated with the presence in the diet of fermentable carbohydrates, particularly those that cling tenaciously to tooth surfaces where they provide raw materials from which bacteria in dental plaque produce acids which attack tooth enamel. Proper brushing and flossing, the avoidance of sticky carbohydrate foods and regular professional dental care provide the best protection against caries among mature and elderly adults.

The role of refined carbohydrates, particularly sucrose, in the pathogenesis of cardiovascular disease is controversial. Controversy has been increased by promulgation of *Dietary Goals for the United States* which recommends increasing total carbohydrate consumption to 58 per cent of diet Calories but reducing consumption of refined carbohydrates to 10 per cent of diet Calories. While the controversy rages, all children, adolescents and adults including the elderly can take advantage of the various presentations to become more knowledgeable, sophisticated and discriminating about good nutrition, a general principle of which is that no one nutrient is solely responsible for such complex, multifactorial pathologies as are represented among the cardiovascular diseases.

Carbohydrates' roles in the management of renal disease are largely related to their ability to limit gluconeogenesis and prevent ketosis.

While high-carbohydrate, low-protein regimens are involved in the pathogenesis of kwashiorkor in infants and small children, excessive intakes of carbohydrate in the presence of negligible protein intake are rare among nonfaddist elderly persons.

Carbohydrate, once described as the "Cinderella of nutrition",[499] has become in recent decades, in the view of some, one of the ugly sisters. Cane sugar in particular has been called everything from a drug of addiction[500] to a prime cause of myocardial infarction, obesity, peptic ulcer and diabetes.[501] For persons concerned with health and aging, carbohydrates appropriately integrated into a total dietary regimen can move many parameters in directions now perceived to be indicative of improved health status.

Sweetness of carbohydrates — particularly of sucrose — have been the centuries-old reason for their popularity on which the "sweet tooth" of many Americans of all ages has developed. While so-called artificial sweeteners (saccharine, *e.g.)* have been condemned,[465] fructose with sweetness exceeding that of sucrose has entered the market place at a reasonable price as a result of the development of production techniques for the enzymatic isomerization of glucose to fructose.[502] Fructose-sweetened foods and beverages lower in Calories and in refined carbohydrate than their sucrose-sweetened equivalents have resulted. Here is a classic example of how a science — in this case enzymology — can serve in bridging the gap between acquired human tastes and the health needs of some individuals.

-9-

Minerals and Trace Elements

CLASSIFICATION OF DIETARY MINERALS AND TRACE ELEMENTS

Minerals with Structural and Biochemical Functions

Calcium (Ca), magnesium (Mg) and phosphorus (P) are major components of bone and tooth structure but also participate in many physiological and biochemical reactions.

Minerals with Primarily Biochemical Functions

Sodium (Na), potassium (K) and chloride (Cl) are present but less involved in bone and tooth structure but are major participants in physiologic and biochemical reactions and particularly in the homeostasis of acid-base balance. Iron (Fe) is traditionally associated with erythropoiesis and oxygen transport but also functions in numerous other biochemical reactions such as those involved in muscle function,[503] immunity and resistance to infectious disease.[504] Arsenic (As), boron (B), bromide (Br), cadmium (Cd), lead (Pb), lithium (Li), mercury (Hg) and strontium (Sr) are also found in living matter but are important to man largely because of their pharmacologic properties when prescribed or their toxic properties when ingestion or exposure is excessive.

Trace Elements Essential to Life

Essential trace elements are those whose concentrations per gram of wet organ weight are measured in minute quantities — micrograms

(10^{-6}), nanograms (10^{-9}) or picograms (10^{-12}) — and whose presence is required for biochemical reactions necessary for life. They include cobalt (Co.), copper (Cu), chromium (Cr), fluoride (F), iodine (I), manganese (Mn), molybdenum (Mo), nickel (Ni), selenium (Se), silicon (Si), tin (Sn), vanadium (V) and zinc (Zn).[505]

ROLES OF DIETARY MINERALS AND TRACE ELEMENTS

Roles of Calcium, Phosphorus and Magnesium

Calcium and phosphorus are major components of the hydroxyapatite crystals of which bone and teeth are composed. Magnesium accounts for 0.5 to 0.7 percent of bone ash, and somewhat over half of the body magnesium content has been shown to be in bone.[506] In bone and to a comparatively minuscule extent in teeth,[507] calcium, phosphate and magnesium enter and leave bone in quantities determined in normal human beings by a complex homeostatic system involving the dietary intake of the minerals themselves; the serum calcium, phosphate and magnesium concentrations; the pH of the system; the plasma concentration of $1{,}25(OH)_2$ vitamin D_3; the plasma concentrations of parathyroid hormone, calcitonin, estrogens, androgens and adrenocortical hormones; and the physical stresses to which the skeleton is subjected. While magnesium is an important component of the hydration shell of the hydroxyapatite crystal of bone,[508] its biochemical functions including its role in the regulation of serum calcium, phosphorus and potassium concentrations are of even greater significance. Similarly, calcium plays biochemical roles in coagulation, in nerve impulse transmission and in cardiac and skeletal muscle contraction. Phosphorus is an ubiquitous participant in the storage, liberation and transfer of energy, in the intermediary metabolism of carbohydrate and in the structure of phospholipids, nucleic acids and nucleotides.

Roles of Minerals with Primarily Biochemical Functions

Sodium: As the principal extracellular cation, sodium plays a major role in acid-base balance. Although 25 percent of total body sodium is thought to be in the water phase of the hydration shell and crystal surface of bone,[508] its quantity in the body at any given time is usually proportional to total body water, giving regulation of total body sodium a paramount role in the management of diseases characterized by anasarca.

Potassium: As the principal cation in intracellular fluid, potassium fills innumerable roles in biochemical reactions. It joins sodium as a major cation in acid-base homeostasis. Total body potassium is a widely used parameter proportional to lean body mass. Serum potassium concentrations in a relatively narrow range are essential for proper function of cardiac and skeletal muscle.

Chloride: As the principal extracellular anion, chloride plays a major role in acid-base homeostasis. As a component of gastric hydrochloric acid, it participates in the digestion of foodstuffs.

Iron: As a component of hemoglobin, iron plays an essential role in erythropoiesis and subsequently in oxygen transport from the lungs to all tissues of the body. Iron is found in myoglobin, the hemoglobin of muscles. It is a component of certain respiratory enzymes (cytochromes, peroxidase and catalase) which are found in virtually all cells throughout the body.

Roles of Elements Found in Tissue Which Are Not Essential to Life

Arsenic, Boron, Bromide, Cadmium, Lead, Mercury and Strontium: These elements are of concern because of their toxicity when their ingestion by or exposure of human beings is excessive. Arsenicals were used extensively in the preantibiotic era in the management of syphilis. Boron is a component of boric acid used widely in solution form as an antispetic and detergent in the management of dermatologic and ophthalmologic problems. Bromides, previously prescribed and used for nervous tension, for asthma and as analgesics, were, when taken in excess, responsible for clinical bromism. Cadmium accumulates in human and animal kidneys even after very low levels of exposure. Persons with hypertension have greater concentrations in their kidneys than those who do not. Lead poisoning is common among young children with pica whose habit may lead to clinical symptoms in situations where they have access to old paint containing lead.[509] Adults scraping lead containing paint while using unapproved methods may also become clinically ill from the same source.[510] In addition, in some communities with acid water supplies, lead derived from century-old lead water mains may lead to excessive ingestion of lead by persons of all ages. Mercury enters the environment as an industrial pollutant and as such may be transmitted to man by fish which enter the food chain. Discovery of high mercury levels in fish found in ancient Egyptian tombs suggests that natural sources of mercury pollution may exist. Strontium toxicity has achieved prominence in the atomic age, since it may substitute for calcium in bone. When radioactive, it therefore may become relatively fixed in bone for long periods of time during which its radiation may induce neoplastic disease.

Lithium: Lithium is not now known to be essential to life. However, its use in the early post-World War II era as a component of salt substitutes and the present widespread use of lithium carbonate in the management of manic-depressive psychoses[511,512] among adults of all ages justify a few comments regarding both lithium therapy and lithium toxicity.

Lithium carbonate in most effective is modulating the manic phases of manic-depressive bipolar psychoses. While a minority of patients have found that lithium obviates depression, most patients require mood elevators to manage the depressed aspects of the cycle.

The therapeutic range of plasma lithium concentrations is from 1.0 to 1.5 mEq per liter during acute manic episodes and from 0.6 to 1.2 mEq per liter during long-term control. Lithium toxicity, which is far more likely to occur in elderly persons, may involve one or more signs and symptoms indicating neuromuscular, central nervous system, cardiovascular, gastrointestinal, genitourinary, dermatologic, autonomic, thyroid, electroencephlographic, electrocardiographic and a variety of miscellaneous abnormalities. Regular monitoring of both the plasma lithium concentrations and the clinical state of the patient is absolutely essential and particularly imperative among the elderly.

Roles of Trace Elements

All of the trace elements mentioned in the classification above have been found to be essential for life. They function as components in biochemical enzymatic reactions which are slowed when trace element tissue concentrations are low and are reduced to activity levels causing serious disability and death under those conditions (found only in the laboratory) when the experimental animals have none of the trace elements under study available from diet, water or air.

While all essential trace elements are important dietary components, those which are of special interest to the biology of aging are chromium, copper, fluoride, iodide, selenium, vanadium and zinc. They will be discussed in more detail below.

QUANTITIES OF MINERALS AND TRACE ELEMENTS IN THE DIET

Historical Perspective

Major Minerals: Calcium is now being consumed in technically developed societies in amounts greater than at any time in history. The production, distribution, availability and safety of dairy products high in calcium are largely responsible. Studies in technically underdeveloped societies who have not developed dairy industries or devised other means of adding calcium to their food supplies reveal calcium consumption levels relatively unchanged through recorded history. Whether even the historical highs in calcium consumption in countries like the United States are high enough or well enough distributed among aging adults will be discussed below.

Phosphorus consumption in the technically developed world has grown rapidly in the twentieth century. In part, this has been due to the marked rise in the consumption of meat and in part to the equally marked rise in the consumption of carbonated beverages high in phosphorus. This rise in phosphorus consumption has outstripped the rise in calcium consumption with a resulting marked reduction in the calcium: phosphorus ratio, a serious matter whose implications will be discussed later.

Magnesium content of the traditional occidental dietary is considerably lower than that of the traditional oriental which includes large amounts of soybeans, vegetables and rice, all foods high in available magnesium. Temporal changes over the years in the amounts of other ingredients in the occidental dietary — increasing quantities of calcium, protein, vitamin D and alcohol, all of which interfere with the retention of and hence increase the requirement for magnesium — suggest that today the average citizen of a technically developed society may be receiving far less magnesium daily than the RDA of 300 mg per day for women and 350 mg per day for men. This is particularly true among consumers of low Calorie diets, since the magnesium content is generally proportional to Calorie intake. Furthermore, the lower the cost of a diet, the less magnesium it is likely to contain. Many occidentals make up for some of the deficiency by consuming magnesium salts as antacids, as laxatives and as dietary supplements.

Sodium has long been a desired component of human food because of the flavor imparted by sodium chloride — common salt. Primitive societies living far from salt water are known to devote enormous effort to the extraction of sodium salts from green plants. Salt has been used extensively in food preservation for centuries. Examples of such foods are salt cod, corned beef, saurkraut and ham. In modern food technology, processed foods such as soups, catsup, stews, frozen vegetables, etc. have salt added primarily to meet taste preferences of consumers which in turn are determined by habits ingrained in childhood by family practices and media pressures. However, ongoing investigations supported by the National Institutes of Health among the newborn have suggested a preference for salt and sugar; the implications of these preferences for the development of food consumption patterns in later life are being pursued. The average American diet has been reported to contain from 6 to 18 gm of salt daily, or from 100 to 300 mEq of sodium.[513] While some of this is derived from processed food, much is added by consumers themselves to fresh meats, fresh vegetables, cereals and dairy products. These consumers may be influenced by the almost ubiquitous presence of salt in recipes found in major cook books. Some consumers are so conditioned to the use of salt that they even reach automatically for the salt shaker before tasting the food. The sodium content of modern foods has also been increased by the addition of compounds like sodium glutamate in the processing and cooking of many foods to enhance their flavor. In oriental cooking, highly salted soy sauce used in meal preparation and at the table increases the sodium content of such cuisine. In brief, the sodium content of modern diets has reached a new high, even though the need for salt as a food preservative has diminished with the advent of modern technology.

Chloride, the anion accompanying sodium in common salt, has an historical perspective essentially similar to that of sodium.

Potassium intake throughout history has been sufficient to supply the minimum needs of healthy human beings. With the widespread application of flame photometry since World War II to the measurement of potassium in body fluids, information has accumulated revealing in disease and during therapy with drugs and hormones both potassium deficiency and potassium excess. Either condition may be managed effectively by prescription of potassium-containing foods and solutions or their prescription in forms minimizing potassium intake.

Iron contents of human dietaries have varied historically for a variety of reasons: analytical methods used in the analyses of diets for iron; quantities of iron-containing contaminants in the food supply; the shift away from iron utensils used in the preparation of foods for consumption; the presence or absence of iron fortification in foods; the rising red meat content of diets in some countries; and the deliberate prescription of ferrous salts in the management of increased iron requirements occasioned by normal menstruation and pregnancy in women and pathological blood loss such as that from parasitic infection. The available iron in human dietaries has also varied depending on whether dietary iron was in the heme or nonheme form, whether — in the case of the latter — it was in the ferric or the reduced ferrous state and whether it was bound to phytates or to fiber thereby becoming unavailable. The availability of nonheme iron also depends on whether it is being consumed in the presence of such adjuvants as meat or ascorbic acid. It also depends on the level of iron stores in the persons under study, those with low stores absorbing more than those with high. The available iron content of the American diet is probably at an all time high among those who spend much on meat containing heme iron daily. For others, it is undoubtedly lower than in past decades by virtue of food processing changes, shifts away from iron utensils in food preparation and the higher costs of animal protein. Many at special risk receive ferrous iron by prescription or foods fortified with iron compounds. Controversy over increased iron fortification of widely used foods such as bakery products is holding in abeyance one method of making available iron more prevalent in the American diet. Data derived from the U.S. Department of Agriculture's Spring 1965 Survey of Food Consumption, from the Ten State Nutrition Survey (1968-1970) and from the Health and Nutrition Examination Survey

(HANES) (1971-1974)[99,514,515] all indicate that the elderly surveyed had iron intakes per 1,000 Calories of food consumed well above the 6 mg per 1,000 Calories usually recommended. However, their Calorie intakes were so low that their total iron consumption barely exceeded (males) or fell slightly below (females) the 10 mg RDA for iron recommended in both the 1968 and 1974 editions of Recommended Dietary Allowances.[516,92] These data are based on survey data collection methods and may not reflect either iron consumed or available iron. The data do suggest a gradual decrease in total iron intake over the decade covered by the three surveys but a gradual increase in the iron intakes per 1,000 Calories, consistent with the gradual decrease in total Calories intake over the same period of time but suggesting also that the elderly are becoming better selectors of foods with high densities of iron.

Nonessential Elements: Improved analytic methods and higher indices of suspicion arising in part from extensive epidemiologic and toxicologic studies have provided data which have enabled health industry workers to identify in the past half-century a number of nonessential elements which are toxic to man if ingested in the food or water supply or inhaled with air. When atomic explosions in the atmosphere were frequent, radiostrontium contamination of the lands on which dairy cattle were pastured provided the route by which radiostrontium entered the food chain and eventually the bones of man. Arsenic, once a component of arsenicals used in the treatment of syphilis, has since the antibiotic era become a problem for man because of its presence in herbicides and pesticides. Bromide has entered man's internal environment largely through improper self-medication of bromide containing drugs used as sedatives and analgesics. Boron as a component of borax (sodium borate) and of boric acid (H_3BO_3) is found in many homes and health-care institutions. When accidently administered into the gastrointestinal tract as a formula for infants or a gavage feeding for disabled adults, boric acid can be life-threatening. When used as a dusting powder for skin hygiene inside diapers of infants and of incontinent adults, boric acid may be absorbed and just as life-threatening. Boron hydrides were extensively used as rocket fuels when the National Aeronautics and Space Administration (NASA) focused on one-time-use rockets. Diborane, a gas extremely irritating to the pulmonary tree, and pentaborane, used either in liquid or solid form, were highly toxic compounds which have been used infrequently in recent years because of their hazards to workers and machines in the NASA program and their adverse impact on the environment.

Cadmium, a bivalent metal, is widely used industrially in metal plating and in the manufacture of alloys, vapor lamps and storage batteries. Human exposure is largely environmentally related. Since cadmium is readily soluble in acids, acid foods and beverages prepared and stored in cadmium-plated containers *(e.g.,* certain ice cube trays) may become sufficiently contaminated to cause acute poisoning. However, from the point of view of aging, cadmium is of greatest interest because of its age-related pattern of ever-increasing accumulation in kidneys through middle age and its declining concentration in kidneys during old age (as determined by cross sectional studies).[517] In longitudinal studies in animals, over-all mortality was greater among cadmium-fed animals, but this difference disappeared among those who survived into old age.[518] In addition, extensive studies in man and animals[519] have shown statistically significant relationships between cadium concentrations in renal tissue and prevalence rates for moderate hypertension. The most accepted theory on cadmium's mechanism of action in producing hypertension is that it induces sodium retention. The known relation between low prevalence rates for hypertension and the hardness of the water supply have been related to the higher cadmium content found in soft waters.[520] In historical perspective, the effects of cadmium at first would seem to be a by-product of industrialization. However, the highest mean renal cadmium concentrations found in a geographic survey[521] were among Mongoloid peoples from the Far East. This suggests — together with the low cadmium concentrations found in cross sectional studies of the kidneys of the very old — that some genetic influence may moderate the impact of cadmium on man as it has been shown to do in rats.[522]

As noted above, mercury in significant quantities was found in mummified fish in the tombs of ancient Egypt. In modern times, alkyl mercury compounds (methyl and ethyl mercury), not being biodegradable, have become significant environmental hazards. Methyl mercury has been found in tuna and swordfish taken from mercury-contaminated waters. Alkyl mercury compounds are used as antifungal agents in the treatment of seed grains which, when accidently diverted into the food chain, have caused serious epidemics in Japan. Phenyl mercuric propionate, incorporated into some house paints to prevent mold growth, has also created mercury toxicity in man and should be used, if at all, only outdoors. From the point of view of aging, mercury is especially important because it is used in many forms for health-related reasons. Trade names such as merthiolate, mercurochrome, mercuzanthin and mercuhydrin are but some of a large number which are used as virtually household terms by members of the health industry. In addition, corrosive sublimate ($HgCl_2$) is commonly found in homes, hospitals and industries. Other mercury compounds such as mercurophen are widely used powerful antiseptics and germicides. Calomel, HgCl, used extensively as a purgative throughout the lifetimes of many older persons, may be toxic *per se* but also may set the stage for later hypersensitivity reactions. Ammoniated mercury ointments are widely used in the treatment of some dermatoses and are readily absorbed through the skin. Some teething powders and diaper rinses contain absorbable mercury. While much progress has been made in eliminating industrial and environmental sources of chronic mercury poisoning, little attention has been paid to the potential and real hazards posed by the use of mercury compounds in the health industry. Among the elderly, this is particularly important, since many signs and symptoms of mercury poisoning may be overlooked, being regarded as a product or normal aging or of the diseases prevalent in old age. Almost any central nervous system and behavioral symptom or sign may be mimicked by chronic mercury poisoning. Patients suspected of exposure to mercury-containing compounds should have their urine checked for its mercury concentration. Concentrations > 0.1 mg per liter are considered evidence of toxicity.

Lead poisoning, commonly seen among children with pica who live in old dwellings whose lead-containing paint is flaking off, is no stranger to adults. Sources of lead include old water systems comprised of lead mains and new water systems in which white lead has been used in sealing joints of the pipes; the use of pewter tableware; the use of gasoline containing tetraethyl lead for cleaning purposes; the ingestion of foods, wines and distilled liquors containing soluble lead salts; the consumption of whiskey made in stills improvised from auto and truck radiators; and a wide variety of occupational exposures. Insomnia, restlessness, irritability, memory loss, hallucinations and confusion — all found in many old persons — may characterize the encephalopathic form of the condition. Bowel colic, constipation, nausea, vomiting and weight loss are prevalent in the alimentary form. Neuromuscular abnormalities including paralysis may also be present. Anemia may be present. Chronic renal failure may result. Since lead diminishes the renal clearance of uric acid, so-called saturine gout may occur, particularly among those persons who have been consuming large quantities of whiskey distilled in radiators. When suspected on the basis of history, lead poisoning should be ruled out or confirmed by urine lead mesurements; when urine is properly collected and analyzed, concentrations > 0.1 mg per liter should be regarded as indicative of dangerous exposure. Historically speaking, much has been done in the past decade to protect the public from lead toxicity. Diagnostic methods are available in most state and city public health laboratories, widespread educational campaigns have been conducted and methods of treatment have been introduced. Environmental control measures such as the use of lead-free gasoline in all new cars has aided in the reduction of risk. Nonetheless, particularly among the elderly, lead poisoning may be overlooked unless a high index of suspicion is constantly maintained and questions regarding possible exposure are included in the taking of every clinical history.

Lithium: Lithium was first recognized for having useful properties in the treatment of manic-depressive psychoses in 1949. Since then, much work has been done to evaluate its effectiveness, to study its mechanism of action and to explore other therapeutic properties. Whether used in managing bipolar psychoses, the treatment of inappropriate secretion of antidiuretic hormone[523] or increasing the total circulating neutrophil mass and accelerating neutrophil production,[524] the proximity of the therapeutic plasma concentration range to the toxic range generates the need for careful clinical and laboratory monitoring of each patient. Particularly among the elderly, in whom the half-life of lithium may be double that found in middle aged adults, therapeutic ranges may be achieved on half the usual dose of lithium carbonate.[525] As in the case of mercury and lead poisoning, lithium toxicity signs and symptoms (tremors, drowsiness, slurred speech, choreoathetoid movements, confusion and nystagmus as well as hyporeflexia, coma and a pitressin resistant diabetes insipidus-like syndrome) may readily be confused with those often associated with old age or the diseases thereof. The prevalence of manic-depressive psychoses among the elderly and the popular faith in lithium therapy stimulated among the laity by two best-selling paperback books[526,527] have made lithium toxicity a matter of constant concern for those who care for older patients.

Trace Elements: Quantification of trace elements in the dietary is a relatively new science. In 1974, the Food and Nutrition Board included a trace element — zinc — in its widely distributed table of Recommended Dietary Allowances (92), although discussions of trace elements have appeared in the texts of earlier editions.[516,528]

Tables of nutrient composition of foods will contain virtually no information on trace element contents. While more information is being collected and will appear in future publications of the U.S. Department of Agriculture's Food Analysis Laboratory and the Department's Data Bank, as well as elsewhere, little specific information is currently available which has programatic significance in planning meals for the elderly or others who are aging.

From an historical standpoint, the changes with time in the quantities in the diet of trace elements now known to have some impact on aging — chromium, copper, fluoride, iodide, vanadium and zinc — are with certain exceptions difficult to evaluate because little information is available from data collected in previous decades. The widespread introduction in the sixties of the atomic absorption spectrophotometer to analytical laboratories has assisted greatly in improving the information base, as have better analytical techniques for measuring the nonmetallic elements.

Certain public health practices introduced since World War II have increased the amount of fluoride and iodide in the water and food supply. Fluoridation of public water supplies for the prevention of dental caries, particularly in young children, is widespread.[529] Fluorides have been described as possible deterrents to osteoporosis and have been used extensively in the treatment of that disease.[530,531] Iodides, once so lacking in inland regions of North America that thyroid goiter was endemic, are now believed to be in excess supply because of the extensive use of iodine-containing compounds in required sanitation practices in the dairy and food processing industries where they become incorporated into human foods.[532]

Modern food preparation practices may influence adversely the trace element content of foods served in the home, in institutions, in restaurants and by commercial caterers.[533] Soaking and cooking foods in large quantities of water which are then poured off as waste removes from foods so treated many trace elements and also increases the waste and destruction of labile vitamins.

The incorporation of trace elements into the formulas of multivitamin preparations and into foods fortified with trace elements has introduced another and highly variable (among individuals and population groups) source of trace elements into the human dietary. The high cost at retail outlets of such products[534] prevents their use among lower income elderly persons, and the frequent lack of compliance by elderly persons with instructions concerning their use limits their effectiveness in any but certain institutional environments. Even there, high cost, insufficient personnel and lack of staff education frequently vitiate the objective of adequate trace element nutrition.

Geographic Perspective

In modern industrial societies like the United States, there are no longer true geographic differences in the availability of major dietary minerals, thanks to nation-wide food distribution networks which make major minerals as well as other nutrients available virtually everywhere. The same may be said for trace elements with the exception of a few pockets of high fluoride concentrations in water supplies. The distribution of nonessential elements with potential for toxicity depends on the source, the exposure to the source of specific persons and the vigor with which environmental protection laws and regulations are enforced.

Among members of technically less developed societies, marked geographic differences in the availability of major minerals and trace elements do occur. Some Peruvians were found to be consuming less than one-quarter of the RDA for calcium.[535] Among Guatemalan aborigines, calcium in the diet was greater as a result of the practice of soaking corn in lime water reaching levels equal to the RDA.[535a] In milk-drinking countries in Asia and Africa, calcium is abundant in the dietaries of those who have access to a supply of milk. Trace elements may be low as a result of combinations of soil conditions and dietary practices. Iodine deficiency results in endemic goiter in vast areas of

Asia and Latin America. The introduction of iodine into the food supply and in some instances directly into the bodies by injection of persons living in these regions has been a major goal of the World and Pan-American Health Organizations. Zinc has been found to be so deficient in the dietary in parts of Iran as to produce a classic deficiency syndrome in young men.[536]

Among the elderly, geography in a less global and more intimate sense may lead to mineral and trace element deficiencies, among others. Relatively short distances from food shopping centers or from restaurants or from sites of the Nutrition Program for Older Americans (NPOA) may serve as deterrents to adequate nutrition among older persons whose disabilities, fears or economic status keep them homebound. These geographically isolated aged have been singled out as target populations for programs like NPOA. However, the high costs of outreach, escort, transportation and primary health care for such isolates has made reaching them with approriate health and nutrition services extremely difficult. As a result, many hundreds of thousands of elderly persons do exist on diets composed of ingredients which have long shelf lives, are easily prepared (often without heating) and are low in cost. Such regimens are almost invariably low in calcium, magnesium and many essential trace elements, as well as vitamins and well-balanced proteins. They are classic examples of dietaries comprising high percentages of "empty Calories" uncompensated for by extra quantities of protective nutrients.

Economic Perspective

As mentioned frequently above, calcium, magnesium, iron and many essential trace elements are present in recommended or suggested appropriate quantities daily when dietary regimens are carefully planned, contain foods which are relatively high in cost or contain less costly foods fortified with minerals and trace elements (among other nutrients) or are supplemented by minerals in the form of mineral-trace element-vitamin tablets, capsules or elixirs. Since educational attainments are directly proportional to income in most societies, poorly educated persons who have difficulty learning the complexities of modern nutrition are usually among the low income groups. Many millions of elderly in the United States fall into this category. They have not acquired the knowledge essential to comprehending the need for high-nutrient-density foods, for fortified foods or for dietary supplements nor would they be able to afford them if they were deliberately prescribed by knowledgeable health industry personnel.

Among better educated and more affluent elderly persons, the quantities of minerals and trace elements in dietary regimens is usually greater; however, much of this group's expendable income may be nutritionally wasted through their purchases of costly foods and costly supplements promoted via mass media commercial advertising, through purchases of even more costly products of food faddism and through unwarranted avoidance of certain low cost foods engendered by consumer activist organizations.

Regardless of economic status, elderly persons frequently retain dietary practices learned during their younger years. Their education in modern, scientifically designed, clinically proven nutrition practices is inadequate, frequently because uninformed educators assume that the elderly can not be reconditioned to abandon former practices and adopt new ones.

Health and nutrition education for all age groups at all economic and educational levels can do much to improve nutrition practices. Such education is required not only by obvious target populations such as those elderly who are impoverished and poorly educated but also by many persons employed in the bureaucracies of provider networks and by some of the principle provider figures — physicians, dentists, nurses, dietitians, nutritionists and social workers, among others — themselves.

Within the NPOA network, several examples may be found where persuasive, informed leadership has altered longstanding dietary beliefs and practices through combinations of education, counseling, example setting and organized peer pressure. While the monetary cost has been low in these projects, so also at the Federal, State and local levels in general has been the motivation by leadership to implement the successful actions in the several projects referred to above.

MINERALS OF MAJOR CONCERN IN AGING

Calcium

For persons already old, dietary calcium serves primarily to prevent further bone loss. The quantity needed daily to accomplish this objective remains controversial. Greater requirements for the aged than for younger persons have been reported.[537,539] No differences have been found by other investigators.[540,541] In one study,[540] calcium was not stored although large amounts of nitrogen and phosphorus were retained. Similarly, calcium was not stored by old men at high and low levels of protein intake with and without injections of a potent synthetic androgen in spite of their retention of large quantities of phosphorus and nitrogen in all phases of the study.[173] After an analysis of data collected from seven sources, Harrison[542] concluded that the efficiency of calcium absorption varied little among old men, young adults and older children, although he did find among infants exceptionally high efficiency of calcium absorption.

Much data in regard to calcium requirements for older persons have been derived from studies of the disease osteoporosis, although it is by no means synonymous with osteopenia observed with physiological aging. Modern therapy for osteoporosis has included increased intake of calcium,[543,544] the prescription of sodium fluoride,[545,547] the use of strontium salts[548] and various forms of vitamin D *(v.i.)*. The hypothesis of Reifenstein and Albright[549] that osteoporosis is associated with lack of an adequate protein matrix which may be restored by appropriate hormonal therapy is now regarded as but one of many contributing to an understanding of the disease.

Considerable disagreement exists in regard to the role of dietary calcium in the bone loss which accompanies physiological aging. Garn in studies measuring the calcium content of metacarpals in 14 different populations between ages 25 and 45 and 45 and 85 has found no relation between losses of bone and levels of calcium intake.[550,551] Exton-Smith[552] on the basis of Garn's studies[550,553] believes that bone loss in old age has no relation to adult calcium intake but rather that the quantity of bone present in old age is directly related to skeletal mass at maturity.

Hegsted, since observing very low calcium requirements during studies performed in Peruvian adult male prisoners,[535] has promoted the concept that the RDA of 800 mg daily is too high and too impractical to apply.[554] Most convincing of Hegsted's arguments are those illustrating the inability of investigations using calcium balance techniques to produce data which is accurate and unbiased in favor of high requirements;[554] the evidence from human[555] and animal[556,557] studies that adaptation to very low levels of dietary calcium may occur; and the evidence derived from Garn's[551] anthropologic data that cortical bone loss is not correlated with calculated calcium intake between ages 25 to 85.

Relating Hegsted's proposals to calcium requirements among older humans deserves consideration of the fact that he is suggesting needs lower than the 1974 RDA based on data collected during studies on ambulatory, healthy persons many of whom have adapted to low intakes of dietary calcium. Such needs may certainly be used as parameters on which to develop recommendations for national nutrition policies, especially for countries in which calcium is in short supply and found largely as a component of high nutrient-density, costly foods.

However, factors such as diminished exposure to sunlight;[558] less performance of heavy physical work;[559] increased frequency of corticosteroid hormone[560] and drug[561] intake; and more stresses from illnesses, accidents, surgery, and radiation therapy — all of which increase bone loss among the elderly — are not prominent among the statistical weights influencing Hegsted's suggestions.

In contrast to Garn's studies,[551] Albanese[562] and Albanese, *et al.*,[563] using methods which quantify radiographically bone losses in longitudinal studies over time in digital phalanges and alveolar ridges (methodology similar to that used by Garn), have shown in controlled dietary studies as high as 30 percent increments in coefficients of bone density when supplements containing 750 mg of calcium and 375 i.u. of vitamin D daily were consumed over periods of one to four years by domiciled but healthy women averaging 80.2 years of age and in-hospital personnel aged 36 to 69 years of age. The supplements increased the total daily calcium intake to about 1200 mg. These investigators, therefore, are urging adoption of a higher RDA — 1100 mg or more — for calcium for all age groups.

The data of Albanese, *et al.* support concepts developed by Lutwak and various colleagues who have presented data suggesting that bone resorption may be prevented and even reversed at any age and in a variety of physiological states such as immobilization if calcium intakes of at least the RDA or higher are consumed daily.[564,567] Their suggestions have been born out in the nutritional management of paralyzed victims of spinal cord injury who showed less bone resorption, less heterotopic bone formation, fewer renal and vesical stones, and lower urinary calcium excretion ratios when ingesting diets containing up to two grams of calcium daily.[81] Persons of any age with traumatic cervical fractures and quadriplegia are victims of "instant aging", since in the few milliseconds of the trauma they acquire the metabolic, skeletal, physical, psychological, economic and nutritional problems usually associated with very advanced old age.

In seeking a policy with regard to recommendations for calcium intake and aging, it is well to remember that bone metabolism involves not only calcium but also phosphorus, magnesium, fluorine, protein, vitamin D and its metabolites, vitamin C, physical activity levels, and the presence or absence of hormone and drug therapy and of stress. However, assuming such factors are relatively standardized, present consensus among investigators suggests that middle-aged and older persons should consume at least the RDA of 800 mg, if not more, calcium daily, unless very specific contraindications confirmed scientifically, not by folklore, exist. In many societies, this implies consumption of dairy products, sometimes unpopular among the aged. Such unpopularity is readily overcome, as demonstrated repeatedly in the experiences of the Nutrition Program for Older Americans (NPOA), by dairy product availability, peer example and appropriate education. The related issue of cost can be moderated by encouraging the use of nonfat dry milk. For those who absolutely can not tolerate milk products, other calcium-containing foods and supplements (calcium carbonate and gluconate) may be used.

Since dairy products are major readily available sources of calcium, recommending their consumption by the elderly frequently raises the issue of whether lactase — the enzyme in the small intestinal mucosa which hydrolyzes the disaccharide lactose, the principal carbohydrate in milk — diminishes to the point of inducing lactase deficiency syndromes in adults as they become old. Present evidence to support a relation between the acquisition of lactase deficiency as a function of aging is insufficient to warrant concern. While persons of African, Oriental, Jewish, Arab and Cypriot ancestry have high prevalence rates of some degree of lactose intolerance,[568,569] even these persons can tolerate moderate amounts of dairy products daily.

A Mayo Clinic study using the presence of $\geq$ 0.20 ml/ minute of respiratory hydrogen (H_2) two hours after a 50 gm lactose load as evidence of lactase deficiency found that eight out of 30 osteoporotic women averaging 65.2 years of age and only one out of 31 women without osteoporosis averaging 61.8 years of age were lactase deficient.[570] All subjects were white and of northern European family background. Those with lactase deficiency indicated smaller but by no means negligible dairy product consumption, an observation suggesting to the authors that lactase deficiency and its related clinical symptoms may lead to less intake and possibly less absorption of calcium, thereby contributing to the pathogenesis of osteoporosis. Similar findings had previously been reported by Birge, *et al.*[571].

International agencies responsible for improving health and nutrition among technically underdeveloped nations have concluded that the nutritional value of dairy products far outweigh the risks of mild symptomatology created by lactase deficiency.[572]

A similar attitude seems appropriate for recommendations among the elderly. During the acceptability trials of Limited Use Supplemental Food (LUSF) by NPOA participants,[534] almost 95 percent of the 6,000 persons involved found LUSF, a nonfat dry milk-based product, acceptable, even though persons of Negro, Native American and Oriental backgrounds were among those recipients to whom the product was acceptable. Hence, as a major source of dietary calcium, dairy products may be recommended for consumption by the elderly, subject only to the usual caveat in regard to individual idiosyncrasies.

Phosphorus

Dietary phosphorus content, according to the RDA,[92a] should equal or be less than dietary calcium content, yielding a calcium/phosphorus ratio of 1.0 or higher. Such ratios are uncommon in modern industrial societies for two principal reasons: (a) the great popularity of red meat, high in phosphorus and low in calcium; and (b) the large quantities of soft drinks imbibed by persons of all ages, drinks which are high in phosphorus and negligible in their content of calcium. Diets high in phosphorus should be used with caution by the elderly in view of the linear decrements in discrete renal functions which occur after age 30. This becomes especially important for persons with a history of renal disease.

Hyperphosphatemia accompanies azotemia in renal failure. Its management includes administration of low phosphorus, low protein, high carbohydrate diets. If these are unacceptable and dialysis either is not indicated or unattainable, hyperphosphatemia may be controlled by the patients' ingesting frequently repeated doses of aluminum hydroxide gel which binds and makes unabsorbable phosphorus in ingested food and gastrointestinal fluids. Such therapy will reduce urinary phosphorus to zero[560] and help maintain serum phosphorus in the normal range. In far advanced renal failure, aluminum hydroxide alone may not control serum phosphorus, necessitating the addition of a low phosphorus diet to the management regimen. Such nonabsorbable antacids, however, are double edged swords. They are practically the only causes of the true phosphorus deficiency syndrome in man.[574] The syndrome is characterized by muscular weakness, anorexia, malaise and pain in the bones, the severity of the symptoms correlating with the decrease in serum phosphorus. The presence of hypophosphatemia and hypercalcuria in a patient consuming large quantities of aluminum gels should not mistakenly be diagnosed as hyperparathyroidism.

Increased dietary phosphorus has been recommended[575] as a result of rodent and primate studies suggesting that it might protect children and adolescents from dental caries and even might improve bone structure. While no completely comparable studies have been performed in elderly humans, Goldsmith, *et al.*[576] have reported that one gram daily supplements of phosphorus significantly reduced demineralization and the time needed for clinical union in patients of a variety of ages with femoral, ankle and wrist fractures. These results led Epstein to suggest the need for a prospective study of the value of phosphates in the management of senile osteoporosis.[577]

Such a prospective double-blind controlled study of phosphate therapy in recurrent nephrolithiasis gave little support to the value of phosphate supplements in the management of that condition.[578]

In an exemplary physiologic animal model, Slatopolsky and Bricker[579] showed that restricting dietary phosphorus prevented secondary hyperparathyroidism (restriction maintained serum phosphorus, serum parathyroid hormone, and serum calcium in the normal range) in dogs subjected to staged reductions in renal mass. Their observations suggest the desirability of limiting dietary phosphorus, prescribing aluminum hydroxide gels, or both, to elderly patients with diminished renal function occasioned by physiologic aging[183] compounded by advanced chronic renal disease.

Gray, *et al.*[580] have observed an inverse correlation between serum phosphate and plasma 1,25$(OH)_2$-vitamin D_3 concentrations in normal subjects and in patients with recurrent calcium nephrolithiasis or with primary hyperparathyroidism. Low phosphate diets led to increases in plasma 1,25$(OH)_2$-vitamin D_3. This stimulation of renal synthesis of 1,25$(OH)_2$-vitamin D_3 by dietary phosphate restriction is significant in view of age-wise reduction in 1,25$(OH)_2$-vitamin D_3 synthesis and that reduction's possible relation to aging-associated osteopenia *(v.i.)*.

A phosphorus-containing drug — disodium etidronate (EHDP), a diphosphonate — has been studied extensively in Europe[581,582] and investigated in both animal and clinical studies in the United States.[583,584] This compound — chemically named disodium ethane-1-hydroxy-1,1 diphosphonate — alters the crystalline structure of hydroxyapatite, making it more refractory to dissolution by immobilization and other factors contributing to bone loss.

However, clinical studies[584] in ideopathic osteoporosis not only have been disappointing but also have suggested that treatment with EHDP may be contraindicated. Hyperphosphatemia, increased total but diminished ionized serum calcium, increased serum parathyroid hormone, failure to diminish bone resorption, increased bone loss, and increased unmineralized osteoid tissue suggested in two male and two female patients (average age, 65.2 years) with primary osteoporosis that EHDP produced morphologic osteomalacia.

Although EHDP was also proposed as an effective tool in the management of Paget's disease of bone,[585] later studies revealed mineralization defects and excessive osteoid during its use. Using lower doses of EHDP combined with synthetic human calcitonin, Hosking, *et al.*,[586] have reported effective treatment without complications of associated with higher doses of either agent administered alone.

In summarizing current consensus in regard to phosphorus as a nutrient in relation to aging, virtually all investigators agree that far more research in man is required. Phosphorus deficiency syndromes exist only when nonabsorbable aluminum hydroxide gels are used in the absence of supplemental phosphorus. Restrictions of dietary phosphorus may be indicated when aluminum hydroxide gel therapy alone fails to control hyperphosphatemia in advanced renal failure. Except for the inverse relation between serum phosphate and plasma 1,25$(OH)_2$-vitamin D_3 concentrations, dietary phosphorus seems to have little proven relation to osteopenia from physiologic aging or from osteoporosis. The high phosphorus contents of modern diets in industrialized societies are potentially hazardous and should be avoided through proper menu planning and the avoidance of high-phosphate soft drinks. EHDP is not effective in the management of osteopenia or alone in the management of Paget's disease of bone.

Magnesium

In relation to aging, magnesium deficiency is an important and commonly overlooked syndrome. The syndrome may appear as a result of low dietary magnesium intake, impaired gastrointestinal absorption, defective renal tubular absorption or incorporation of magnesium into lean body mass or into the skeleton during episodes of rapid metabolic repair. Among the elderly, factors contributing to magnesium deficiency include parenteral alimentation, use of certain diuretics, use of certain antibiotics, excessive use of enemas, alcohol ingestion, malabsorption syndromes and the syndrome of inappropriate secretion of antidiuretic hormone (SIADH).

Common manifestations of magnesium deficiency are hypocalcemia and hypokalemia. Since serum magnesium is measured far less frequently than serum calcium and serum potassium, magnesium deficiency in the pathogenesis of hypocalcemia and hypokalemia is often overlooked. Hypocalcemia from magnesium depletion has been attributed to peripheral resistance of bone and kidney to parathyroid hormone, to interference with parathyroid hormone release from the parathyroid glands in response to hypocalcemia, or to both.[587] From a practical standpoint, no matter what the underlying mechanism, the magnesium-deficiency-related hypocalcemia is rectified within hours by the parenteral administration of magnesium salts. In hypocalcemic and hypokalemic elderly parsons, consideration of hypomagnesemia in the differential diagnosis is mandatory and may be life-saving.

The relation of magnesium deficiency to diseases and their treatments and the high prevalence rates for such diseases and treatments among the elderly suggest the critical importance of individualized diagnoses and replacement therapies in addition to the 300 mg of dietary magnesium suggested by the RDA.

Sodium

Sodium is a natural component of many foods and is added to other foods by processors or by the ultimate consumers during meal preparation or at the table. Common salt (sodium chloride) is the most widely used condiment, but sodium is also consumed as monosodium glutamate (MSG), sodium bicarbonate, disodium phosphate, sodium caseinate, sodium citrate, sodium saccarinate, sodium benzoate and dioctyl sodium sulfosuccinate, to mention only a few. Many common drugs — including antibiotics — contain sodium in relatively high concentrations. Because of sodium's ubiquitous distribution, sodium deficiency from insufficient dietary intake is virtually unknown among healthy adults.

An exception to this generalization is the case of healthy adults performing strenuous physical work in hot, humid environments where the workers perspire profusely and have not been acclimatized. Since perspiration under such circumstances may exceed ten liters daily and since the sodium concentration in such perspiration may range from 30 to 90 meq per liter,[598] sodium losses sufficient to induce symptoms (confusion, intense headache, exhaustion, muscle cramps) may occur, especially when the workers assuage their thirst with sodium-poor fluids. Their symptomatology is relieved by administration or consumption of fluids containing sodium chloride.

Among the elderly, heat exhaustion arising from losses of water, sodium and chloride may occur in the absence of hard physical work if older persons are subjected to high environmental temperatures and humidity so abruptly that compensatory increases in adrenocortical hormone secretion characteristic of acclimatization have not taken place.[589,590] Heat exhaustion is best treated by relief from high temperature and replacement of water, sodium and chloride as indicated by laboratory monitoring.

Great care must be taken to distinguish elderly persons with relatively simply treated heat exhaustion from those with the more malignant syndrome of heat stroke where priority must be given to the immediate reduction of body temperature. Heat stroke may be associated with early hypophosphatemia followed in 24 to 48 hours by hypocalcemia, the result of a hyperventilation-caused respiratory alkalosis which in turn induces increased phosphofructokinase activity creating an intracellular demand fulfilled by extracellular fluid inorganic phosphate.[591]

The complexity of heat-related syndromes and the heat-associated mortality (reported rates often in excess of ten per 100,000 per annum) among the elderly strongly suggests that age *per se* (not to mention the diseases associated with old age) is a major risk factor in high ambient temperatures. The need for sodium chloride replacement therapy in heat cramps in muscles and in heat exhaustion contrasts with its contraindication because of the danger of pulmonary edema in heat stroke. Diagnosis and management by trained health professionals is essential in all heat-related syndromes.

Hypo-osmolar hyponatremia is never occasioned by dietary sodium deficiency and is rarely due to excessive water intake. It almost invariably suggests the presence of a debilitating disease or an unfortunate response to drug therapy. Except for those situations in which the patient's loss of sodium from the body can be corrected, the patient with hypo-osmolar hyponatremia has an ominous prognosis.

Among the elderly, the principal sodium-related nutritional need is that of meeting the demand for sodium-restricted dietary regimens. This demand is undboubtedly inflated, since drug therapy for hypertension and other cardiovascular conditions has sharply reduced the need for rigorous sodium restriction and since the prevention of hypertension requires sodium restriction beginning early in life. Nonetheless, patients with congestive heart failure, cirrhosis of the liver with ascites, and other conditions associated with excessive extracellular fluid retention may benefit from dietary sodium restriction as may those patients for whom drug therapy of hypertension *per se* is inappropriate.

For patients who have specific indications for sodium restriction, many difficulties arise. If they dine in restaurants or with others who do not practice sodium restriction, they find it virtually impossible to adhere to a low sodium regimen. Secondly, virtually all processed and convenience foods contain large quantities of sodium and those that do not are produced in such small volume that their prices are high. Finally, low sodium regimens have low levels of palatability. Among the elderly this last mentioned difficulty may lead to reduced food intake and, with time, to deficiencies of other essential nutrients.

These problems may be resolved by education directed at training patients to recognize and to consume low sodium, low cost foods and to prepare them in such combinations and with such condiments low in sodium that their palatability is high. Just as important are careful, periodic reappraisals of the indications for sodium restriction in specific patients. If drug therapy can be effectively used,[592] moderate sodium restriction may be substituted for the more rigorous variety, thereby increasing compliance with dietary instructions. Among the elderly, constant monitoring is necessary to assure compliance with instructions regarding the dosage and timing of drug therapy as well as constant observation to detect drug sensitivities and side effects.

Hypernatremia is a condition seen often in obtunded, tube-fed patients. It is preventable by attention to nutritional detail based on an understanding of the pathogenesis of the problem.[593] Many formulas for tube feeding are high in protein and salt. Their use augments the load of urea and salt for excretion. Obligatory renal water loss required to handle this excretory load is increased sufficiently to produce a negative water balance and hypernatremia.

The hypernatremia syndrome itself comprises confusion, neuromuscular excitability, seizures or coma. Since the most likely victims of the syndrome are those whose tube feeding was occasioned by their being obtunded or comatose and therefore unable to respond appropriately to sensations of thirst, observations of the developing symptomatology are rarely worthwhile.

What is essential for the prevention of hypernatremia is planning in advance the fulfillment of the water requirement for the obligatory renal water loss, the insensible water loss, the fecal water loss, the loss through perspiration, and losses through pathological or surgical fistulae.

Should hypernatremia occur in spite of or in lieu of careful advanced planning, appropriate treatment is the administration of water sufficient to add four percent of body weight in kg for each ten mEq per liter increase in serum sodium above normal.[594] Correction of hypernatremia should be carried out over an interval of 12 to 24 hours to avoid cerebral edema which can be caused if an osmotic gradient favoring movement of water into cells is allowed to develop by too rapid a reduction in serum osmolality.

Potassium

The wide distribution of potassium among natural foods virtually eliminates primary potassium deficiency as a cause of malnutrition in healthy man. In healthy man, the renal excretion of potassium is so efficient that excessive potassium intake rarely creates problems.[595] However, both hypokalemia and hyperkalemia may occur in the presence of disease, the former in conditions characterized by excessive potassium losses via the gastrointestinal tract and the latter, by deficient potassium excretion during renal insufficiency. The diagnosis of either condition is aided by a high index of suspicion but should be confirmed by objective laboratory measurements.

Hypokalemia is readily treated by the administration of potassium-containing solutions parenterally or orally or by ingestion of potassium-containing foods by mouth. Hyperkalemia is a more challenging therapeutic problem. When time permits, it may be treated by the administration of pure Calories in the form of fat and carbohydrate supplemented with vitamins and trace elements, a regimen which reduces potassium intake virtually to zero and minimizes breakdown via gluconeogenesis of body tissue, an endogenous source of potassium. When time is of the essence, hyperkalemia may be treated by the administration of glucose and insulin, a therapy designed to move potassium intracellularly, or, when time is not a critical factor, by oral administration of sodium polystyrene sulfonate, a cation-exchange resin which sequesters potassium *(in vivo,* approximately 1 mEq potassium per gm) first from the small but in greatest quantity from the large bowel and hence in sequence from the extracelluar space. Dialysis may be resorted to when other measures are not appropriate.

Meneely and Battarbee[596] have reviewed the protective effect of potassium in the presence of chronic sodium toxicity, a state they believe afflicts virtually all civilized societies. Encouraged by the report of McQuarrie, *et al.*[597] and later by the earlier report of Priddle[598] that the addition of potassium to dietary regimens lowered blood pressure in man even though sodium intake remained high, Meneely, *et al.*[599] showed in rats that potassium protected the animals even though chronic sodium intake continued. Later Meneely and Ball[600] reported dramatically enhanced survival with prolongation of the median duration of life by two to six months when rats consuming excess sodium chloride were given extra potassium. The greater longevity was observed even though the blood pressures of the rats with and without extra dietary potassium were the same. These findings suggest that the rice diet,[40,601] although low in sodium, may have achieved some of its desired effect by virtue of its high potassium content (about 100 mEq daily of potassium and less than 2 mEq of sodium) attributable to the large quantity of citrus fruits and fruit juices it contained. In concert with this idea, Sasaki[602] found a low incidence of stroke and relatively low blood pressures in Japanese who consumed a high-potassium fruit-containing diet even though the diet was also high in sodium derived from other components.

The information about high-sodium, low-potassium intake societies reviewed by Meneely and Battarbee,[596] although written primarily to indict sodium, strongly suggests the need for additional investigations of potassium as a nutrient. They believe evidence overwhelmingly indicates that a diet low in sodium and higher in potassium "would increase both the duration and quality of life for many millions of people." They conclude their review with the question: "Would such a strategy have as much to offer for longevity in humans as it clearly does in the rat?"

Chloride

Chloride is the principal anion in extracellular fluid. It plays a major role in acid-base homeostasis. Since it is a component of gastric hydrochloric acid, any disease or condition causing loss from the body of gastric contents will lead if continued for long to hypochloremia. However, hypochloremia *per se* may also signal the presence of potassium deficiency, since, as potassium leaves the intracellular environment, it is replaced by sodium, while chloride is excreted by the kidneys as potassium chloride. The resulting metabolic alkalosis requires for its correction the replacement of lost potassium.

From a nutritional standpoint, chloride is abundant in food either as sodium or potassium chloride. Specific chloride deficiency may develop during protracted vomiting or during therapy with rigid and successful restrictions of dietary sodium chloride. Potassium chloride supplements may be used as replacement therapy if not contraindicated.

Hyperchloremia and particularly hyperchloremic acidosis is a condition encountered among patients with a variety of clinical conditions. It is found among patients whose ureters have been implanted in their large bowels which then serve as substitutes for urinary bladders which have been surgically removed, usually for cancer. It may be found in patients with alkali loss associated with chronic diarrhea and bowel fistulae. It is observed in patients with renal tubular acidosis. It may be caused by consumption of ammonium chloride or of such organic acidifying salts as arginine hydrochloride. It may be a problem in parenteral feeding comprising synthetic amino acid mixtures. In these, the excess of cationic amino acids (arginine, histidine and lysine) contribute H^+ and Cl^- to body fluids as they are converted to urea or incorporated into peptides, producing a hyperchloremic metabolic acidosis. This may be prevented by adding sodium bicarbonate rather than sodium chloride to the infusion when synthetic amino acid mixtures are administered. Hyperchloremic acidosis may be managed by the administration of Schohl's solution,[603] a mixture of citric acid and sodium citrate dissolved in water. If potassium is required, potassium citrate may be mixed with the citric acid and half the amount of sodium citrate.

As this brief discussion of chloride suggests, the management of disorders of acid-base balance is complex. It requires knowledge of fundamental biochemistry and physiology and also a wealth of experience. Successful management requires the services of a reliable laboratory. Here is an excellent example of the necessity of integrating nutrition, medicine and gerontology into the nutrition-health-aging (NHA) triad.

Iron

If pathologic blood loss is excluded, adult males and postmenopausal females lose about one mg of iron daily. Men aged 60 contain an average of about 3500 mg of iron and women aged 60, about 2500 mg, *i.e.*, about 50 mg per kg of body weight.[604] In one year, therefore, older men lose about 10 percent and older women, about 15 percent of their total body iron. On the average, about ten percent of dietary iron is absorbed. Hence, even excluding pathological losses, the need for dietary available iron is apparent.

The Recommended Dietary Allowance (RDA) of 10 mg per day is based on the assumption that a well-balanced diet contains six mg iron per 1,000 Calories, of which ten percent is absorbed. If the diet contains little highly available heme-iron from animal red meat and little ascorbic acid (which increases absorption from nonheme iron[921a]) from citrus fruits, the absorption of nonheme-iron is minimal. In view of the cost of a well-balanced diet containing animal red meat and citrus fruits, the wisdom of the ten mg daily RDA may be questioned. Since many elderly have gastric achlorhydria, which alone can decrease the absorption of ferric iron by 50 percent,[605] an even stronger case may be developed for a higher RDA for iron for elderly persons.

Increasing the iron content of the diet may not be, however, the only answer. In view of the limited Calorie intake of many elderly persons, increasing the quantity of dietary available iron may be a more effective measure, even though more costly. Fortification of common inexpensive foods has not been entirely satisfactory, since some iron salts used are absorbed far less well than even the other nonheme-iron in the diet.[606,607]

Anemia is a very late manifestation of long-standing dietary iron deficiency. Anemic elderly persons should be assumed to be bleeding and a search instituted to identify the pathology associated with that bleeding before attributing the anemia to dietary iron deficiency.[603]

Earlier stages of iron deficiency are detectable using modern, more sensitive parameters of iron status. Plasma ferritin concentrations are proportional to the body's mobilizable iron reserves (found in ferritin and hemosiderin) and hence give useful measures of iron status.[609] Plasma transferrin binding capacity rises in iron deficiency. Transferrin saturation — *i.e.*, plasma iron divided by the total plasma iron binding capacity — diminishes in iron deficiency. In iron deficiency, serum ferritin itself decreases, while simultaneously the efficiency of iron absorption from the gut rises.

In later stages of iron deficiency, when mobilizable iron stores are exhausted, plasma iron falls and red cell protoporphyrin concentrations rise. Even in this stage of impaired erythropoiesis recognizable anemia may not be evident.

The final stage is reached when overt iron deficiency anemia characterized by microcytic hypochromic erthrocytes is found in peripheral blood.

It would seem evident that future evaluations of aging to aged populations for nutritionally created iron deficiency should emphasize collecting data on plasma ferritin, transferrin, iron and transferrin saturation and on erythrocyte protoporphyrin to obtain earlier evidence of mobilizable iron store depletion and iron deficiency. Lesser degrees of iron deficiency than those associated with anemia may manifest themselves clinically by abnormalities in immune responses, resistance to infection and muscle dysfunction, all familar disorders among the elderly. Such tissue responses to iron deficiency need investigations[610] which could be conducted with high probabilities of generating useful applications among the elderly.

Chromium

Chromium metabolism is one of the most complex of any trace element, primarily because in performing its major function — that of potentiating the peripheral action of insulin — chromium is thought to be effective only when it is a component of substances having the generic term glucose tolerance factor (GTF). GTF probably serves as an insulin cofactor, facilitating the binding of insulin to cell membranes by forming a ternary complex among chromium, insulin and insulin receptors of cell membranes. In foods, GTF is most abundant in brewer's yeast and also is found in nonfish animal protein and in foods made from whole grain.

GTF has tentatively been identified as a low molecule weight substance which is water soluble, is heat stable in solution and absorbs at 262 nm. While its exact structure in the biologically active form has not been determined, it seems probable that it is a tetra-aquo, dinicotinato chromium (III) complex.[612] Since this dinicotinic acid-chromium complex is unstable at an alkaline pH, it is also probable that the coordinated water molecules are replaced *in vivo* with glycine, glutamic acid or sulfur-containing amino acids.

Whereas less than one percent of simple trivalent chromium compounds are absorbed, from ten to 25 percent of chromium present as GTF is absorbed.

Pertinent to elderly persons with carbohydrate intolerance[364,367] is the fact that GTF, but not simple chromium compounds, does equilibrate promptly with the physiologically important chromium pool which is the source of the sharp increase in plasma chromium occurring in response to increases in circulating insulin. Elderly persons may have marginal chromium deficiency states as suggested by agewise decrements in tissue levels[613] and by markedly lower concentrations of total, nonvolatile and volatile chromium concentrations in the urine of elderly when compared to the concentrations in the urine of younger subjects.[614] Elderly and middle-aged adults given 150 to 250 μgm supplements of trivalent chromium as $CrCl_3 \cdot 6H_2O$ showed improvement in glucose tolerance when impaired glucose tolerance had previously been present.[615,617] However, when elderly persons with impaired glucose tolerance were fed supplements of GTF-containing brewer's yeast,[618] even more dramatic improvements in glucose tolerance were observed. When $CrCl_3 \cdot 6H_2O$ comprised the supplement, improvement in glucose tolerance was evident only after several days or weeks of chromic chloride ingestion, whereas GTF-containing supplements could induce improved glucose tolerance rapidly. These observations suggest the necessity of endogenous GTF synthesis when poorly absorbed chromic compounds are prescribed.[612]

The complexities of GTF metabolism together with difficulties in standardizing analytic procedures for both chromium and for GTF have left meaningful recommendations for a chromium RDA yet to be devised. A minimum daily requirement for man of about ten μmg is frequently mentioned. This is based on observations that about seven to ten μgm of chromium are found daily in the urine of healthy adults.[619] This amount increases when blood chromium concentrations are increased following a glucose load in persons with adequate chromium nutrition but fails to change in those whose biologically active stores of chromium are exhausted.

In view of the very poor absorption of simple chromium compounds and the long delay in their becoming biologically active, the critical need at present is the development of reliable, inexpensive assays for chromium and for GTF which may be applied to available foodstuffs. If accompanied by the development of readily applicable assays for chromium and GTF in biologic tissues and fluids, investigations unraveling the enigmas of GTF metabolism may be accelerated and a rational RDA for chromium established.

Hexavalent chromium has a special affinity for red blood cells. This makes it a tool of special value when bleeding is suspected but difficult to locate and to quantify. Chromium in hexavalent form may be incubated with either the patient's own cells or a donor's compatible cells and injected into the blood stream of the person suspected of bleeding. Identification of ^{51}Cr-labelled red cells in aspirates of gastrointestinal tract fluids, in urine or in other biologic fluid of the recipient may reveal the presence and location of previously undetected bleeding. In addition, by relating the ^{51}Cr label's concentration in the fluid sample with that present (after mixing) in the blood, an estimate of the ^{51}Cr clearance through the pathologic lesion may be obtained, suggesting the magnitude of the hemorrhagic process. This technique is particularly valuable in elderly persons whose anemias must always be assumed to be caused by bleeding before other possible causes are investigated.[608]

Cobalt

Cobalt is essential to man only because of its presence in the vitamin B_{12} molecule. Vitamin B_{12} will be discussed below in the chapter dealing with water soluble vitamins.

Copper

Copper, while ubiquitous, is particularly important in the biochemistry of the hematologic, cardiovascular, skeletal, dermatologic, nervous, genitourinary and gastrointestinal organ systems. In spite of its essentiality in the enzymes of so many organ systems, copper deficiency in healthy adult man as a result of insufficient dietary copper intake has not been observed and is regarded as highly unlikely to occur.[620] Hypocupremia, however, is observed frequently in association with diseases.

Curiously, one of these — Wilson's disease, also known as hepatolenticular degeneration, an autosomal recessively inherited disease — is characterized not only by decreased serum copper and ceruloplasmin *(v.i.)* concentrations but also by increased copper absorption, decreased biliary copper excretion, increased tissue deposition of copper particularly in the liver, the basal ganglia of the brain and in Descemet's membrane at the limbus of the cornea (where it produces the brown or green Kayser-Fleischer ring pathognomonic of the disease), and increased urinary excretion of copper. The most probable hypothesis attributes these findings to a gene responsible for decreasing the synthesis of ceruloplasmin, the alpha$_2$-globulin blue in color to which 98 percent of serum copper in normal man is bound. This diminished ceruloplasmin synthesis, in manners not yet understood, increases copper absorption, diminishes biliary excretion and creates conditions favoring the deposition of excessive amounts of copper in tissues. Nonceruloplasmin copper is bound loosely to albumin. In Wilson's disease, its concentration in serum is much higher than that in normal man. Almost all copper is transported from the gastrointestinal tract to the tissues in this loosely bound form. The higher concentration of the albumin-bound copper accounts for the increased urinary excretion.

Treatment of this condition requires a low copper diet, as close to one mg per day as possible as opposed to the 2.0 to 5.0 mg range found in average diets.[620] Diets containing close to one mg of copper daily are difficult to devise unless so severly restricted in Calories as to be unacceptable. Since about 32 percent of ingested copper is absorbed,[621] the ingestion of potassium sulfide with meals to reduce copper absorption has been advocated. However, even diets low in copper and combined with potassium sulfide ingestion failed to provide a pragmatic, lifesaving therapeutic regimen.

In 1951, the introduction of British Anti-Lewisite (BAL), an agent capable of chelating copper *in vivo* and dramatically increasing its excretion in the urine, revolutionized the therapy of Wilson's disease and the life expectancy of its victims.[622,623] Copper concentrations in liver decreased as did damage to liver cells and cells of the brain which prior to BAL therapy had derived their copper from dead hepatocytes. However, the required intramuscular administration of BAL with its attendant local induration and occasional abscess formation as well as other undesirable side effects resulted in its being regarded a therapy less than ideal.

In 1956, an orally administered compound with relatively few side effects, penicillamine (beta, beta-dimethylcysteine), supplanted BAL as chelating agent of choice.[624] When used in its dextro-isomeric form, penicillamine in doses of one to two gm (depending on body weight) results in very high urinary copper excretion, decrements in tissue copper, and falls in the serum copper and ceruloplasmin concentrations below their already low levels. D-penicillamine therapy prevents disability and prolongs life.[625] Whether persons with clinically evident disease will survive to true old age as a result of penicillamine therapy is not yet known. Nonetheless, since one in 500 persons is thought to be heterozygous for the Wilson's disease gene,[626] and since, as an exercise in prudent prevention medicine,[625] treatment is recommended for any asymptomatic patient's sib — no matter how asymptomatic that sib may be — who displays low serum ceruloplasmin and elevated hepatic copper concentrations,[627] there exists the possibility that appropriately treated patients with the disease may reach old age. Certainly the Wilson's disease story illustrates perfectly the necessity of viewing nutrition, health and aging as an integrated triad, not as separate unrelated entities.

With the exception of patients with Wilson's disease and of Wilson's disease heterozygotes, hypocupremia in man is a valid manifestation of copper depletion and one of its earliest detectable manifestations.[620] Hypocupremia in adult man is synonymous with hypoceruloplasminemia which may develop from deficient ceruloplasmin synthetic capacity by or excessive ceruloplasmin loss from the body. Inadequate ceruloplasmin synthetic capacity could arise from lack of sufficient available copper or, in the presence of available copper, from inability to synthesize ceruloplasmin's protein portion (apoceruloplasmin) because of a specific genetically determined metabolic defect (as in Wilson's disease) or by generalized protein deficiency. Loss of ceruloplasmin may occur across the intestinal walls, in the urine or via the bile. While chronic blood loss results in loss of copper-containing erythrocytes, iron loss becomes limiting long before copper depletion from this source alone is of significance.

Hypocupremia and hypoceruloplasminemia have been reported most frequently in infants and children. They have been observed when these infants and children have received for long periods of time dietary regimens comprising low copper milk, food and water.[628] They have been reported in infants with cystic fibrosis of the pancreas who were fed soya protein.[629] They have been found in children with kwashiorkor.[630,633] They have accompanied a syndrome in infants characterized by microcytic, hypochromic anemia, edema, hypoproteinemia and hypoferremia, presumably due to iron deficiency.[634,635]

Hypocupremia and hypoceruloplasminemia from dietary deficiency of copper have not been reported in adults. However, diseases creating one or more of the conditions leading to hypoceruloplasminemia do result in hypocupremia in adults. Among these are the proteinurias such as those associated with the nephrotic syndrome;[636,637] tropical[638] and nontropical[620] sprue; celiac disease; and the protein-losing enteropathies[639-641] whose pathogeneses are multiple.[642,643] Hence, copper depletion occurs in adults, even though it may not be related directly to a deficient intake of dietary copper.

Such depletion is pertinent to physiologic aging because copper serves as a biocatalyst in the biochemistry of every organ system. As metalloproteins, copper-dependent enzymes are involved in iron absorption and mobilization prior to hemoglobin synthesis in erythropoiesis. Hence, experimental copper deficiency has led to anemia identical to iron-deficiency anemia in swine[620] and in infants.[644] A copper metallo-enzyme, lysyl oxidase, is essential for the crosslinking and maturation of collagen and elastin.[645] Crosslinking of both collagen and elastin is required for the integrity of the cardiovascular system. In its absence, rupture of the aorta, other major vessels, and of the heart itself occur in experimental animals. Subcutaneous hemorrhages, presumably from defective collagen in smaller vessels, also have been observed. Copper treatment of copper-deficient ataxic lambs increases the concentrations of dopamine and norepinephrine in specific areas of the affected lambs' brains.[646] While the role of copper in maintaining dopamine levels is obscure, the conversion of dopamine to norepinephrine is known to be catalyzed by the copper metallo-enzyme, dopamine-beta-hydroxylase. Relating these findings to aging humans requires only recognition of the fact that dopamine concentrations are low in the basal ganglia of patients with Parkinson's disease, the paralysis agitans characterized by dyskinesia similar to that observed in experimental lambs. The copper metallo-enzyme tyrosinase catalyzes the formation of melanin from tyrosine. In its absence in copper deficiency, skin demonstrates a lack of appropriate pigmentation.

All copper metallo-enzymes contain both copper and zinc and possess superoxide dismutase activity. This enzyme catalyzes the reaction $2(O_2^-) + 2H^+ \rightarrow H_2O_2 + O_2$. The superoxide anion, (O_2^-), appears during biological oxidations like the xanthine oxidase reaction. Superoxide dismutase functions in the catalysis of (O_2^-)'s decomposition, thus protecting aerobic cells from damage by the accumulation of free radicals. Anaerobes unable to survive in the presence of oxygen contain no superoxide dismutase. In view of the role free radicals may play in aging as a biologic process *(v.s.)*, this aspect of copper's role in human nutritional biochemistry is worthy of more extensive investigation. Furthermore, studies in subhuman species have shown diminished cytochrome oxidase activity and decreased adenosine triphosphate (ATP) and phospholipid synthesis in mitochondria from cells of copper deficient animals. Such mitochondria are described as becoming more fragile and more susceptible to aging.[647]

The confluence of copper with zinc in the metallo-enzymes brings to mind another physiologic interaction of copper and zinc which may have relevance to the occurrence of atherosclerotic vascular disease, the leading cause of death among middle aged and elderly Americans. Klevay[648] and Murthy, *et al.*,[649] have presented data from studies in rats which show a significant direct relation between the ratio of zinc to copper in the diet and the concentration of cholesterol in the sera of the rats. Klevay[650] has combined these data with extensive epidemiologic data to propose the hypothesis that the incidence of coronary heart disease is directly related to the ratio of zinc to copper in blood serum.[650]

Factors increasing or decreasing the zinc/copper ratio correspond to those believed to increase or decrease the serum concentration of cholesterol. These include consumption of cow's milk (+); consumption of human milk (−); diets high in fat and refined carbohydrates and low in fiber (+); the "protective" effect of liver cirrhosis (−); supplementation of diets with calcium and magnesium (−); muscle and bone anabolism from physical work (−); administration of calcium disodium ethylenediamine tetra-acetate (EDTA) (which selectively chelates more zinc than copper) (−); viral infections such as infectious hepatitis (increases zinc loss) and sandfly fever (conserves copper) (−); sweating (sweat contains about 16 times as much zinc as it does copper) during exercise (−); ingestion of excessive doses of ascorbic acid (+); pregnancy (+); bone destruction during chronic renal disease (large amounts of zinc are released from bone during demineralization) (+); nephrotic syndrome (+); histidinemia (+); hypertension (+); drinking hard water (−); chronic hemodialysis (+); and consumption of bread (containing phytic acid which reduces the availability of dietary zinc (−). In a study comparing the tissue concentrations of 26 trace elements in undamaged myocardial tissue from victims of myocardial infarctions with similar mycardial tissue from accident victims, Wester[652] found higher zinc/copper ratios in the tissues from myocardial infarction victims.

The information reviewed above suggests that, with the exception of patients with Wilson's disease, dietary copper should be maintained in the two to five mg daily range. Unfortunately, relatively little information is available in regard to the copper content of foods. Almost every author discussing copper metabolism cites nuts, some shellfish, liver, kidney, corn oil margarine and dried legumes as the richest sources of dietary copper, a list repeated in the Ninth Edition (1980) of the Recommended Dietary Allowances (RDA) (92a). The data of Schroeder, *et al.,*[653] on institutional diets, of White[654] on diets of college and secondary school females, and of Price, *et al.,*[655] on adolescent females from low income families are frequently used as estimates of the copper content of the American diet. These values produce means with huge variances. Furthermore, the availability of dietary copper[656] is an additional variable worthy of consideration. Finally, copper nutrition may be influenced by the presence or absence of copper in the pipes supplying water to specific persons.

In regard to copper metabolism and its role in aging, it may be well said that the past is prologue.

Fluorine

When drinking water provides (either naturally or by controlled fluoridation) a concentration of one part per million (one mg per liter) of fluoride, children under five drinking such water will be protected from dental caries during the susceptible childhood and adolescent years.[529,657,659] Their teeth will be available for use in adulthood, late maturity and old age.[660] Scientific evidence backing contentions of certain antifluoridation groups that fluoridation of public water supplies is harmful has not been published.

Epidemiological evidence[530] and clinical investigations by metabolic balance study and bone density techniques[661,665] have suggested a role for fluoride in the prevention and treatment of the disease osteoporosis. However, some investigators have found the favorable effects to be transient or negligible.[531,666] The principal salt used in therapy, sodium fluoride, may produce toxic manifestations such as anorexia, epigastric pain, ectopic calcification, optic neuritis and retinal damage,[666,667] suggesting the need for regularly scheduled medical supervision of such a treatment regimen. Symptomatic osteoporosis is now managed in some clinics by combination therapy consisting of 50 mg of sodium fluoride and one gm of calcium as calcium carbonate daily and 50,000 IU of vitamin D twice weekly.[547] Dietary calcium in adequate amounts throughout life remains the key ingredient in the prevention of osteoporosis, while the combination therapy just mentioned is reserved for treatment of symptomatic disease.

Since whole fish flour has been proposed as an inexpensive source of high quality protein and of calcium in diets for the elderly, it is important to note that the potential hazards of the fluoride content of the bones incorporated into such flour have been investigated.[668,669] No toxic effects of importance to man have been observed in these studies.

Iodine

Iodine is an essential micronutrient because it is a component of the thyroid hormones, thyroxine (T_4) and diiodothyronine (T_3). Dietary iodine deficiency may lead to simple goiter but is not the sole cause of that condition. Susceptibility to simple goiter is determined by genetic factors in the individual leading to defective thyroid hormone synthesis. Prevalence of simple goiter may also be conditioned by the presence of goitrogenic compounds in the food supply. These are estimated to contribute about four percent to the world incidence of goiter.[670] Most active are the goitrins derived from (R)-2-hydroxy-3-butenylglucosinolate found in brussel sprouts, broccoli, kale, kohlrabi, cabbage, cauliflower, turnips and rutabagas, in the oil seed meals from rape and turnip and from the corresponding (S)-glucosinolate in crambe.[671] Infectious agents and bacterial goitrogens in water supplies may also contribute to the incidence of simple goiter. The susceptibility to goiter caused by such factors may be revealed in the presence of iodine deficiency, whereas in the absence of such deficiency it would not become evident.[672]

The Food and Nutrition Board[673] has estimated that the dietary requirement for iodine is approximately one mg per kg per day in healthy human beings. Iodine content is highest in seafoods, edible seaweed, bread in whose production iodate has been added and in foods which have been seasoned (usually not in processing but in the kitchen or at the table) with iodized salt. Fruits contain very little iodine. Vegetables, grains and animal products vary in iodine content depending on their proximity to the sea's salt spray and the iodine content of fertilizers applied to fields and of the pasturage and the feeds ingested.

Whereas iodine deficiency goiter was once endemic in inland North America, data collected during the Ten State Survey[674] suggested no relation between the prevalence of goiter and the dietary intake of the communities studied. The disappearance of goiter based on iodine deficiency was achieved through the introduction of iodized salt following the research of Marine and Kimball[675,677] in Akron, Ohio in the early part of the century. In fact, in recent years, the use of iodine in animal feeds and medications and as a component of bactericidal agents used in food and dairy product processing has introduced exogenous iodine into the food chain[532] to the extent that the mean amount ingested daily per person is well in excess of the 100 to 300 μgm daily recommended by the Food and Nutrition Board.[673]

This increased iodine intake is not an inconsequential matter. Excess iodine intake on the order of 200 mg and up daily has been found to produce hypothyroidism and "iodide" goiter, particularly in persons with preexisting thyroid disorders.[678] Furthermore, in northern Japan, an endemic form of iodide goiter in many residents of the area has been related to ingestion of an iodide-containing seaweed "kombu".[679] The early efforts to stamp out endemic goiter with iodized salt were vigorously opposed because many goitrous individuals in iodine-deficient areas became hyperthyroid when iodine therapy was instituted. This condition was called Jod-Basedow's disease, literally Basedow's disease (exopthalmic goiter) created by iodine.[680]

While the quantities of iodine required to produce these syndromes caused by excessive iodine intake may seem so large as to be unworthy of serious consideration, it should be remembered that human susceptibility is quite variable. In addition, iodine-containing drugs for the treatment of nonthyroid pathology and for roentgenographic diagnoses are commonly used. Hence, iodism in various guises may be found among all persons and especially among the disease- and self-medication-prone elderly as a result of the increased quantities of iodine entering the food chain.

This discussion of the trace element iodine again highlights the interrelations of science, medicine and public health.

Selenium

Selenium is an essential component of the mammalian and avian enzyme, glutathione peroxidase.[681] Selenium toxicity in animals[682] was recognized well before selenium was identified as an essential nutrient.[683,684] Toxicity in man, even in the same areas where animal toxicity was endemic and even among men with urinary selenium excretion in the same range as that of toxic animals, has never been demonstrated.[685,687] However, among the 111 persons receiving complete physical examinations as part of the investigation of the rural population under study,[686,687] a high incidence of dental caries was observed. Over a decade later, even lower level exposure to selenium was reported to facilitate development of caries in Oregon school children.[688]

As in the cases of copper metalloenzymes *(v.s.)* and of vitamin E *(v.i.)*, part of selenium's potential role in biologic aging may be inferred from its ability to inhibit lipid peroxidation. Selenium and selenium-containing amino acids assist in decomposing hydrogen peroxides and scavenging free radicals. In this way, they help stabilize the lipid-containing biologic membranes of subcellular components such as mitochondria, microsomes and lysosomes.[689]

When experimental animals ingest diets containing appropriate amounts of selenium, their erythrocytes contain the selenoprotein glutathione peroxidase which utilizes reduced glutathione as an electron donor for the reduction of peroxides.[690] In selenium-deficient animals, erythrocytes do not contain glutathione peroxidase. This observation has provided a basis for further studies of selenium metabolism in aged humans.

In New Zealand, whose soil is low in selenium,[691] selenium concentrations in the blood of man have been found to be highly and directly correlated with glutathione peroxidase activities. More recently, selenium concentrations in the whole blood, erythrocytes and plasma of twelve control subjects (mean age 25 years) were compared with concentrations found in 48 elderly New Zealanders (mean age 78 years).[693] Selenium concentrations among the young subjects were consistently more than 140 percent of the concentrations among the elderly. (Concentrations in all New Zealand subjects ranged from 22 to 31 percent of the 0.22 μgm/ml of whole blood regarded as normal for North Americans.[694] When glutathione peroxidase activity per ml of erythrocytes and per gm of hemoglobin was measured in the same 12 young adults and in 28 elderly persons, the young adults again had about 140 percent of the activity found in the elderly. The correlation between selenium concentrations and the glutathione peroxidase activities in the erythrocytes of the elderly was high ($r = 0.80$). Since cell death is a postulate in biologic aging and since glutathione peroxidase is essential for the integrity of cell membranes, it is reasonable to attribute to selenium nutriture a role in aging as a biologic process.

In animals, a concentration of 0.1 μgm/gm in the dietary prevents selenium deficiency. This concentration is present in the average mixed American diet.[695] No RDA for man has yet been established (92a).

The reasons underlying the lower selenium and glutathione peroxidase concentrations in the blood of elderly New Zealanders have not been adequately identified. While lifelong ingestion of New Zealand foods containing low concentrations of selenium might be a contributing factor (in the same sense that consumption of iodine-deficient foods may disclose latent genetically determined defective thyroid hormone synthesis), evidence presented to date does not exclude dietary selenium deficiency among the elderly contrasted with adequate (for New Zealand) dietary selenium intake among the younger subjects. Nonetheless, the analogy with the metabolism of certain other trace elements, the selenium story suggests the need to explore agewise changes in the synthesis of the protein portion of glutathione peroxidase.

The selenium story provides again the comment that more effort must be made to focus the resources devoted to nutrition, to health and to gerontology combined on single objectives such as explaining the agewise decrement in selenium and glutathione peroxidase concentrations suggested by the New Zealand studies. The word suggested is used advisedly, since the variances about the mean concentrations among the elderly were greater (in spite of larger n's) than in the younger subjects.[683] These data reconfirm the fact that variances of almost any parameter increase with age. They also suggest that the physiologic ages of the elderly subjects may have varied far more than their chronologic ages. Comparisons based on estimates of physiologic ages among the elderly themselves could shed more light on the selenium-aging phenomenon.

Two recent reports of myocardiopathy associated with selenium deficiency[695a,695b] and a report of deficient serum concentrations of selenium in patients with alcoholic cirrhosis[659c] suggest that clinical manifestations of selenium deficiency in human beings are less rare than commonly believed. This is particularly true among persons receiving prolonged parenteral alimentation.[695a] Goldman and Kantrowitz[695d] have suggested that congestive alcoholic myocardiopathy's progression may be accelerated in selenium deficiency because of the decreased protective activity of glutathione peroxidase on myocardial cells as Aaseth, *et al.*,[695c] proposed might occur in liver cells of cirrhotics undergoing rapid deterioration.

Since so-called senile myocardiopathy is found unassociated with known causes among older persons[695e-h] and since older persons may receive prolonged parenteral alimentation during illness or after surgery, the possibility that selenium deficiency will reduce glutathione peroxidase activity certainly exists. Its presence in hospitalized older persons can be readily determined and if found to be present in substantial numbers should stimulate a broader evaluation of selenium nutrition in relation to aging *per se.*

Vanadium

Vanadium was originally discovered in Mexico in 1801 where it was named erythronium for the red color acquired by its salts on their being heated. In 1830, the metal was rediscovered in Sweden where it was given the name vanadium after Vanadis — an Old Norse name for Freya, the goddess of beauty and youth — reflecting the beautiful colors of its compounds in solution. Vanadium is widely distributed among various minerals, in coal and in petroleum. It is not surprising, therefore, that vanadium was recognized as an essential nutrient only after studies in which the experimental animals were housed under conditions guaranteeing strict control of metallic contamination from the environment.[696,698]

Vanadium is the first member of subgroup 5b of the periodic table of elements. It possesses four oxidation states (+2, +3, +4, and +5). It also has a strong tendency to form coordination complexes. These characteristics make it a highly reactive element in biologic systems.[699] In animals and in plants, vanadium seems to function as a biocatalytic element attached to organic compounds as part of the catalytic machinery of the organism.

Vanadium's relation to aging was first investigated prior to proof of its essentiality when Curran and various colleagues[700,703] published data suggesting that vanadium added to total dietary regimens depressed synthesis of cholesterol from labeled acetate in rat livers by inhibiting the microsomal squalene synthetase enzyme system, reduced *in vivo* cholesterol biosynthesis in rabbits made atherosclerotic by a high cholesterol diet, mobilized more cholesterol from rabbits' atherosclerotic aortas than was mobilized in nonvanadium-fed controls, and inhibited cholesterol synthesis in normocholesterolemic young men.

After vanadium had been shown to be an essential nutrient for the rat, Hopkins and Mohr[704] found that vanadium-deficient chicks had lower plasma cholesterol concentrations at four weeks of age, but higher at seven weeks. Nielsen and Ollerich[705] later reported reduced plasma cholesterol concentrations in four week old chicks. Hopkins and Mohr[706] subsequently observed significantly elevated plasma triglyceride concentrations in vanadium-deficient chicks four weeks of age. Over a decade after the initial reports,[700,703] Curran and Burch[707] presented data indicating stimulation of cholesterol biosynthesis in 500-600 gm rats when they were fed vanadium.

Meanwhile, two other groups[708,709] found in old persons and in younger persons with hypercholesterolemia or ischemic heart disease no lowering of serum cholesterol concentrations with vanadium administration.

One of these groups[710] subsequently studied the effect on serum cholesterol concentrations in rats of vanadyl sulfate at a concentration of five mg of vanadium per liter in double-deionized drinking water to which zinc (50 mg/liter), manganese (10 mg/liter), copper (5 mg/liter), cobalt, molybdenum and trivalent chromium (all at 1 mg/liter) had been added. The basic diet contained 3.24 μgm vanadium per gm. Total intake was estimated to be 54.44 μgm/100 gm body weight per day. From these complex investigations, the author concluded that trivalent chromium was the trace element most responsible for lowering cholesterol concentrations and that the vanadium effect was antagonistic to that of chromium. Female rats (whose cholesterol concentrations were lower when drinking vanadium-containing water) were excluded from the author's conclusions, since female rats were shown to require 5.0 mg/liter of chromium in drinking water (as opposed to 1.0 mg/liter for males) for the chromium-based cholesterol-lowering effect.[710]

These contradictory and often inexplicable findings led to an abandonment of vanadium as a useful model for inhibition of cholesterol biosynthesis. However, the same lack of understanding also led to more recent studies which have shed much needed light on the influence of pharmacologic doses of dietary vanadium on cholesterol and fatty acid synthesis and turnover, at least in growing chicks.[711] Chicks in the experimental group consumed the control chicks' basal diet to which 100 mg/kg of vanadium had been added. The data from these investigations suggest that dietary vanadium enhanced hepatic lipogenesis while simultaneously reducing the turnover of plasma total lipids and plasma fatty acids, actions which accounted for the increase in plasma total lipids observed in the vanadium-fed chicks. Furthermore, the rate of hepatic cholesterol synthesis was greater in the vanadium-fed chicks, providing an explanation for the higher fresh liver and plasma cholesterol concentrations. While the rate of turnover of the rapidly equilibrating cholesterol pool was insignificantly increased by vanadium feeding, the half-life of cholesterol in the slowly equilibrating pool was about 12 percent shorter than that observed in the control chicks.

The authors attribute their findings to the uncoupling of oxidative phosphorylation resulting from the accumulation of reducing NADH (reduced nicotinamide-adenine dinucleotide) in the cytoplasm occasioned by its vanadium-induced failure of transfer into mitochondria. The accumulation of the reducing equivalence of NADH in cytoplasm could be transferred to $NADP^+$ (nicotinamide-adenine dinucleotide phosphate) by an enzyme pathway to generate NADPH (reduced nicotinamide-adenine dinucleotide phosphate), required for lipid synthesis. The authors suggest that the availability of NADPH enhanced fatty acid and cholesterol synthesis in vanadium-fed chicks.

The search for vanadium's role in biologic aging has extended beyond its influence on endogenous cholesterol synthesis. Studies in deficient animals have revealed that vanadium has a role not yet defined in the mineralization of bones and teeth.[712,713] While some have related caries prevention to this mineralization stimulating effect,[714] Underwood[715] on reviewing the evidence found inconclusive any beneficial effect of vanadium on the incidence of dental caries. No studies in older animals have been reported.

More pertinent to biologic aging *per se* are the studies of Schroeder, *et al.*.[716] They studied vanadium's impact on the survival and longevity of rats. Vanadyl sulfate (5 mg/liter) was added to drinking water of rats from weaning until death. All received the basal diet and other additions to drinking water described above.[710] The survival curves for the vanadium-fed rats showed female rats to have lower mortality rates than their controls until they were 36 months of age. In other words, vanadium consumption moved the survival curve to the right in the direction of an idealized type of curve.[717] Survival curves for vanadium-fed male rats differed little from those of their controls and depicted higher mortality rates than vanadium-fed females throughout the study. The average age at death of the last ten percent of surviving animals and the age at death of the ultimate survivor was lower in vanadium-fed animals of both sexes than in their controls.

This four year study involving 603 rats showed no vanadium-related advantage for males. The significance of the advantages reported for females is made less clear by virtue of the fact that the females did not receive the five mg/liter of trivalent chromium believed to be essential for normal serum cholesterol concentrations in female rats.[710] In spite of the presumed antagonism between tetravalent vanadium and trivalent chromium, the vanadium-fed females receiving only 20 percent of their required chromium had serum cholesterol concentrations not only far lower than their controls (also deficient in chromium) but also far lower than male vanadium-fed rats and twelve percent lower than male controls. Resolving this enigma is made more difficult by discrepancies in the ages at which blood samples were acquired in the tables reporting data on the same animals.[710,716]

Subsequent studies from the same laboratory[718] on interactions of zinc, chromium, copper, and manganese with 13 other elements, including vanadium, in mouse and rat tissues attributed no statistically significant role to vanadium. However, inspection of the data from rats indicates that vanadium in drinking water (5 mg/liter) resulted in higher concentrations (mg/kg dry weight) compared to control values of copper, manganese and zinc in liver, lung, heart, kidney and spleen tissue. In mice, the same was true for zinc concentrations.

While vanadium is present in abundance virtually everywhere, Hopkins and Mohr[706] have raised the issue of its possible low intake by animals because of its low concentration in naturally occurring feeds. Pointing to its extremely low concentrations in milk, liver, meat, and fish, and its possible low concentration in highly refined foods, they also raise the question of its marginal deficiency in human diets. This latter possibility seems remote, since most human food is prepared for consumption in contact with some vanadium-containing metal or compound. In fact, the probability of studying the impact of vanadium deficiency in man is very remote largely by virtue of the enormous cost involved in procuring vanadium-free foods and liquids and assuring a vanadium-free environment acceptable to human subjects.

The vanadium story in relation to nutrition and aging is confusing and somewhat sad in view of the quantity of sophisticated information regarding vanadium in the field of metallurgy where it plays an extremely valuable role in the production of alloys. It exemplifies the extremely complex problem of how to investigate the mechanisms by which trace elements influence human health. Variables to be controlled in the case of vanadium include species, sex, dose, the vanadium compound used,[698] the toxicity of some vanadium compounds,[719] vanadium's concentration in feed or meals, the concentration of other elements in food and fluid, and the subject's access to metal cages or implements.[697]

The vanadium story suggests the waste in time and resources and the potential hazards associated with quick acceptance of vigorously promoted new concepts in nutrition before they have been grounded in fundamental understanding of the biochemistry involved. In terms of the future, it suggests again the need for basic scientific investigation followed by clinical studies and then broad application, only if indicated. Perhaps most important is commmunicating with the public *pari passu* with the conduct of the investigations so that the status of essential nutrients in human health may be available to concerned consumers. The vanadium story also indicates the potential for vanadium's role in the pathogenesis and in the prevention and treatment of disease, opening the door to further exploration at clinical levels by medicine and its allied professions.

Zinc

Since zinc was found to be an essential nutrient for rats in 1934,[720] it has been more extensively investigated and reviewed than other true trace elements. Recently added to its accolades was its incorporation into the widely distributed table of Recommended Dietary Allowances (RDA) (92, 92a) where its quantity for mature and aged adults has been set at 15 mg daily.

In human nutrition, primary zinc definciency was first observed by Prasad, *et al.*,[721] in 1958 in Iranian youths manifesting a syndrome characterized by anemia, hepatosplenomegaly, hypogonadism, dwarfism, rough and dry skin, mental lethargy and geophasia. Subsequent investigations in Egypt established zinc deficiency as the cause of the syndrome.[722,723] Supplemental zinc resulted in growth and sexual maturation.[724,725]

Overt primary zinc deficiency is virtually never seen in the United States. However, marginal zinc deficiency has been inferred from improved wound healing[726] and from improved taste acuity[727] observed in adult humans when zinc intake was deliberately increased. The etiologies of conditioned zinc deficiencies are numerous among persons of all ages and particularly among the elderly. Since only 15 to 20 percent of ingested zinc is absorbed under the ideal circumstances afforded by diets high in animal protein, dietary components (calcium, magnesium, phosphorus, vitamin D, phytate, fiber, amino acids, fat and alcohol), medications (chelating agents like EDTA and penicillamine), and pathology (causes of steatorrhea and of massive losses of gastrointestinal fluids, inflammatory bowel disease, protein-losing enteropathies, genetic or toxic failures of renal tubular reabsorption of zinc, proteinurias, neoplasms and extensive burns) may reduce the effective zinc intake well below that needed for optimal function of zinc-dependent metallo-enzymes.

Although possibilities for marginal zinc deficiencies are certainly numerous, proving that marginal zinc deficiency is present in a given person is difficult. Plasma zinc concentrations, even when bloods are properly drawn and processed and zinc analyses are accurately performed, may not reflect zinc deficiency, since the plasma zinc may have been shifted to another tissue. Favorable response to zinc therapy is probably the most accurate means of diagnosing zinc deficiency currently available. However, even this method is fraught with uncertainties. This was demonstrated in adult humans in a double-blind Veterans Administration Cooperative Study[728] of the treatment of pressure ulcers of the skin, a problem common among bedridden elderly and among victims of spinal cord injuries of all ages. The study failed to demonstrate the value of supplemental zinc but failed also to show zinc to be valueless. The failures were attributable to the enormous variances of measures of healing of the lesions and of zinc nutriture of the patients. Even though the cooperative study involved several hundred patients, no conclusions could be reached.

As has been noted above, zinc is associated with copper in almost all copper-containing metallo-enzymes. In experimental studies, zinc deficiency has been correlated with enzyme deficiencies in tissues sensitive to lack of available zinc but not in all tissues. The differences are attributed by Prasad[729] to differences in zinc-ligand affinity of zinc metallo-enzymes and in their turnover rates in cells of affected tissues. Enzymes in man whose activities seem dependent on dietary zinc include thymidine kinase, alkaline phosphatase, lactic dehydrogenase, carbonic anhydrase, alcohol dehydrogenase, and carboxypeptidase. Ribonuclease, however, is increased in zinc deficiency, in inverse correlation with RNA/DNA ratios which decline.[730] DNA synthesis is directly related to zinc-dependent thymidine kinase activity.[731] The growth-inhibiting effect of zinc deficiency is probably related to this. Zinc deficiency is also directly associated with DNA-dependent RNA polymerase activity.[732] In view of the roles nucleic acids play in biologic aging, these observations make obvious the potential impact of zinc alimentation on aging from time of conception to death.

Animal protein is the principal source of zinc in the American diet. Liver, meat, eggs and seafood (oysters being especially high in zinc) represent major foods of this type. Dairy products fall next in line. Finally, whole grain products such as whole wheat or rye bread, oatmeal or whole corn complete major items providing zinc. A review of these foods suggests that elderly persons on limited incomes may have difficulty in obtaining sufficient zinc to meet the 15 mg daily recommended allowance. When the various etiologies of conditioned zinc deficiencies and their prevalence among the elderly are considered, the possibility of marginal zinc deficiencies among older persons certainly exists. Unfortunately, the diagnosis of such marginal states is presently difficult. Adding to the problem is the fact that elderly persons in need of high nutrient density dietaries frequently lack not only adequate zinc but adequate quantities of amino acids, vitamins, minerals and other trace elements in their diets. Hence, the arguments used for supplementing the diets of elderly persons with zinc could be applied to a variety of other nutrients. Since the elderly human being can only rarely be studied with the precision applied to investigations in laboratory animals, evidence supporting any public health-level recommendation in regard to zinc supplementation is not yet available. Until it arrives as a result of improved scientific methods, highly individualized management remains the key to assuring optimum zinc nutrition for man.

EPILOGUE ON MINERALS AND TRACE ELEMENTS AND AGING

If nothing else, the preceding discussion demonstrates that no single mineral nor trace element can be considered as a dietary ingredient without concern for other factors involved in the proper nutrition of man or woman. First, each must be related to other nutrients in the diet: calcium to phosphorus and magnesium; iron to copper; iodine to goitrogens and to bactericidal agents used in food processing; zinc to copper; etc. Second, each must be related to the genetic, toxic, traumatic and disease factors which influence the nutrient requirements of each person. Finally, each must be considered with respect to the vehicle or the compound or the format through which it will be ingested and metabolized by the human being. The phytate content of a food, the oxidation state of a compound and the quantity of fiber in the carrier will influence the availability and the toxicity of given minerals and trace elements.

Since socio-economic and health-related factors influence the dietary intake of millions of older persons, the availability of low cost, acceptable dietary supplements is often advocated. The experience of the Nutrition Program for Older Americans (NPOA) in evaluating the acceptability of Limited Use Supplemental Food (LUSF) (732a-c), a nonfat dry milk-based product to which vitamins, trace minerals and a small quantity of corn syrup solids had been added, revealed the impossibility of evaluating the effectiveness of a dietary supplement without objective measures at the disposal of the investigators. The number and variety of positive health-related events following consumption of LUSF by 6,000 elderly volunteers reporting subjectively could only be viewed as classic examples of the Hawthorne phenomenon.

Unfortunately, the cost of large scale objective evaluations of dietary supplements which would pass muster before a board of scientists is beyond reach. More unfortunately, this lack of objective data allows exposure of the entire population, and especially the elderly who can least afford it, to the promotion of dietary supplements by faddists and by commercial interests. The gravity of this problem will become even more evident in the discussion of vitamins in the ensuing chapter.

-10-

Vitamins

Vitamins comprise a large number of organic compounds essential for life which neither provide energy nor serve as structural components of tissue. Present in minute quantities, vitamins catalyze and regulate metabolic reactions. If not synthesized by the host or available to the host following their synthesis by microorganisms harbored by the host, vitamins essential for the life of the host must be provided by foods ingested by the host.

Foods vary greatly in the concentrations of nutrients, including vitamins, per unit of Calories.[733] The term "empty Calories" applied to a food implies that that food contains energy only and is devoid of other nutrients, including vitamins. Carbonated beverages exemplify this type of food.[734] The nutrient density of a given dietary is a matter of great concern in planning adequate nutrition for all age groups but particularly so for the elderly. Most elderly persons perform less physical work and consume fewer Calories than younger adults.[266] Unless the foods they consume have higher nutrient densities than those consumed when, as younger adults, they habitually ingested more Calories, their total daily consumption of many vitamins (and also amino acids, minerals and trace elements) will fall well below the Recommended Dietary Allowances (RDA) (92a).[735] Furthermore at least one-quarter of the American elderly have incomes at or below the official poverty level and can not afford to purchase high nutrient density foods, the better known examples of which retail at prohibitively high prices for those on limited incomes. Unless they select with extreme care among the commonly used, less expensive high nutrient density foods, the elderly will be unable to meet their RDA (92a). The ability to exercise such extreme care is derived from in-depth knowledge of modern nutrition. Unfortunately this knowledge is lacking not only among the impoverished elderly but also among those with incomes well above the poverty level. Finally, the high cost of dietary supplements[534,736] usually eliminates their use in meeting the challenge to the elderly posed by their consumption of too small quantities of foods with low nutrient densities.[737]

Many reliable investigators have postulated and several have sought data to prove deficiencies of vitamins among the elderly as a class. They have based their investigations on hypotheses regarding deterioration with age of capability to absorb, transport and/or utilize vitamins assumed to be present in ingested food or dietary supplements. As will be documented *(v.i.)* such hypotheses remain generally unsupported. Among the elderly, factors associated with diseases, medications, insufficient education and deplorable socio-enomic conditions are far more prevalent and potentially more remediable causes of vitamin deficiency syndromes.

The diagnosis of clinical deficiencies of vitamins is still an inexact as well as costly art, despite improved methodology in the science of nutrition. This has led to the conviction, widely held by many and especially by those concerned about persons in late maturity and old age,[738] that so-called subclinical deficiency states may adversely influence human physical and mental performance.

Procedures used to quantify the nutritional status of man with respect to vitamins have been published.[739,740] These include: (1) measurement of concentrations of vitamins or their metabolites in blood and urine; (2) measurement of blood concentrations and urinary excretions of vitamins after administration of standardized doses of the vitamins under study, the assumption being made that low tissue "saturation" with the vitamins will result in tissue capture of the administered vitamins leading to lower than normal rises in blood concentrations and/or urinary excretions; (3) measurement of vitamin concentrations in tissue biopsies; (4) microscopic studies of the histopathology of various tissues; (5) measurement of physiologic impairment, *e.g.*, dark adaptation in vitamin A deficiency; (6) measurement of characteristic metabolic abnormalities in deficiency syndromes, *e.g.*, hypocalcemia, hypophosphatemia and increased serum alkaline phosphatase activity in vitamin D deficiency; (7) evidence of successful therapy with specific vitamins, *e.g.*, prompt relief of peripheral neuropathy on administration of thiamin; (8) evaluation of various arrays of clinical signs and symptoms; and (9) evaluation of dietary intake.

Under ideal circumstances, several of these methods of evaluation of vitamin nutriture should be used simultaneously, since each suggests the state of vitamin nutriture at a chronologically different time. Dietary intake studies, properly conducted, suggest only the vitamin intakes at the time of investigation. Blood and urine chemistries give an indication of vitamin nutriture in the recent past — weeks to a few months. Clinical signs and symptoms suggest the state of vitamin nutriture over a longer span of time — several months to years.

In application of such methodology to the elderly, clinical signs and symptoms combined with available biochemical parameters are most useful and cost-effective. Diet history taking is less accurate and far more time consuming. However, since the technique is noninvasive and can be carried out without investment in extensive scientific and medical training and costly laboratory supplies and equipment, it has become a very popular means of estimating vitamin nutriture among older people. Unfortunately, the diet history technique reveals, even when exceptionally well done, only the intake of vitamins presumed to be in various foods, a presumption often unjustified. Since most older persons have many chronic illnesses and are taking many prescribed or self-administered drugs, other clinical and biochemical parameters must be measured if the true state of vitamin nutriture of the elderly is to be evaluated.

FAT-SOLUBLE VITAMINS

Vitamins A, D, E and K are the major components of the fat-soluble category of vitamins. The term fat-soluble indicates that historically these organic compounds were first characterized as unidentified components of dietary lipid fractions whose absence led to anatomic and physiologic pathology in animals and man. Other fat-soluble organic compounds (ubiquinone and thioctic acid, *e.g.)* have vitamin-like properties but are either so widely distributed or so little studied as to have relatively little practical significance in human nutrition. Essential fatty acids, sometimes called vitamin F, are occasionally included among taxonomical classifications of fat-soluble vitamins. Their role in human nutrition has been discussed above *(v.s.,* Chapter 7).

While the original fat-soluble designation may seem anachronistic in view of the fact that the vitamins have been synthesized and their biochemical functions elucidated, the terminology still serves a useful clinical function. Since lipids are the vehicles transporting vitamins into the gastrointestinal tract, appropriately functioning physiologic fat absorption mechanisms are essential if these vitamins are to gain access to the internal milieu of the animal body. Diseases resulting in long-standing steatorrhea may produce fat-soluble vitamin deficiency syndromes. Unsupervised consumption of low fat diets may also preclude effective absorption of both naturally occurring and supplemental fat soluble vitamins.[741] Among victims of chronic constipation, habitual use of mineral oil as a laxative may make unavailable for absorption sufficient fat-soluble vitamins to induce clinical deficiency states.[561,742]

Cholestyramine, the chloride salt of a basic anion exchange resin, is widely used in the management of primary type II hyperlipoproteinemia.[743] The resin absorbs and combines with bile acids in the intestine to form an insoluble complex which is excreted in the feces, resulting in a continuous, partial removal of bile acids from the enterohepatic circulation by preventing their reabsorption. This increased loss of bile acids induces more rapid oxidation of cholesterol to bile acids which in turn leads to decreases in serum low density lipoprotein and cholesterol concentrations. While these reductions are usually deemed desirable, cholestyramine has additional effects which may lead to fat-soluble vitamin deficiency syndromes.[561]

Several investigations[744,746] have demonstrated that cholestyramine in doses ranging from 12 to 36 gm daily increases fecal fat excretion to quantities comparable to those found in patients with active sprue.[747] By interfering with normal fat absorption, cholestyramine interferes with the absorption of all fat soluble vitamins. Hence, when given over long intervals, cholestyramine should be accompanied by supplementary vitamins A and D in water-miscible form or administered parenterally. Bleeding associated with hypoprothrombinemia from vitamin K deficiency may also result and may be treated with parenterally administered vitamin K_1.

Although cholestyramine is used successfully in the management of bile acid diarrhea in patients with ileal resections up to 100 cm in length,[745,746] such patients benefit from diminished water and electrolyte losses but continue to have increased fat losses leaving them at risk for fat-soluble vitamin deficiencies.

Fat-soluble vitamins A and D are capable of producing clinical toxicity syndromes when taken in excessive amounts. Since the human body is from 15 to 50 percent fat by weight, excessive vitamin A and D may be stored in large quantities making recovery from toxicity a slow process even after excessive intakes of the vitamins have been discontinued. While vitamin E toxicity has not been reported, synthetic naphthoquinone derivatives with vitamin K activity have caused hemolysis in persons with G6DP (glucose-6-phosphate dehydrogenase) deficiency and in others receiving very large doses. Unlike many of the water-soluble vitamins, fat-soluble vitamins do produce toxicity and may be lethal when consumed in excessive amounts. Among the elderly who often practice self-vitaminization, the dangers of overdosage are particularly great. Since symptoms of toxicity may resemble other pathology in the elderly, fat-soluble vitamin toxicity deserves consideration in differential diagnoses.

Vitamin A

Vitamin A, as its name implies, was the first-named of all vitamins. Since its identification in 1913 as "unidentified dietary factor fat soluble A," the vitamin A story has gradually unfolded with progress toward more complete understanding of its functions and metabolism continuing in the seventh decade since its initial identification.

In the human diet, vitamin A is found preformed as vitamin A_1 alcohol (retinol), vitamin A_2 alcohol (3-dehydroretinol), the aldehyde derivatives of retinol (retinal) and dehydroretinol (dehydroretinal), and various esters of both compounds called retinyl esters. These last-mentioned compounds are the major source of dietary preformed vitamin A. Some are hydrolyzed in the lumen of the small intestine by pancreatic retinyl ester hydrolase, while the remaining esters are hydrolyzed by an enzyme in the brush border of the intestinal mucosa. The resulting retinol is rapidly reesterified in the intestinal mocosal cells to saturated retinyl palmitate and stearate and smaller amounts of retinyl oleate and linoleate.

Other dietary sources of vitamin A include the so-called provitamins, naturally occurring pigments found in carrots, sweet potatoes, dark green leafy vegetables, winter squash, broccoli, apricots, pumpkins, tomatoes, and yellow corn. Preeminent among these provitamins is beta-carotene which on hydrolysis in the small intestinal mucosa by beta-carotene 15, 15′-dioxygenase yields two molecules of retinaldehyde (retinal). These are converted to retinol by a nonspecific retinaldehyde reductase. The retinol is then reesterified with fatty acids. These esters then travel in chylomicrons through the lymphatic system to the blood and thence to storage sites in the liver. Other carotenes such as alpha-carotene and gamma-carotene containing one beta-ionone ring form only one molecule of retinol on hydrolysis in the gut. Some carotenes are absorbed directly without cleavage in the gut. They account for the carotenemia frequently associated with the ingestion of large amounts of carotene-containing foods. This carotenemia may lead to carotenosis, a condition of which the skin, especially the soles of the feet and the palms of the hands, (but not the sclera) becomes deep yellow. Carotenosis also occurs in some patients with diabetes mellitus and with myxedema, apparently from a defect in conversion of carotene to vitamin A. Carotenosis, deliberately induced by administration of beta-carotene, is used to protect against the deleterious effects of photosensitization in human erythropoietic protoporphyria. When used for this purpose in such patients, the daily dose may range from 30 to 300 mg daily. Several weeks of therapy may be needed for enough beta-carotene to accumulate in the skin to produce the desired protective effect. However, beta-carotene has not been demonstrated to be an effective sunscreen in normal individuals.

In the liver, vitamin A is stored in lipid droplets as a mixture of long-chain retinyl esters. Prior to release from the liver, a liver enzyme hydrolyzes the retinyl esters to retinol. The free retinol circulates in human plasma bound to a specific transport protein, called retinol-binding protein (RBP). Purified human RBP has a molecular weight of 21,000, shows alpha-mobility on electrophoresis, and contains one binding site for each molecule of retinol. In plasma, RBP circulates as a highly specific protein-protein complex with prealbumin. Prealbumin is a stable tetramer comprising four identical subunits each containing 127 amino acids. It has a molecular weight of 55,000. This RBP-binding prealbumin is the same protein which transports thyroxin. In man less than one percent of the total prealbumin molecules circulates with bound thyroxin. Prealbumin's major role in man appears to be vitamin A transport. The RBP-prealbumin complex decreases the glomerular filtration of the much smaller RBP molecules, hence reducing the rate of removal of retinol and RBP from circulating plasma by the kidney.

A third form of vitamin A is retinoic acid. In general it represents a small proportion of total body vitamin A. Less than ten percent of the retinaldehyde formed from beta-carotene cleavage is oxidized in the intestine to form retinoic acid. Whereas retinol and retinyl esters are transported through the lymphatic system, retinoic acid is transported by way of the portal vein probably bound to serum albumin. It is rapidly metabolized and excreted in the urine and in bile where its major metabolite has been identified as retinoyl beta-glucuronide.

L.M. DeLuca has prepared a detailed review of the chemistry and physiologic functions of vitamin A and its metabolites.[747a]

Major Functions of Vitamin A: Although vitamin A was historically the first of the vitamins, a biochemical basis for its physiological function has been defined solely in the visual system. George Wald was awarded the Nobel Prize in Medicine in 1967 for his discoveries of the role of vitamin A in vision. The following year he completed a review of the entire subject.[748]

The retina of the eye contains two distinct photoreceptors. The cones deal with acute perception, and the rods are concerned with visual acuity in dim light. A combination of retinal and a protein, opsin, called rhodopsin is the photosensitive pigment of the rods. In the cones the protein moiety is different and is called iodopsin. Inadequate intake or impaired utilization of vitamin A can cause impairment of dark adaptation and night blindness. Such rod disfunction, one of the earliest signs of vitamin A deficiency, can be detected by dark adoptometry, rod scotometry, or electroretinography.

The other physiological functions of vitamin A have been described but are not completely understood. Nonetheless, it has long been known that vitamin A deficiency produces growth retardation, increased susceptibility to infection, xerosis of the bulbar conjunctiva, corneal xerosis, corneo-caretomalasia, liquefaction of the cornea, rupture and extrusion of the eye contents, and subsequent shrinking of the globe (phthisis bulbi). A version of this pathology comprises anterior bulging with ectasia of the cornea and stapholomas. Blindness in any case is a common result. Were the mortality rate in vitamin A deficiency not so high (50% and greater) among young victims of this form of xerophthalmia, the prevalence of vitamin A deficiency-created blindness among living adults would be far higher than that reported today.

Since death is the ultimate endpoint in vitamin A deficiency, it seems evident that vitamin A performs some very essential functions common to many biochemical systems and tissues. Much evidence has pointed toward a function of vitamin A in regulating membrane structure. Abnormalities in RNA metabolism and protein synthesis have been reported in vitamin A deficiency. Deficient animals have been shown to have an increased incidence of cancer. From a clinical standpoint, the physical sign of follicular hyperkeratosis suggests an important function of vitamin A in maintaining the integrity of the epithelium. In animals, reproduction in both males and females has been adversely affected by vitamin A deficiency. Male synthesis or release of androgen by the testis may be diminished. Either resorbtion or growth retardation and death of the fetus may occur early in pregnancy apparently due to placental injury. Deficient animals display several abnormalities of bone and teeth. These result apparently from alterations in the activities of osteoblasts and osteoclasts. In some animals there is a decrease in the inside dimensions of the skull and reduction of the marrow cavities of long and flat bones.

Animal experiments, clinical investigations and data from human epidemiologic surveys have suggested that vitamin A deficiency impairs the synthesis of hemoglobin. In studies of human volunteers consuming diets providing all essential nutrients except vitamin A, Hodges, *et al.*[749] observed a significant anemia and have concluded that this anemia is a consequence of an inadequate intake of vitamin A. Repletion with either carotene or vitamin A while the subjects were consuming the test diets led to prompt and complete recovery. These authors also observed comparable anemias in vitamin A deficient rats. In addition, they reviewed the dietary intake and the hemoglobin and plasma vitamin A levels of persons in eight countries selected for the adequate iron intake of their populations (evaluated during nutrition surveys conducted by the Interdepartmental Committee of Nutrition for National Defense [ICNND]). This review showed hemoglobin and vitamin A to be positively correlated, and observation already made in the original report of the ICNND survey of Paraguay.[750] Similar studies[751] of hemoglobin and plasma retinol in Central America reveal positive correlations.

Hypervitaminosis A: Most vitamin A functions have been analyzed through studies of vitamin A deficiency in animals or in man. Toxic manifestations from acute or chronic ingestion of large doses of vitamin A are impressive and should be considered in differential diagnosis of varied and bizarre symptomatology. Early Arctic explorers developed drowsiness, irritability, headache, and vomiting, followed by peeling of the skin after ingesting several million units of vitamin A in polar bear or seal liver.[752] Acute poisoning resulting from the administration of a single dose of 300,000 international units has been reported in an infant.[753] More common is chronic poisoning which occurs after 100,000 or more units have been taken for many months.[753a] Coarse, sparse hair, alopecia of the eyebrows, dry, rough skin, and cracked lips appear early, while severe headache and generalized weakness develop later in the course of the phenomenon. Arthralgia, hard tender cortical thickenings over the radius and tibia, splenomegaly, hypoplastic anemia and leukopenia may also be found. Fortunately prognosis, once a diagnosis has been established, is excellent. Signs and symptoms disappear within one to four weeks after cessation of vitamin A ingestion.

The signs and symptoms of hypervitaminosis A have been related to increased levels of serum retinyl esters circulating in association with serum lipoproteins and not bound to retinol-binding protein (RBP). Clinical toxicity may be found when RBP's capacity to transport vitamin A is exceeded and excessive vitamin A is presented to cell membranes in a form other than that bound to RBP.[754] Even while patients are toxic the concentrations of plasma retinol-binding protein and prealbumin are normal and continue to be normal in the post-toxic period after cessation of vitamin A administration. Serum lipoproteins are the principal vehicles transporting retinyl esters in vitamin A toxicity. They nonspecifically deliver vitamin A to biologic membranes. Surface-active properties of the vitamin lead to increased lability to biologic membranes. It seems apparent that RBP may function to protect tissues from the surface-active properties of the vitamin as well as to regulate the supply of the retinol to the tissues.

Vitamin A and Aging: The above discussions suggest many ways in which intake of vitamin A — too little or too much — may produce pathology in childhood which may be carried over as extreme disability or disease to youth, middle and late maturity, and old age. However, little evidence has been found relating old age *per se* to vitamin A deficiency syndromes in the United States. Kirk and Chieffi[755] could find no age-wise decrements in vitamin A or carotene in the plasma of human subjects. Yiengst and Shock[756] found no decrement with age in the absorption of vitamin A from the small intestine. Birren, *et al.*[757]

did find a significant decrement in light threshold related to aging but could demonstrate no correlation with serum vitamin A concentrations and no improvement in light threshold measurements with the administration of 100,000 international units of vitamin A daily for as long as 76 days.[758] Follicular hyperkeratosis, traditionally associated with vitamin A deficiency, is frequently seen among the elderly but, more often than not, is related to poor personal hygiene and is not necessarily an outcome of vitamin A deficiency.

While age *per se* may not be related to vitamin A deficiency, the intake by elderly persons of numerous pharmaceuticals which influence vitamin A absorption provides a potential source of vitamin A deficiency. As previously noted, mineral oil extracts carotene and vitamin A from the diet, carries them through the intestinal tract and eliminates them with the feces. The antibiotic neomycin inhibits vitamin A absorption by decreasing secretion of pancreatic lipase, inactivating bile salts and causing mucosal damage in the small intestine. Cholestyramine combines with bile salts which are essential for the absorption of vitamin A, thereby diminishing the quantity absorbed. Excessive intake of alcohol can impair the conversion of retinol to retinal by preferentially utilizing alcohol dehydrogenase required in the oxidation process of the retinol to retinal conversion. Alcohol may also interfere with the hepatic synthesis of retinol-binding protein (RBP).

The symptoms of vitamin A toxicity may be confused with a variety of more common problems associated in general in the elderly with mental confusion. The availibility of high potency vitamin A capsules and their use by some dermatologists in the treatment of some disorders like psoriasis suggest that vitamin A toxicity is a potential hazard to be considered in the differential diagnosis of otherwise unexplained ailments among the elderly. Food faddists - of whom there are many among the elderly - who ingest larger amounts of vitamin A as part of their daily regimen may also manifest vitamin A toxicity.[759]

Vitamin D

Although the antirachitic properties of codliver oil had been demonstrated in 1824[760] and the antirachitic action of sunlight suggested in 1890,[761] McCollum and associates in 1922[762] conclusively demonstrated that the antirachitic properties of codliver oil could not be attributed to the presence of the previously identified factor vitamin A, since the antirachitic factor was stable to heat and aeration and the vitamin A factor was not. McCollum named the factor vitamin D.[763] Two years later Steenbock and associates[764,765] showed that antirachitic activity could be induced in certain foods and in animals by ultraviolet irradiation.

The natural and active precursors of the D vitamins, *i.e.*, the provitamins, are cyclopentanophenanthrene derivatives or steroids. Provitamin D_2, ergosterol, is found in plants, while provitamin D_3, 7-dehydrocholesterol, is found in animals. Ergosterol is converted by ultraviolet light to vitamin D_2 or activated ergosterol. 7-dehydrocholesterol, itself derived from cholesterol, is converted by ultraviolet light to vitamin D_3 or activated 7-dihydrocholesterol.

Real progress in understanding metabolism of vitamin D *in vivo* came in the late sixties and seventies. In 1968 Blunt, *et al.*[766] identified 25-hydroxyvitamin D_3 as the predominant D_3 derivative in blood. Following absorption from the jejunum and ileum, the active forms of vitamin D are transported to the bloodstream as chylomicrons via the lymphatic system. They are then concentrated in the liver where they are hydroxylated to 25-hydroxyvitamin D_3 (25-OH-D_3). This compound is transported next to the kidney where it is converted to 1,25-dihydroxyvitamin D_3 (1,25-$(OH)_2D_3$) which appears to be a true sterol hormone that mediates calcium transport in such target tissues as intestine and bone.

During the seventies, a more complete understanding of the intermediary metabolism of vitamin D was developed through numerous laboratory and clinical investigations.[761,773b] Clinical applications of the knowledge acquired in these investigations mushroomed toward the end of the decade. Progress in the clinical field was delayed by lack of reliable quantification of the various vitamin D metabolites in the plasma and other tissues of man. While competitive protein-binding radioassays and ultraviolet absorption of high pressure liquid chromatography eluates offer considerable hope for the future, the simplest and most widely used assay of the adequacy of vitamin D therapy and the presence of either vitamin D deficiency or vitamin D excess has been that for 25-OH-D_3.[774] This assay also permits measurement of the absorption of 25-OH-D_3.[775]

Low levels of 25-OH-D_3 in plasma have been noted in pregnant women, patients with advanced hepatocellular and renal disease, thyrotoxicosis, gastric and small bowel operations, and in patients subjected to long term anticonvulsant therapy, high-dose glucocorticoid therapy, sunlight deprivation and/or nutritional inadequacies.

Unfortunately the assays for 1,25-$(OH)_2D_3$ are technically complicated and satisfactorily performed in very few laboratories. Production of 1,25-$(OH)_2D_3$ in the kidney is stimulated or depressed relatively rapidly by hormonal and ionic factors, particularly by alterations in mineral homeostasis,[776] especially when compared with the stable plasma concentrations and long half-life of 25-OH-D_3. When compared to vitamin D, 1/1000 as much 1,25-$(OH)_2D_3$ can correct hypocalcemia of human hypoparathyroidism.[776]

In one respect, assays for 25-OH-D_3 are more useful in that they provide a sensitive index of vitamin D deficiency or intoxication. Low levels have been reported in patients receiving anti-convulsant medications and elevated values, in patients with hypervitaminosis D. Plasma 1,25-$(OH)_2D_3$ concentrations, on the other hand, have been found to be normal in both clinical conditions.

Clinical investigations in small numbers of patients have suggested an inverse correlation between plasma concentrations of 1,25-$(OH)_2D_3$ and age.[778] The enzyme 25-OH-D_3-1 alpha-hydroxylase which catalyzes the transformation of 25-OH-D_3 to 1,25-$(OH)_2D_3$ is produced in the kidney. Preliminary evidence suggests that bone loss in women over forty and men over fifty[779] may correlate with decrements with age in nephrons.[780,782] The wisdom of such a suggestion is corroborated by data from studies of patients with renal disease. In them, when glomerular filtration rate falls below 30 ml/min.,[783] bone disease becomes clinically apparent. There is a linear correllation between renal impairment and calcium absorption by the small intestine.[784] Undetectable plasma concentrations of 1,25-$(OH)_2D_3$ have been observed in patients with end-stage renal disease and in those who have been nephrectomized.[785,786] When such end-stage patients are treated with 1,25-$(OH)_2D_3$, calcium absorption from the small intestine is increased and parathyroid hormone activity is suppressed. The same results may be achieved with 1 alpha-$(OH)D_3$, a synthetic analog of vitamin D_3 which *in vivo* is rapidly converted to the natural hormone 1,25-$(OH)_2D_3$. This analog is easier and less expensive to synthesize than the natural hormone. In addition its future is especially bright because it is converted quickly and efficiently into 1,25-$(OH)_2D_3$ by the widely distributed 25-hydroxylase enzyme. The rate-limiting kidney enzyme 25-hydroxyvitamin D_3-1 alpha-hydroxylase (1 alpha-hydroxylase) is circumvented.[787,788]

Often confused with the osteopenia of aging is the disease osteoporosis. Gallagher *et al.*[789] have observed that patients with osteoporosis have lower plasma 1,25-$(OH)_2D_3$ concentrations than do their age-stratified controls.

These various observations suggest new techniques for the management of osteopenia, whether associated with aging alone or with the disease osteoporosis. Hypervitaminosis D, or vitamin D toxicity, is a problem far more serious than hypervitaminosis A, since irreversible renal damage results from long-term hypercalcemia even with concentrations no higher than 11 mg per 100 ml.[790] This seeming paradox is especially likely to be seen in patients with hypoproteinemia. Since about 0.8 mg of calcium is bound to each gram of protein, the remainder is ultrafilterable and includes ionized calcium plus calcium complexed with phosphate and citrate. Such pathogenetic hypercalcemia may also be seen in acidemia during which the increase in ionized calcium may occur independently of any change in total calcium concentration.

The syndrome associated with vitamin D toxicity includes metastatic calcification, hypercalcemia, azotemia, weakness anorexia, visual disturbances, anemia, dermatitis and inflamation of fatty deposits in the sclera. At one time very high potency vitamin D capsules were used in the management of rheumatoid arthritis and led to many reported cases of vitamin D intoxication.[791,793]

The toxicity of vitamin D is ample evidence that vitamins deserve the same respect as other therapeutic drugs when given in pharmacologic doses.

Vitamin E

"Vitamin E" is a generic term including many tocol and tocotrienol compounds, the most active of which is alpha-tocopherol. Since data on the content of the tocopherols in food was insufficient, only alpha-tocopherol was considered in dietary calculations (92). Previously (92), one International Unit (IU) of vitamin E was defined as the activity of 1 mg of dl-alpha-tocopherol acetate. Free synthetic dl-alpha-tocopherol has a potency of 1.1 IU/mg. The activity of naturally occurring alpha-tocopherol, d-alpha-tocopherol, is 1.49 IU/mg and its acetate, 1.36 IU/mg (92).

Whether expressed on the basis of mgs of d-alpha-tocopherol equivalents (92a) or in the previously used International Units (IU) (92), all forms of vitamin E have the same activity.

In calculating the vitamin E activity of mixed diets, mgs of beta-tocopherol should be multiplied by 0.5, of gamma-tocopherol by 0.1 and of alpha-tocotrienol by 0.3. These three are the only vitamers with significant activity present in United States diets. When these are added to the mgs of alpha-tocopherol, the sum of the total is alpha-tocopherol equivalents (alpha-TEs). If only the alpha-tocopherol of a mixed diet is given, the value in mgs should be increased by 20 percent, by multiplying by 1.2, to account for the other tocopherols present, thereby giving an approximation of the total vitamin E activity as mgs of alpha-TEs.

The 1980 RDA (92a) expresses the vitamin E allowance in terms of mgs of these (alpha-TEs). In these terms, one alpha-TE is equivalent to one mg of d-alpha-tocopherol. For adult males 51 years of age or older, the RDA is 10 alpha-TEs; for adult females 51 years of age or over, the RDA is 8 alpha-TEs. These values may be compared with the 15 IU for males 51 years of age and over and the 12 IU for females 51 year's of age and over in the 1974 RDA (92) where the total vitamin E activity was estimated to come 80 percent from alpha-tocopherol and 20 percent from other tocopherols.

One alpha-TE represents approximately 0.667 IU. This conversion arises because one mg of d-alpha-tocopherol is equivalent to 1.49 IU *(v.s.)* which when rounded off is 1.5 IU. Therefore, one alpha-TE equals 0.667 IU. Hence, the 1980 RDA for vitamin E (92a) is identical to that of the 1974 RDA (92).

In contrast to vitamins A and D, vitamin E has been and continues to be a topic of great controversy. Agreement has not been reached even in regard to the toxicity of pharmacologic-sized doses. In 1975, Farrell and Bieri[794] reported finding no disturbances in liver, kidney, muscle, thyroid gland, erythrocytes, leukocytes, coagulation parameters or glucose — let alone clinical signs or symptoms of toxicity — in twenty-eight adults ingesting from 100 to 800 IU of alpha-tocopherol per day for an average of three years. In 1977, an Expert Panel on Food Safety and Nutrition and a Committee on Public Information of the Institute of Food Technologists issued a special report on vitamin E maintaining that no evidence existed that tocopherols are toxic even in large doses.[795] Later that year Herbert[796] pointed to evidence reported by Hayes and Hegsted[797] that symptoms of headache, nausea, fatigue, giddiness and blurred vision were observed in six of thirteen patients receiving three hundred mg of vitamin E per day. The same authors cite disruption of gonadal function from the intake of four to twelve grams by men for prolonged periods. They also noted that two to four grams per day for three months produced slight creatinuria, chapping, chylosis, angular stomatitis, gastrointestinal disturbances and muscle weakness in one case in whom the signs and symptoms ceased within two weeks when vitamin E was discontinued. They also mentioned that hypoglycemia and depressed prothrombin levels had been reported. Corrigan and Marcus[798] observed a coagulopathy associated with vitamin E ingestion. Briggs[799] has also listed a number of studies leading him to conclude that published evidence of potential hazards from ingestion by man of megadoses of vitamin E make the present lack of definitive information disturbing. In 1978, Scott,[800] following an extensive review of the literature, concluded that vitamin E supplements produced no toxic side effects.

Tsai, *et al.*[801] disturbed over the large number of reports dealing with undesirable side effects of vitamin E[798,802,805] performed a controlled study in two hundred two healthy college student volunteers aged 18 to 35. Volunteers were measured for general health, prothrombin time, total blood leukocyte count, serum creatine phosphokinase activity and the serum concentrations of vitamin E, cholesterol, triglyceride and the thyroid hormones, T_3 and T_4. This double-blind study compared those students receiving 600 IU of dl-alpha-tocopherol acetate daily with those receiving a placebo for 28 days. The megavitamin E supplementation had no effect on work performance, sexuality and general well-being and did not cause muscular weakness or gastrointestinal disturbances. It had no effect on prothrombin time, leukocyte count or serum creatine phosphokinase activity. It was associated with slightly elevated cholesterol concentrations in the serum of both males and females. Similar slight increases in serum triglyceride were noted in males, but statistically significantly elevated levels were associated with megavitamin E supplementation in females. Significantly elevated concentrations of vitamin E itself were noted in both females and males, the high levels being found in females. It significantly decreased serum T_3 and T_4 concentrations in males and in those females not using steroid oral contraceptives. On the basis of the changes observed in T_3 and T_4 concentratons and in the concentrations of serum triglycerides in females, the authors concluded that further studies were desirable.

In reality the controversy regarding the toxic properties of megadoses of vitamin E is but a small segment of the overall dispute over the necessity for supplemental vitamin E in the American diet. Since megadoses of E have been proven to be no adjuvant to health but at the same time no definite menace, the vitamin has become popular among faddists but also a source of dispute in the scientific community.[806] If any consensus exists at all, it is in agreement with the views of Tappel[807] who has pleaded for more investigations on the grounds that no one benefits from the present standoff between the proponents and detractors of vitamin E. This attitude has been expressed more recently by others.[799;800]

The calls for more investigations of the vitamin E conundrum are particularly cogent for older Americans among whom the present uncertainty adds to the economic burden they face. One hundred 400 mg capsules of dl-alpha-tocopherol have been selling in Florida retirement communities at prices ranging from seven to ten dollars, the specific price depending on the packager. Even when ordered by physicians through discount mail order houses, one hundred 400 IU capsules of d-alpha-tocopherol cost more than four dollars. At retail, sold as nonprescription items, these capsules are readily available to all, including older persons. They are usually ingested without their consumers having the benefit of professional counseling. Considering their cost which represents a serious drain on limited economic resources of the older persons who buy them, their potential toxicity and the fact that no conclusive evidence of their value has yet been published, the need for additional investigations is apparent.

The evidence that vitamin E plays any role in the pathogenesis of heart or other vascular diseases is a classic example of present day lack of conclusive information pro or con. Since the original reports of Vogelsang and Shute in 1946,[808] evidence supporting[808a,809] and denying[810,814] its effectiveness has appeared in the clinical and scientific literature. Authoritative reviews[795,807] and unbiased authorities[815] commenting on the situation have generally concluded vitamin E is ineffective in treating or preventing heart disease or that "the discrepancy between the results of advocates and skeptics may be attributed, in part, to the greater degree of placebo effect evoked by the enthusiasts".[815] While such preventive and therapeutic skepticism is completely justified on the grounds that no conclusive evidence is available supporting a role for vitamin E, the commentary of Scott[800] provides an explanation and also holds out an improved basis for evaluating vitamin E's role in the future. Scott maintains that in the half-century since vitamin E was discovered "research on the many interrelationships existing between this vitamin and other dietary factors has led to such confusion that a number of researchers and clinicians have tended to relegate vitamin E to a position of little importance." Fortunately, some order is infiltrating the confusion through research suggesting the mutual relationships of vitamin E, selenium and sulfur-containing amino acids in protecting vital phospholipids from peroxidation.[795,800,816,817] Since such findings have possible links to the pathogenesis of cardiovascular diseases, a better understanding of vitamin E's role in maintaining a healthy cardiovascular system may soon evolve.

While vitamin E's role in managing angina pectoris is dubious, more general agreement has been found in its use in the management of intermittent claudication.[818,821] However, the failure to use a double-blind protocol in the most recent study[821] and the fact that exercise *per se* is regarded as the most effective treatment for intermittent claudication[822] suggest that the reported success of vitamin E may be related to increased exercise among those persons under study (the Hawthorne effect).

The elucidation of vitamin E's antioxidant properties were followed shortly by proposals that vitamin E could slow the process of biologic aging.[823,824] The principle evidence favoring a positive role for vitamin E in aging derived from Tappel's observation[807] that mice receiving for one year pharmacologic doses of supplemental vitamin E had at sacrifice half the amount of "aging" pigment found in controls. Unfortunately, the decrements in age pigments were not associated with any slowing of mortality or deceleration of the normal decline in performance due to aging in the mice under study. With the development of a quantitative method for the determination of organic solvent soluble age pigments in animal tissues,[825] a reevaluation of the effect of dietary vitamin E on tissue age pigment concentrations became possible. Csallany, *et al.*[826] studied the concentrations in uterus, lungs, spleen, kidney, liver, heart and brain in mice sacrificed at one, four, eight, eleven and seventeen months after the initiation of diets with and without supplementation with d-alpha-tocopherol acetate. The vitamin E supplements resulted in lower age pigment concentrations in the liver at two, five, nine, twelve and eighteen months of age. However, in all other tissues measured in eighteen month old mice, dietary vitamin E did not lower the concentration of age pigment. Furthermore, although liver age pigment concentrations were suppressed by vitamin E in all age groups, a dramatic increase in age pigment had still occurred by eighteen months of age.

Grinna[827] conducted in rats a study designed to investigate the age of an animal as a factor in the induction of tocopherol deficiency, the modification of age-related changes by alpha-tocopherol and the modification of subcellular membrane composition and function by alpha-tocopherol. He observed that the older the rat the more difficult it is to produce signs of deficiency or to deplete the liver of its store of alpha-tocopherol. No age-associated functional and compositional changes were modified by alteration of the dietary level of alpha-tocopherol. Jager[828] reported finding no increase in mortality of rats fed a diet deficient in vitamin E for 22 months. Tappel, *et al.*,[829] have reported a number of physiological parameters not improved over those of controls in aging rats fed a diet containing over 2.7 gm of d-alpha-tocopherol per kg of diet for seven months. These studies suggest that supplements of vitamin E to the average diet will have little influence on biologic aging.

An interesting controversy arose from reduction in the vitamin E 1974 RDA[92] to 12-15 mgs daily from the 1968 RDA of 10-30 mgs.[516] The 1980 RDA,[92a] as noted above, has been changed only in unitage, not in the quantitative amount of the vitamin recommended in the 1974 Revision. The reduction was justified because dietary vitamin E far in excess of the minimum daily requirement of 3-6 IUs was assured by the high consumption of vegetable oils and hydrogenated vegetable shortenings and margarines used in the American diet today. However, the vitamin E requirement rises in proportion to the polyunsaturated fatty acid (PUFA) content.[830] Ratios (mg/gm) of alpha-tocopherol to PUFA of about 0.4 have been recommended as satisfactory.[831] If followed, this recommendation would fix 4.6 mg of vitamin E as the requirement for a man consuming a 2600 Calorie diet containing 40 percent fat energy, ten percent of which is PUFA. The reduction in the RDA of vitamin E came at a time when the United Kingdom and Canada had not committed themselves to a recommended intake.[817,807] Their reasons included the difficulty in evaluating dietary intake, vitamin E's wide distribution in nature, the lack of reliable analytical information on its content in foods and the fact that there are at least eight known chemical forms (four tocopherols and four tocotrienols) and widely differing biologic activities. The 1974 reduction in the RDA therefore put the United States more in line philosophically with other industrialized countries.

Strongly opposing the reduced allowance, Horwitt[806] maintained that persons consuming diets virtually devoid of PUFA require a minimum of 4 mg vitamin E daily for protection against lipid peroxidation. He cites evidence that the requirement rises appreciably on diets high in PUFA.[832] Horwitt estimates the human daily requirement by the formula:

$$\text{alpha-tocopherol equivalent} = 0.25(\%\text{PUFA} + \text{gm PUFA}) + 4 \text{ mg}$$

In the man cited above consuming a 2600 Calorie diet containing 40% fat Calories, 10% which are PUFA, Horwitt's formula yields a minimum daily requirement of 9.4 mg. Doubling this requirement would yield an RDA of 18.8 mg, an amount well within the 10-30 mg daily d-alpha-tocopherol suggested by Horwitt.[832]

In concluding this discussion of the role of vitamin E in maintaining health in the face of aging, it is important to acknowledge that the processes inhibited by tocopherols produce tissue changes in man that can be evaluated in no less than thirty years, given present scientific knowledge of biologic aging.[806] The involvement of vitamin E in disease processes and in biologic aging is intuitively felt by many scientists.[800,807,817] The need for more basic investigation in the role of vitamin E in both normal and pathologic aging is evident. At the present time, a genuine issue in the scientific community concerns the differences between the proponents of the 15 and 30 mg maximums for the RDA. Since the evidence for assigning merit to pharmacologic doses of 400 mg and more daily is lacking, the public in general and the elderly in particular should not waste resources on megavitamin E therapy which in more than three decades has yet to produce anything but scientific disappointment.

Vitamin K

Vitamin K was discovered by Henrick Dam who christened it after the German word *Koagulation* as well as because it was the first letter of the alphabet not already in use to describe some existing or postulated vitamin activity.[833,833a] The vitamin prevented a hemmorhagic diathesis in chickens fed a diet extracted with nonpolar solvents.[834] It is now known to be essential for the synthesis of prothrombin and three other blood clotting factors in the liver.

The nomenclature of vitamin K used at the present time[835] uses "vitamin K" as a generic description for 2-methyl-1,4-naphthoquinone and all derivatives thereof which show antihemmorhagic activity in animals fed a vitamin K deficient diet. "Vitamin K_1" or "phylloquinone" is described in chemical terms 2-methyl-3-phytyl-1,4-naphthoquinone and is found primarily in plants. "Vitamins K_2" are derived from animal and bacterial sources and comprise a series of vitamin K's with unsaturated side chains called "multiphrenylmenaquinones" or "menaquinone-n." The parent compound, 2-methyl-1,4-naphthoquinone (once called "vitamin K_3") is now known as menadione, a synthetic product which is also the progenitor of many water-soluble analogues.

The vitamin K story is a classic example of the mutual relationships among nutrition, health and aging in the United States. With the exception of newborn infants *(v.i.)*, primary vitamin K malnutrition, *i.e.*, malnutrition from the absence of vitamin K in the dietary, is virtually unknown. However, secondary vitamin K malnutrition, *i.e.*, secondary to disease or iatrogenic factors, is a frequent occurrence. This situation arises not only from the fact that vitamin K is abundant in most American diets (300 to 500 micrograms/day [836]) but also from the fact that vitamin K is synthesized by intestinal microflora, providing therefore two sources of the vitamin estimated to be of approximately equal physiologic significance.[837] In addition, since vitamin K is fat soluble, it shares with other fat soluble vitamins the possibility of malabsorption from diseases interfering with the delivery of bile or pancreatic secretions to the small intestine *(e.g.*, obstructive jaundice, biliary fistulas and pancreatic cystic fibrosis), from consumption of antibiotics or bile sequestrating agents such as cholestyramine, from excessive ingestion of mineral oil, from surgical resection of portions of the small intestine and from a variety of other diseases such as tropical and nontropical sprue, pellagra, regional enteritis, ulcerative colitis and celiac disease. Antibiotics not only may interfere with its absorption but also may diminish the growth of intestinal micro-flora, thereby reducing the availability of vitamin K from that particular source.

In newborn infants, whose intestinal microflora have yet to develop, hemorrhagic disease of the newborn remains a problem for the first five to eight days of life unless they are given supplemental vitamin K at the time of birth. This problem occurs both in breast fed infants and in those fed formulas deficient in vitamin K. Premature infants are particularly susceptible because the premature liver is often unable to secrete enough bile to adequately absorb orally administered vitamin K and to produce vitamin K-dependent blood coagulation factors.

In mature adults, primary dietary vitamin K deficiency may rarely be found in persons with extremely bizarre eating habits.[838,840] One clinic[841] has suggested that many elderly persons have hypoprothrombinemia which improves on the administration of oral vitamin K. Since hypoprothrombinemia may have many etiologies, such reports must be viewed with considerable skepticism.

Among the elderly, a major use of vitamin K is in the correction of hypoprothrombinemia induced iatrogenically by excessive doses of vitamin K antagonists such as 3,3'-methyl-*bis*-(4-hydroxycoumarin) (Dicumarol[R]) and other 4-hydroxy-coumarins known under a variety of trade names. All of these have been used extensively to prevent intravascular clotting after myocardial infarcts and other diseases involving immobilization, problems very common among the elderly. The hypoprothrombinemia which may develop in persons receiving excessive doses of 4-hydroxycoumarins may be rapidly corrected by the parenteral administration of vitamin K.[842] Water soluble menadione is ineffective in the management of 4-hydroxycoumarin toxicity since its conversion to physiologically active menaquinone-4 is too slow to attain pharmacologically effective concentrations.[843,844]

The exception to the correction of hypoprothrombinemia with vitamin K occurs in patients with severe hepatocellular disease. When parenteral administration of vitamin K fails to correct hypoprothrombinemia within 2-3 hours, severely impaired function of the recipients liver is strongly suggested (the Koller test[845]).

Vitamin K deficiency may also occur in patients who have received total parenteral or enteral nutrition devoid of vitamin K. Such patients are often on antibiotics which have diminished the production of vitamin K by the intestinal micro-flora. Such iatrogenically induced vitamin K deficiency states have been utilized with some success to estimate the actual requirements of man for the vitamin. Frick, *et al.*[846] estimated the vitamin K requirement of starved, debilitated patients fed intravenously and receiving antibiotics to decrease intestinal synthesis of vitamin K. They interpreted their data to indicate that the minimum daily requirement for man was approximately 1 microgram/kg/day. Doisy[847] fed a chemically defined diet combined with mineral oil and antibiotics to two normal subjects and reduced prothrombin concentrations 50% in about 20 weeks. The prothrombin time in these subjects returned to normal following administration of 0.5 micrograms of vitamin K/kg/day, leading Doisy to conclude, as had Frick, that 1 microgram/kg/day was sufficient to maintain normal clotting factor synthesis in healthy adults. O'Reilly,[848] following a study in four normal volunteers who received a diet containing 25 micrograms of vitamin K per day plus antibiotics, reported that as little as 0.5 micrograms of vitamin K/kg/day would maintain normal prothrombin concentrations. Such studies have led to the conclusion that 0.5-1.0 micrograms of vitamin K/kg/day are the appropriate range for the vitamin requirement for a human being.

While this amount of vitamin is present in almost any reasonable diet, the possibility of vitamin K deficiency must be considered in differential diagnosis, particularly in the elderly whose capacity to suffer from a variety of diseases and of iatrogenic conditions is legendary.

Research in bacteria has indicated a role for vitamin K in electron transport systems.[849,851] Studies in animals have indicated the presence of another vitamin K-dependent plasma protein.[852] Perhaps of even greater interest is the research indicating nonplasma vitamin K-dependent proteins, particularly those associated with bone.[853,854] While these observations hold considerable promise of further insight into the physiological and biochemical role of vitamin K, they have not yet reached a point where clinical applications are feasible.

Vitamin K, in common with other fat-soluble vitamins, may be toxic when used in pharmacologic doses.

Excessive doses may lead to hyperbilirubinemia in newborns (especially in premature infants) which may be sufficient to result in kernicterus with its many ramifications (brain damage) for the welfare of the infant in future life. Because of this risk, the Committee on Nutrition of the American Academy of Pediatrics[855] recommends that the administration of vitamin K_1 to all infants (but especially to those who are premature) should be limited to a single dose of 0.5-1.0 mg of phytonadione, MSD, U.S.P. (aqueous colloidal solution of vitamin K_1).

Although used to treat hypoprothrombinemia, vitamin K analogs like menadione given in large, repeated doses may produce bromsulphalein retention and prolongation of prothrombin time.

In patients with a genetic deficiency of glucose-6-phosphate dehydrogenase (G6PD) in their red blood cells, menadione and its water-soluble analogs may induce erythrocyte hemolysis.

Since excessive doses of vitamin K used to counteract iatrogenic hypoprothrombinemia may lead to temporary refractoriness to further anticoagulant therapy, the patient may again face the clotting hazards that led to anticoagulant therapy, *viz.*, the possibility of thromboembolic phenomena. Hence, dosages should be as low as possible to produce prothrombin times in the desired range.

Used intravenously, aqueous colloidal solutions of K_1 (phytonadione, MSD) may produce severe, even fatal, reactions resembling hypersensitivity or anaphylaxis, including shock and cardiac and/or respiratory arrest.

These examples reconfirm the often-repeated warning about the dangers of fat soluble vitamins when used as pharmacologic tools in medical practice.

In conclusion, vitamin K is a classic example of a nutrient available in food and produced by microflora in the gastrointestinal tract of normal man in such quantities that primary malnutrition from vitamin K deficiency is virtually unheard of. It is also the classic example of a nutrient whose deficiency, caused by disease and iatrogenic factors, creates secondary malnutrition in large numbers of persons, particularly among the elderly. Management of such secondary malnutrition requires all the skill of health professionals well-versed in the mutual relationships of the nutrition-health-aging triad.

WATER-SOLUBLE VITAMINS

As their name implies, the water-soluble vitamins are those which in their unbound form may be dissolved in aqueous solutions. Prominent among the water-soluble vitamins is the so-called vitamin B complex group. These include the water-soluble substances thiamine (B_1), riboflavin (B_2), nicotinic acid (niacin), nicotinamide (niacinamide, nicotinic acid amide), the vitamin B_6 group (pyridoxine, pyridoxal, pyridoxamine, alpha-pyrocin, beta-pyrocin), biotin, pantothenic acid, folic acid, possibly para aminobenzoic acid, inositol, vitamin B_{12} and possibly choline. Numbered vitamins not listed above include vitamin B_3, a water-soluble growth factor for pigeons; vitamin B_4, a water-soluble factor from yeast that prevents specific paralysis in rats and chicks; vitamin B_5, a factor necessary to maintain growth in rats and growth in pigeons; vitamin B_8, adenylic acid, a decomposition product of nucleic acid occurring in muscle, blood corpuscles, yeast and other nuclear material; vitamin B_{10} and vitamin B_{11}, compounds allied to folic acid which have an influence on feathering and on growth in chicks; vitamin B_{14}, a compound isolated from urine said to check the reproduction of cancer cells and to act as an antipernicious anemia factor; and "vitamin B_{15}" and "vitamin B_{17}", *trade names*[855a,855b] for pangamic acid and laetrile, respectively. In addition, many water-soluble compounds known under other names have been given designations such as vitamin B_c for folic acid, vitamin B_x for para aminobenzoic acid and vitamin B_t, a vitamin necessary for the nutrition of a mealworm, for carnitine. Vitamin C, ascorbic acid, belongs to the water-soluble group. Vitamin P, formerly called vitamin X, is a flavone factor in lemon juice and Hungarian red pepper, deficiency of which is thought to increase permeability of capillary walls.

As noted above in the introductory comments about vitamins in general, socioeconomic, educational, disease and iatrogenic (drug and diet therapy) factors are primary causes of water-soluble vitamin deficiency signs, symptoms and abnormal objective biochemical parameters among older persons. Truly substantial evidence relating water-soluble vitamin deficiency problems among the elderly to biologic aging *per se* have been unconvincing. Carefully controlled studies by Horwitt, *et al.*[856] failed to reveal in institutionalized subjects differences in thiamine and riboflavin excretion between young and old. Few correlations have been found between age and urinary vitamin excretion in studies during which test doses of various B complex vitamins were administered.[857,859]

These investigations by no means suggest that there is lack of opinion in regard to water-soluble vitamin therapy among older persons. However, because of the influence of the combination of placebo and Hawthorne effects among elderly subjects (effects which tend to produce positive subjective reports from the subject under investigation), obtaining valid documentation of the influence of water-soluble vitamin supplementation by means short of conducting rigidly controlled double-blind studies is virtually impossible. This situation has created an environment in which many older Americans spend scarce financial resources for water-soluble vitamin supplements for whose use there is no scientific or medical indication.

In institutions where much of the information regarding clinical evidence of vitamin metabolism in the elderly has been explored in depth,[860] improper meal preparation practices may lead to loss of labile vitamins as well as minerals and trace elements prior to the meals' being offered to older residents for consumption.[861] When added to the fact that appetites of many elderly are diminished by reduced physical activity, ill-advised use of tranquilizers and lack of sufficient personnel adequately to feed those who can not or will not feed themselves, these practices may lead to clinically manifest water-soluble vitamin deficiency syndromes.[862,864]

The water-soluble vitamin deficiency problem in the elderly is obviously a multifactorial one which can be resolved only by a multifactorial solution. In this solution must be education for the elderly and the personnel charged with serving them. Panaceas in the form of one or more vitamin supplements will not work themselves, although they may provide ingredients for a broader attack on the total problem.

Many investigations have been conducted in which water-soluble vitamins were administered in groups rather than individually. One group of investigators gave B complex vitamins and ascorbic acid to older subjects and reported improved "general vitality and vigor" among those studied.[865] Other investigators also administering B complex vitamins and ascorbic acid reported improvement in symptoms previously attributed to nonspecific senility and cerebral atherosclerosis.[866,867] Influenced by these reports one psychiatrist has attributed to further dietary restrictions superimposed on an already borderline reserve blame for acute psychotic episodes in elderly adults.[868] Rafsky and Newman reported greater ascorbic acid needs,[869] greater quantities of thiamine for "saturation"[870] and lower blood thiamine concentrations and lower urinary thiamine excretion[871] in older persons fed diets qualitatively adequate for young adults.

Some evidence exists that vitamin B_6 requirements increase with age.[872,875] This evidence has been amplified more recently by Rose, *et al.*[876] They examined the effect of age on vitamin B_6 metabolism in 617 community-dwelling men, aged 18-90, who were participants in the Baltimore Longitudinal Study on Aging.[266,270] Of the 617, 203 were consuming on their own initiative vitamin supplements containing pyrodoxine hydrochloride. The remaining 414 took no supplements. Data on plasma pyridoxal phosphate (PLP), the primary criterion for B_6 status, revealed a significant decrease of PLP with age of 0.9 mg/ml per decade among those taking no supplements but no significant decrease with age for those taking supplements. The same authors also measured glutamic-oxaloacetic transminase in plasma (PGOT) and in erythrocytes (EGOT) as well as alpha-EGOT, the ratio of EGOT with PLP stimulation *in vitro* to actual EGOT. PGOT values varied little with increasing age but were significantly higher for the supplemented group. EGOT and alpha-EGOT values decreased slightly with increasing age. The supplemented and unsupplemented groups had statistically significant differences in EGOT and alpha-EGOT values.

While these investigators have compiled the most extensive normative data available on vitamin B_6 status in adult males, they admit that they can not yet establish independent criteria for determining "subclinical" B_6 deficiency states. More correlations of health status with the parameters measured conceivably might provide data needed to determine the adequacy of B_6 intake.

Some evidence has also been reported that older persons use thiamine less efficiently,[856,877] leading to the recommendation in the 1974 RDA[92] which has been repeated in the 1980 Revision[92a] that older persons maintain an intake of 1 mg of thiamine per day even though they consume less than 2000 Calories daily.

The complexities of studying the requirements of people of different ages receiving diets varying in niacin and tryptophan content together with the unavailability of niacin in some foods have made impossible the development of data substantiating any special requirement for niacin among the elderly. Pantothenic acid deficiency is seen in man only when metabolic antagonists such as omega-methylpantothenic acid are consumed.[878] However, possible marginal deficiencies have been reported in malnourished alcoholics.[879] Biotin deficiency has been observed in man only in those individuals consuming large quantities of raw egg white which contains the glycoprotein avidin, a potent inactivator of biotin.[880,882] The fact that 3-6 times more biotin is excreted in the urine than is ingested in food[883] reflects the major contribution made by intestinal microflora and suggests that deficiencies in adult man of any age would be found only in the presence of antibiotic therapy radically changing the microflora of the gut.

All of this information suggests that scientific data on the water-soluble vitamin needs of elderly persons are (a) unavailable, (b) based on studies subject to placebo and Hawthorne effects or (c) based on investigations conducted under such unusual institutional circumstances and outdated laboratory methodology that they contribute little useful knowledge. Perhaps even more important is the fact that most studies have been done among persons aged 60-75 with very few conducted among persons in the age group over 86 where the effects of true biologic aging as opposed to effects related to disease and iatrogenic factors (including institutionalization) are operative.

The outlook for the future does not appear to be particularly bright. Conduct of double-blind studies of individual vitamins would be prohibitively expensive. Conduct of double-blind studies involving the permutations and combinations of water-soluble vitamins themselves and of water-soluble vitamins in conjunction with varying amounts of amino acids, Calories and other nutrients which influence their metabolism is certainly beyond the budgets reasonable for large-scale clinical investigations. Highly selective approaches to specific problems are feasible and, if carried out, may provide some insight into the interrelations of water-soluble vitamin requirements and physiologic aging.

Of the water-soluble vitamins, vitamin C (ascorbic acid) and the folate and vitamin B_{12} groups deserve additional comment. Vitamin C is worthy of special attention because of the notoriety it has achieved as a result of assertions that it favorably influences the morbidity of diseases ranging from the common cold to neoplasia. These claims led innumerable elderly persons, among others, to put themselves at risk by consuming megadoses of the vitamin. The folic acid and vitamin B_{12} groups deserve some additional comment because of their interrelated metabolism and the fact that that metabolism involves elements known to be of significance in the biochemistry of aging itself.

Vitamin C (Ascorbic Acid)

The Nobel Laureate Linus Pauling has been the personality most responsible for promoting the notion that diseases ranging from the common cold[884] to neoplasia[885] may be ameliorated by pharmacologic doses of the vitamin.

Pauling's claims for the value of huge doses of ascorbic acid in the management and prevention of upper respiratory infections have led to extensive scientific efforts which so far have yielded little in the way of positive results. Wilson's review[886] covering data published through 1974 does reveal some statistically significant results in studies dealing with large populations but has little to comfort the individual. Chalmer's conclusions in 1975 after his review[887] of all evidence up to that time is particularly pertinent to the interests of gerontologists. Chalmers concluded that minor potential benefits of lifelong pharmacologic doses of ascorbic acid are worth neither the effort nor the risk, no matter how slight the latter might be. Several examples of increased risks follow.

A very logical risk is that of scurvy when very high intakes of ascorbic acid are reduced to the RDA[92,92a]. Rhead and Schrauzer[888] have found that persons accustomed to high ascorbic acid intakes metabolize and excrete the vitamin more rapidly and have a high incidence of scurvy even though plasma concentrations in the individuals involved differ insignificantly from those of persons not receiving nondietary ascorbic acid.

A second risk is that of falsely negative fecal occult blood tests caused by the ingestion of nondietary ascorbic acid.[889] Among older populations the first diagnostic step in the detection and management of alimentary tract pathology involves testing stools for occult blod. Falsely negative tests associated with the ingestion of pharmacologic doses of nondietary ascorbic acid may lead to delayed detection and erroneous management of the pathology involved.

A third risk was reported first by Herbert and Jacob[890] who claimed that 0.5 gm ascorbic acid would destroy 50-95 percent of the B_{12} content of a meal. Jacob, *et al.*[891] previously had reported low serum vitamin B_{12} concentrations in spinal cord injury victims with neurogenic disfunction of the bladder who were receiving 2.0 gm ascorbic acid daily as a gesture toward acidification of the urine to control urinary tract infections. Hines[892] later reported data from 90 patients who received 1.0 gm daily of ascorbic acid for three or more years of whom three had serum vitamin B_{12} concentrations ranging from 65-100 pg/ml and two of whom had hypersegmented neutrophils and ovalomacrocytes. Herbert and Jacob[890] were challenged by Newmark, *et al.*[893] who attributed the apparent destruction of vitamin B_{12} by vitamin C to methodologic differences. Herbert, *et al.*[894] accepted the challenge and seem to have resolved the differences in a report showing that, using the radioisotope assay in measuring vitamin B_{12}, ascorbate will lower vitamin B_{12} concentrations substantially unless KCN is added to the assay mixture or the ascorbate is added after the boiling step. While conceding a methodological problem, Herbert, *et al.*[894] reaffirmed their belief that adequate interpretation of a low serum vitamin B_{12} concentration requires knowing whether the patient has been taking pharmacological doses of ascorbic acid either by self-medication or by prescription. They also point out that an alkaline pH in the small intestine is needed for the absorption of vitamin B_{12}.[895,896] They urge that further investigation be done to determine if megadoses of ascorbic acid diminish vitamin B_{12} absorption, thereby producing the slowly developing B_{12} deficiency observed by Hines.[892] While this risk is still a matter of some debate, it must be acknowledged that it is a source of diagnostic confusion and potentially a biochemical hazard.

The fourth risk is that of uric and oxalic acid lithiasis in the urinary tract which may result from the marked increase in uric and oxalic acid clearance following single large (4.0 gm) or chronically administered (8.0 gm daily) doses of ascorbic acid.[897,897a] Moreover, by its action on the renal tubule, ascorbic acid reduces serum uric acid concentration and thereby invalidates measurements which may be critical in the diagnosis of gout.

A fifth risk is that of increased erythrocyte hemolysis associated with the ingestion of pharmacologic doses of ascorbic acid.[898] This hemolysis occurs particularly in patients with glucose 6-phosphate dehydrogenase (G6PD) deficiency.[899]

These 5 examples of risk lend great credibility to the conclusions of Chalmers *(v.s.)*.[888]

While controversy has been raging about the promotion of pharmacologic doses of vitamin C, Butt, *et al.*,[900] as part of a large nutrition survey in Wales, have confirmed earlier reports indicating that older persons have lower plasma and leukocyte ascorbic acid concentrations than do those who are younger. Their data demonstrate decline in both sexes with advancing age. They found no correlations between ascorbic acid concentration and the prevalence of chronic disease of old age, the presence of anemias, body weight or skin fold thicknesses. So far, no plausible explanations for their data have been found. Burr, *et al.*[900] are not alone in reporting evidence suggesting inadequate intakes of vitamin C among the elderly.[99,463,900,911] This plethora of reports includes some based on measurements of plasma and leukocyte ascorbic acid concentrations and others based on estimates of dietary intake both among free-living elderly and among those who are institutionalized. The majority suggest that elderly persons do not consume enough vitamin C in the foods they eat. This may be due to lack of education in regard to the value of vitamin C-containing foods, to the cost of such foods and to the fact that meal preparation practices in many institutions lead to destruction of vitamin C. No studies have been reported suggesting that, when fed adequate amounts of vitamin C, elderly persons are not able to absorb or metabolize it properly. Brin and Bauernfeind,[912] in commenting on vitamin deficiencies in general, have expressed a rational approach for an understanding of vitamin C deficiency among the elderly. They note that deficiency is a result of a gradual depletion of body stores secondary to poor dietary habits or to disease. They note that the elderly are particularly vulnerable to deficiency because of the high prevalence of illness and disability among them and because of other problems such as low income, social isolation and depressed appetites.

While the role of vitamin C in the management of the common cold and of neoplastic disease has attracted more attention, a possible role for vitamin C in the prevention of atherosclerosis is a matter of even greater interest re the nutrition-health-aging triad. Considerable evidence has been cited[913] stressing the importance of intercellular glycosamino-glycans in arterial wall metabolism and the important role ascorbic acid plays in the formation of these materials. In ascorbate deprivation, both in human beings and in experimental animals, unsulfated polymers accumulate in arterial walls. These mucoid materials bind plasma lipids and fibrinogen with affinity greater than that of the sulfated polymers. Furthermore, ascorbic acid seems to play a significant role in cholesterol metabolism. In certain animal experiments and some human studies, ascorbate is reported to have a cholesterol lowering effect. Vitamin C seems, therefore, to be involved in two systems: the maintenance of vascular integrity and the metabolism of cholesterol to bile acids.

The hypothesis that vitamin C deficiency may contribute to the pathogenesis of atherosclerosis implies that a prescorbutic state must be a quite common occurrence, whereas overt scurvy is in fact very rare. Krumdieck and Butterworth[913] have reviewed the evidence supporting this hypothesis. Although they feel that considerable experimental evidence is corroborative, they note in summarizing their review that there have been no carefully controlled scientific evaluations in groups of human beings so selected as to result in statistically significant conclusions in regard to the effectiveness or safety of vitamin C in the management of atherosclerosis.

Somewhat less circumspect in his support of the hypothesis is Ginter, who bases much of his argument on the observation[914] that vitamin C deficiency in guinea pigs slows the transformation of cholesterol to bile acids. He has also reported[915,916] that a chronic marginal ascorbate deficiency in guinea pigs leads to hypercholesterolemia, hypertriglyceridemia, a prolongation of the half-life of plasma cholesterol, cholesterol accumulation in blood vessels and atheromatous changes in the vascular system, changes which may be reversed with administration of vitamin C. Ginter has also reported that long-term administration of ascorbic acid to human subjects with low vitamin C intakes depresses hypercholesterolemia and hypertriglyceridemia.[916] Ginter also has made the interesting observation[916] that the production of synthetic ascorbic acid in the United States has risen dramatically since 1966 at the same time that mortality from coronary artery disease has been dropping dramatically.

Bates, *et al.*[917] noted a positive correlation between leukocyte ascorbate levels and high-density lipoproteins (HDL's). Knox[918] has observed lower standardized mortality ratios from ischemic heart and cerebrovascular diseases in those regions of the United Kingdom with traditionally higher intakes of vitamin C.

Findings such as these suggest that the role of ascorbic acid in the pathogenesis of the disease most associated with death and disability in the United States deserves further scientific attention, not further exploitation by faddists.

The question of the vitamin C requirement of the elderly has been reviewed by Irwin and Hutchins.[919] They have noted the imprecision of reported requirement estimates. They comment favorably on the prospect for more precise information on utilization, turnover rates, side reactions, the interactions of various environmental and physiological conditions with vitamin C metabolism, and vitamin C synthesis, all of which they believe may be possible with studies using isotopically labelled ascorbic acid.

One such study[920] observed the time course of radioactivity in plasma and urine after oral administration of a single dose of (1-^{14}C) ascorbic acid in healthy, nonsmoking male volunteers. Subjects were investigated under steady state conditions with regard to ascorbic acid intakes which ranged among subjects from 30 to 180 mg/day. The investigators found that the half-life of ascorbic acid was inversely related to the dosage and that the ascorbic acid total metabolic pool could be increased to about 20 mg/kg body weight by increasing the dosage. The authors concluded that a total turnover of about 60 mg/day of ascorbic acid was an appropriate goal. Since ascorbic acid is incompletely absorbed from the gut,[921] they suggest this total turnover would be reached by an intake in the range of 70-77 mg/day. By adding two standard deviations to these estimates of total turnover (in order to enable 95 percent of the population to reach the desired pool size), they justified increasing the daily intake of 100 mg/day and concluded that a daily intake of 100 mg of ascorbic acid would enable a pool size of 20 mg/kg body weight to be reached in 95 percent of the population.

While these figures are somewhat higher than the RDA, 60 mg,[92a] they in no way support the contentions of those proposing megadoses of vitamin C. The methodology used in these studies in young men could be applied advantageously to similar studies in the elderly. It may be appropriate to note here that the RDA for vitamin C falls within two standard deviations of the mean intake (70 mg/day) recommended for normal, healthy, nonsmoking males. Obviously more investigations in man are needed to supply scientific data upon which to base allowances for vitamin C capable of withstanding all assaults by faddists.

In the 1980 Revision, the Food and Nutrition Board raised the ascorbic acid allowance from 45 mg to 60 mg daily.[92a] While some consideration was given to increasing the body pool size, consensus was reached in the Committee on Dietary Allowances primarily because of evidence published by Monsen, *et al.*, that the absorption of iron is increased when the ascorbic acid content of a meal is 25-75 mg or more.[921a]

Folic Acid and Vitamin B_{12}

Among all water-soluble vitamins and perhaps even among all nutrients, no topic is more complex than that of folic acid and vitamin B_{12}. The topic comprises the independent and the biochemically interrelated activities of the two vitamins. It includes their joint involvement in the synthesis of DNA. Therefore *(v.s.)*, they may play important roles in the biochemistry of aging itself. This segment of the water-soluble vitamin chapter will deal first with folic acid, second with vitamin B_{12} and finally with the interrelations between the two.

Folic acid: Although Castle[922] has reported that Barclay in 1851 had described a death from an anemia probably due to folate deficiency resulting from several pregnancies superimposed on a bad diet, the modern history of folic acid began in 1930 when Wills and Mehta published their first report[923] on the pernicious anemia of pregnancy seen among women of Bombay, India. Subsequently, by feeding to monkeys a diet similar to that ingested by their patients, Wills, *et al.*[924] reproduced the disease and demonstrated curative effects of extracts derived from crude (but not purified) liver and also from yeast and wheat germ. In 1946, Watson and Castle[925] reported investigations clearly establishing that nutritional macrocytic anemias, especially in pregnancy, responded to a substance in liver other than that effective in the treatment of Addisonian pernicious anemia. Ultimately, the so-called "Wills Factor" proved to be the same factor called vitamin M and vitamin B_c in yeast and the *Lactobacillus casei* factor of liver. The active principle was isolated and its structure determined by degradation and synthesis in 1948.[926,928] The term "folic acid" was coined by Mitchell, *et al.*[929] in 1941 after their extracting a highly concentrated and probably nearly pure form of an acid nutrilite from four tons of spinach and finding the material in green leaves of many kinds, including grass (Latin: *folium* = leaf). The many chemists who determined its structure named it "pteroylglutamic acid".[928]

Pure folic acid is a yellow crystal, a pteridine derivative linked through a C^9 methylene bridge to a molecule of para-amino-benzoyl-glutamic acid. In animals it is a nutritionally essential precursor of a large family of compounds (to which the trivial name "folates" is given) which serve as coenzymes for one-carbon transfer reactions in virtually all living systems. While lack of these coenzymes is incompatible with life, compounds interfering with certain aspects of their metabolism or biosynthesis are among the foremost antitumor, antimalarial and antibacterial agents known. For this reason, interest in folates extends far beyond the realm of vitamin deficiency disease.

The nomenclature of folic acid is confusing to the uninitiated. In the words of the International Union of Nutrition Sciences Committee on Nomenclature and the Committee on Nomenclature of the American Institute of Nutrition (IUNSAIN) for identifying derivatives of the monoglutamate, folic acid or pteroylglutamic acid, "...the generic descriptor for folic acid and related compounds exhibiting qualitatively the biologic activity of folic acid..." is folacin.[930] Folacin utilized by *L. casei* without treating the sample with conjugase is referred to as "free folacin." In those cases where conjugase is used, the term "total folacin" is employed. Polyglutamates are the folic acid derivatives in which the glutamic acid residue of the monoglutamate is combined through a peptide bond at its gamma-carboxyl group to one or more glutamic acid residues. The term "polyglutamate" refers to any folacin containing one or more glutamyl residues in the side chain, *e.g.*, pteroyldiglutamic acid, pteroyltriglutamic acid, *etc.*[931]

Pteroylglutamic acid, the monoglutamate, is virtually never found in foods or in the human body in significant concentrations.

Folates occur in nature in very large numbers, greatly complicating a study of the naturally occurring compounds. Moreover, many of these are unstable, and all of them are present in cells in such low concentrations (nanomoles [10^{-9} moles] per gram) that they have been measured, until recently, only by microbiological assays, none of which can utilize pteroylglutamates having more than three glutamyl residues.

Folacin coenzymes function primarily in single carbon transfers and, together with B_{12}, in nucleic acid synthesis. They are also required for the metabolism of amino acids, *e.g.*, the serine-glycine interconversion which is vitamin B_6 dependent, the conversion of homocysteine to methionine, and the degradation of histidine to glutamic acid.

Of three microorganisms used in the microbiological assay of foods and tissues for folic acid, *L. casei* only can utilize most folic acid derivatives and is the only one that can use the methyl derivative, 5-methyltetrahydrofolate, the predominant form in plasma, red cells and liver. However, as noted above, *L. casei* can not utilize folacins containing more than a total of three glutamic acids.

Folacin is present in a wide variety of foods, *e.g.*, fresh green leafy vegetables, fruit, organ meat, liver and dried yeast.

Many foodstuffs prior to cooking are rich in folate which is rapidly destroyed by heat. Hence, persons eating no uncooked fresh fruits or vegetables but only well cooked or processed foods are at risk for folate deficiency. This is particularly true for foods comprised of small particulate matter such as rice, dried beans or peas, bulgur wheat, and a variety of particulate breakfast cereals which require cooking prior to being eaten. Viewed teleologically, the high prevalence rates for folacin deficiency worldwide may reflect the well justified fear that consumption of uncooked or undercooked grains, fruits and vegetables can lead to serious illness. It is easy to understand how elderly persons brought up in traditions of thoroughly cooked grains, fruits and vegetables and consigned by faulty dentition, economic deprivation and social isolation to particulate, low cost, overcooked, easily prepared and masticated foods can easily consume dietaries sufficiently low in folacin to create recognizable deficiency signs and symptoms.

L. casei assays of food prior to and after conjugase treatment have suggested that 25 percent or less of dietary folacin is in the free form. Daily intakes among healthy persons ingesting mixed diets have ranged when measured from 37 micrograms to 297 micrograms of free folacin and may reach as high as 2300 micrograms of total folacin.[932,937] Estimates of need by a variety of techniques have fixed the minimum daily requirement (MDR) at about 50 micrograms of crystalline folic acid per day. Assuming that 25 percent of folic acid activity in a varied diet will be absorbed in a manner similar to that for absorbing crystalline pteroylglutamic acid and allowing for a wide range of availability of the polyglutamate forms, the Food and Nutrition Board has set the RDA for total folacin at 400 micrograms for the adolescent and for nonpregnant, nonlactating adults, regardless of age.[92a] In formulating the RDA for folacin, the Food and Nutrition Board made no specific reference to the influence of diseases and their treatment by various drugs and hormones on the folacin requirements of man. The fact that many of these diseases and their associated therapies are prevalent among the old place the elderly at particular risk for folacin deficiency.

Folacin is absorbed in the proximal small intestine. Hence, any surgical procedure removing or by-passing the proximal small intestine may lead to malabsorption of folate.[938] Although intestinal synthesis of folate available to man has not been demonstrated,[939,940] it is theoretically possible that infection of the gut by microorganisms such as *Streptococcus faecalis* which requires folacin for its own growth could deprive the host of folacin derived from bacterial synthesis.[941] Patients with gluten-induced enteropathy, celiac disease and sprue are obvious candidates for folate malabsorption.[938]

The effect of alcohol on folacin absorption is still controversial.[931] Most evidence suggests that folate malabsorption is caused by poor nutrition as well as by alcohol ingestion.[942] Ingesting beer which is high in folacin is often associated with normal serum or even high red cell folacin values among alcoholics who favor this beverage.[943,944] Folacin deficiency itself initiates a vicious cycle leading to folate malabsorption which may be worsened when alcohol ingestion replaces ingestion of folacin containing foods.[945,946]

Many drugs commonly used in the treatment of elderly patients adversely affect folacin absorption and metabolism.[947,949] Among these, methotrexate and aminopterin are powerful inhibitors of the enzyme dihydrofolate reductase, an enzyme of major importance in the regeneration of tetrahydrofolate, the coenzyme form of folacin central to its numerous biochemical functions. The antimalarial drug pyrimethamine and the antibacterial, trimethoprim also inhibit dihydrofolate reductase. The anticonvulsants diphenylhydantoin (Dilantin), primadone and barbiturates appear to worsen folacin status as evidenced by the fact that epileptics may develop folacin deficiency after taking such drugs for prolonged periods of time. Bile sequestering agents such as cholestyramine and polidexide (Secholex) used in the management of type IIa hyperbetalipoproteinemia adversely affect folate parameters in man.[950,952] Even aspirin has been reported to increase the plasma clearance of ^{3}H-folic acid and to reduce significantly the binding in serum of ^{3}H-folic acid.[953] While of little concern to the elderly, oral contraceptives have been indicted by many investigators for inducing signs and chemical test parameters indicative of abnormalities in folacin absorption and metabolism. However, the differences among investigations are so great that it is impossible to confirm the indictment at this time.[931,954]

The question of the dangers of excessive intakes of folacin is also controversial. No reports of toxicity from excessive intakes of foods containing folacin have been reported. However, one group of investigators found that excessive doses of folacin produced mental changes, sleep disturbances, gastrointestinal symptoms, malaise and irritability.[955] Others using double blind studies could not confirm these observations.[956,957] Others have reported that large doses of folic acid given to persons already taking diphenylhydantoin induced epileptic seizures.[958,959] Still others have warned against giving large doses of folic acid to patients with megaloblastic anemia. One death was attributed to a fall in serum potassium occurring simultaneously with the onset of the reticulocyte response.[960] A specific danger lies in the fact that large doses of folate which temporarily relieve megaloblastic anemia caused by B_{12} deficiency do not prevent the irreversible damage to the nervous system which occurs in B_{12} deficiency.[961,965]

Studies of the folacin requirements of the elderly have been numerous.[931] These have been divided into evaluations of folacin intake, evaluations of folacin concentrations in serum, measurements of the excretions of formiminoglutamic acid (FIGLU) (which is increased on a folacin-deficient diet) before and after folacin therapy, measurements of the standard red blood cell indices, and measurements of folacin concentrations in red cells. Several groups have reported studies suggesting mental dysfunction in folacin-deficient elderly patients.[75,966,974] Unfortunately, the lack of any organized, coordinated approach to the problem in these studies makes an evaluation of their results virtually impossible. Nonetheless, the facts that elderly persons frequently have diseases adversely influencing folate absorption and metabolism, ingest drugs which unfavorably affect folacin status, and consume meals which are low in folacin suggest that folacin malnutrition among the elderly is a potential problem which should be considered in many differential diagnoses of pathology among older persons.

Vitamin B_{12}: Understanding vitamin B_{12} requires knowledge of the history of the chronic disease called "pernicious" anemia. This ailment derived its name because it was once universally fatal even though its course might have been interrupted by remissions and relapses. The first complete description of the clinical features of this anemia was published by Addison in 1855.[975] Biermer contributed an even more complete account in 1872.[976] The disease hence became known as Addison's or Biermer's anemia. In 1880, Fenwick[977] suggested the primary role of the stomach in the anemia's pathogenesis. It was not until the third decade of the twentieth century, however, that Whipple, *et al.*[978,978a,978b] in extensive experiments demonstrating the influences of various foods on hemoglobin production in dogs previously made anemic by blood loss, suggested that the lack of a dietary factor might be a cause of pernicious anemia. A few years later, Minot and Murphy[979] demonstrated conclusively that pernicious anemia could be treated by the administration of large amounts of liver. The amount of hog, beef or calves' liver needed to produce an average reticulocyte response in relief of the anemia and its symptoms was at least 400 grams. Shortly thereafter, Castle[980,980a] demonstrated that an underlying defect was inadequate formation in the stomach of an "intrinsic" factor, as a result of which the absorption of or utilization of an "extrinsic" factor was impaired. During the next two decades, an antianemic principle of whole liver concentrated in liver extracts and of desiccated hogs' stomach[981,982] was found to be an effective remedy.

In 1948, Shorb[983] reported that *Lactobacillus lactis Dorner* required for its own growth and therefore could be used in an assay for the "animal protein factor" (APF) required for the growth of animals fed all-vegetable diets and present in liver extracts in amounts proportional to their ability to treat pernicious anemia. In the same year, pharmaceutical industry research teams at the Merck Corporation in the United States[984] using Shorb's assay and at the Glaxo Laboratories in the United Kingdom[985] using pernicious anemia patients for assay of the vitamin isolated the antipernicious anemia factor of liver in the form of pure red crystals. The Merck team named the crystals vitamin B_{12}.

It was not until 1955, however when the combined efforts of Hodgkin, *et al.*,[986] Bonnett, *et al.*,[987] and Kuehl, *et al.*[988] permitted derivation of the structural formula of vitamin B_{12}. Even though clinical trials by West[989] in 1948 had shown positive responses from three to six microgram doses of vitamin B_{12}, many years passed before vitamin B_{12} was genuinely accepted as Castle's "extrinsic" factor and before it replaced liver extract as the principal therapy in the management of pernicious anemia.

The stable form of vitamin B_{12} crystallizes as dark red needles or prisms of cyanocobalamin *(v.i.)*. The accepted empirical formula is $C_{63}H_{88}O_{14}N_{14}PCo$.[990] From a strictly chemical standpoint, vitamin B_{12} is a compound with a molecular weight of 1355. Molecular weights have measured 1490 $\pm$ 150 determined by the boiling point method and from 1360 to 1575 determined by x-ray crystallography.[990a] The range of molecular weight arises from the variable hydration of the crystals. The official USP cyanocobabamin contains 12 percent absorbed moisture.

The molecule has two major portions: a corrin nucleus and a nucleotide which lies in a plane at right angles to the corrin nucleus. The nucleotide (5,6-dimethyl-benzimidazole) is linked to a cobalt atom which occupies the center of the corrin nucleus by a coordinate bond with one of the nitrogen atoms of the nucleotide. The nucleotide also is joined from its other nitrogen through a gylcosidic linkage to ribose-3-phosphate which in turn is esterified to D-1-amino-2-propanol, the nitrogen of which is in amide linkage with the carboxyl group of the propionic acid side chain of ring D of the corrin nucleus. This relative spacial configuration bears a close but not complete resemblance to porphyrins. The central cobalt atom is linked to four reduced pyrrole rings forming a macroring.

The four reduced pyrrole rings linked together become a macrocylic ring designated "corrin" because it is the core of the vitamin B_{12} molecule. The letters "co..." of corrin are not derived from the fact that B_{12} contains cobalt. All the compounds containing this ring are designated corrinoids. The letters "cob..." do designate that compounds contain cobalt. The cobalamins contain the entire structure. The permissive or trivial term "cobalamin" or "B_{12}" is used to describe the vitamin B_{12} molecule without a cyanide group. The term "cobalamin" is prefixed by the designation of the anionic R group attached to the cobalt. "Cyanocobalamin" is the permissive name for vitamin B_{12} and the term "vitamin B_{12}" without qualification means exclusively cyanocobalamin. However, in much nutritional and pharmacologic literature the term "vitamin B_{12}" is a generic term for all the cobamides active in man. So far, the cobamides found to play a role in human metabolism have been cobalamins.

The two cobalamins currently known to be enzymatically active in man are methylcobalamin and 5'-deoxyadenosyl cobalamin which is also called "coenzyme B_{12}" even though it is only one of the two B_{12} coenzymes with known activity in man. These cobalamins are unstable to light and undergo photolysis with the formation of aquocobalamin (vitamin B_{12b}) or, in the presence of potassium cyanide, cyanocobalamin. The terms "coenzyme B_{12}" and "vitamin B_{12} coenzyme" are not interchangeable. The former means 5'-deoxyadenosyl cobalamin exclusively, whereas the latter applies to any coenzyme form of vitamin B_{12}. Alphabetical congeners of vitamin B_{12} (B_{12a} [hydroxocobalamin]; B_{12b} [aquocobalamin]; B_{12c} [nitritocobalamin]) are believed to be equivalent in the treatment of most B_{12} deficiency states. Since therapeutic doses in clinical practice are always far greater than the minimum B_{12} requirement, all forms of vitamin B_{12} appear to be equivalent when used in greater than the minimal amounts.[991,991a]

Sources of B_{12} are almost exclusively foods of animal origin. B_{12} is synthesized by many bacteria such as *Streptomyces griseus, Streptomyces aureofaciens* and *Bacillus subtilis.* Herbivorous animals obtain vitamin B_{12} from the micoorganisms of their rumens. Bivalves obtain their vitamin B_{12} by siphoning large numbers of the B_{12}-synthesizing micoorganisms in sea water. In general, the most available sources of vitamin B_{12} are liver, kidney, meat and dairy products, listed in the order of decreasing concentraions of the vitamin. Oysters — while less readily available — contain concentrations of B_{12} second only to liver among foods commonly eaten. Vitamin B_{12} is virtually absent from vegetables, fruits and grains. Whatever vitamin B_{12} is obtained from food by truly rigid vegetarians is derived from microorganisms contaminating the food eaten or from those micoorganisms found in the root nodules of certain legumes.

The size and complexity of the B_{12} molecule has made industrial synthesis of vitamin B_{12} difficult and uneconomic. Hence most vitamin B_{12} available through commercial channels is derived from synthesis by microorganisms.

The absorption of vitamin B_{12} occurs by two distinct mechanisms. These are known as the "pharmacologic" and the "physiologic" mechanisms.

The pharmacologic mechanism involves simple diffusion and occurs along the entire length of the small intestine. It may account for the absorption of approximately one percent of any amount of free vitamin B_{12} present in the small bowel. By this mechanism, oral therapy for vitamin B_{12} deficiency because of failure of the physiologic mechanism is possible.

The physiologic mechanism is dependent on Castle's intrinsic factor, a heat-labile glycoprotein having a molecular weight in the range of 50,000 which is produced in the fundal and cardiac parietal cells of the stomach. It removes vitamin B_{12} from its complexes with animal protein, protects it from absorption by bacteria in the upper gastrointestinal tract, attaches it by a mechanism involving a calcium-dependent bond to the intestinal mucosa, and releases the vitamin into the mucosal cells. In addition to ionic calcium, this process requires a pH of intestinal contents above 6. On combining with vitamin B_{12}, two molecules of intrinsic factor and two molecules of vitamin B_{12} join to form a dimer. Through mechanisms that are not yet clear, vitamin B_{12} released from intrinsic factor finds its way across the intestinal mucosal cells into the portal venous blood where it becomes attached to a serum vitamin B_{12}-binding protein. Deficiency of intrinsic factor, the primary defect in Addisonian pernicious anemia, is a gene-linked abnormality which may be due to abnormal immunologic responsiveness in some patients.

Upon entering portal vein blood, vitamin B_{12} immediately is bound to one or more of the B_{12}-binding glycoproteins. Transcobalamin I (TC I), which has the electrophoretic mobility of an alpha globulin, carries largely endogenous B_{12}, while transcobalamin II (TC II), a protein with the mobility of a beta globulin, functions as a carrier of recently administered vitamin B_{12}.[992,994] TC I also appears to be a storage protein for vitamin B_{12} and has a molecular weight in the range of 60,000. The molecular weight of TC II is approximately 35,000, leading to speculation that TC I is a dimer of TC II.

Gottlieb, *et al.*[995] and Mikkonen, *et al.*[996] reported a third B_{12}-binding protein in the plasma of patients with polycythemia vera. Hall and Finkler[997] characterized this third binding protein as having characteristics similar to TC I. Gräsbeck[998] grouped all of the body's B_{12}-binders other than intrinsic factor and transcobalamin II into a category called "R" which initially stood for rapid electrophoretic mobility. Bloomfield and Scott,[999] after demonstrating the presence of a third binder in the serum of 50 normal people, designated the third binder transcobalamin III (TC III). Carmel and Herbert[1000] suggested that granulocytes are the sources of TC III and possibly of TC I. Scott, *et al.*,[1001] have presented data indicating that TC III may not occur in plasma *in vivo* but may be an artifact caused by the release of TC III from granulocytes during or after the blood collecting process. Burger, *et al.*,[1002,1003] isolated and characterized TC I, TC III and the granulocyte-binding protein (GBP). They found TC III and GBP to be identical, leading them to support the hypothesis that TC III is an artifact in plasma derived from granulocytes *in vitro.* However, they believe TC I may not be derived from granulocytes, since their methods separated TC I and TC III.

The precise functions of R-type B_{12}-binding proteins have not been elucidated. Gilbert[1004] has proposed that GBP may serve as a scavenger leaching B_{12} from intra- and extra-cellular bacteria and providing a means by which B_{12} in dying cells is transported directly to the liver where it may be processed and returned to the blood as TC I.

The B_{12}-binding glycoproteins deliver the vitamin to the liver, to the bone marrow and to reticulocytes in a manner similar to that by which intrinsic factor delivers vitamin B_{12} to mucosal cells in the ileum. Binding sites on the surfaces of bone marrow cells and reticulocytes function only in the presence of ionic calcium and a pH greater than 6.

Gastric intrinsic factor and the B_{12}-binding glycoproteins are not identical. Studies in which serum with B_{12} concentrations as high as 24,000 picograms per milliliter from patients with chronic myelocytic leukemia was administered by nasogastric tube to elderly patients with pernicious anemia following its incubation with ^{58}Co-labelled vitamin B_{12} revealed no absorption of the labelled vitamin.[1005]

In myeloproliferative disorders, the abnormally high concentrations of vitamin B_{12} are asociated with comparable elevations in the concentrations of TC I which is incapable of delivering its load of B_{12} to tissues. Acute and chronic liver disease and livers harboring metastases are also associated with abnormally high B_{12} concentrations apparently caused by elevations in a B_{12}-binding protein with beta globulin mobility.[1006] However, Carmel[1007] has reported two patients with metastases in the liver and extremely high TC I plasma concentrations. In Addisonian pernicious anemia, TC II binding capacity is diminished or absent but that of TC I is unaltered.

Still uninvestigated are the possibilities of age-related changes in the binding capacities of TC I, TC II, TC III and GBP or of other as yet undescribed B_{12}-binding proteins. Further studies on B_{12} absorption, plasma transport, metabolism and excretion may provide explanations for the frequently reported low concentrations of vitamin B_{12} in the sera of elderly persons *(v.i.)*. Such studies might also set patterns for better evaluations of nutrition with respect to other vitamins in aging man. With stores of B_{12} ranging between two and five milligrams, of which 50 to 90 percent are in the liver, and with the average daily requirement for exogenous B_{12} being 0.1 microgram, it is evident that many years on a totally B_{12} deficient diet would be required to produce vitamin B_{12} deficiency. This undoubtedly explains how many truly rigid vegetarians who take no vitamin B_{12} supplements are able to survive over prolonged periods of time with negligible B_{12} intakes. There is no significant metabolism of vitamin B_{12} in man. Loss occurs only by excretion, mainly in the bile. There is an entero-hepatic circulation of vitamin B_{12} which has been estimated to be 0.6 to six micrograms excreted in the bile and reabsorbed in the ileum daily.

Vitamin B_{12} functions in man *inter alia*, in normal hematopoiesis and in the synthesis of myelin. In its absence, megaloblastic anemia and so-called combined system disease characterized by parasthesias, diminished virtation and position senses, unsteadiness, poor muscular coordination, moodiness, mental slowness, poor memory, confusion, agitation, depression and dim vision may result. Delusions, hallucinations and even overt psychoses may also occur. Exact mechanisms by which vitamin B_{12} is involved in myelin synthesis are not known. However, vitamin B_{12}'s role in hematopoiesis is certainly related to its role in the synthesis of thymidylate and therefore of DNA. This role in protein synthesis will be discussed under the interrelations of vitamin B_{12} and folic acid.

Studies among the elderly have comprised primarily tolerance tests involving the measurement of vitamin B_{12} appearing in urine at stated intervals after parenteral administration of various doses of the vitamin and, secondarily, the quantification of serum concentrations of vitamin B_{12}. Vitamin B_{12} tolerance tests at four different dose levels showed significantly less excretion or greater retention of administered vitamin B_{12} in old than in young men.[1008] In addition, agewise decrements in B_{12} plasma concentrations have been reported.[1009,1011] None of these findings was related to previous dietary intake which in the patients studied had been adequate in B_{12} for many months prior to the investigations. Agewise decrements in renal function could not account for the differences.[1012] Studies of the renal clearance of vitamin B_{12} indicated that B_{12} glomerular filtration and excretion was proportional to plasma concentration at plasma concentrations over one nanogram (1 X 10^{-9}) per milliliter. Normal B_{12} binding capacity is exceeded at concentrations over one nanogram per milliliter.[1013] While explaining the findings of the renal clearance studies, these B_{12} binding capacity observations do not explain the agewise decrements of B_{12} excretions in tolerance tests or the agewise decrements in B_{12} plasma concentrations.

The meaning of these tolerance test and serum concentration results in older persons in not clear. In view of the decades needed to exhaust liver stores of vitamin B_{12} and in view of the widespread availability of oral and parenteral B_{12} supplements to dietary intake and of B_{12}-fortified foods, it is highly unlikely that aged adults free from gastric or small intestinal disease are candidates for vitamin B_{12} deficiency. Obviously, further investigation is needed. However, in contemplating such investigations, potential investigators must consider many serious problems.

One problem not experienced by earlier investigators arises from the fact that serum B_{12} concentrations may now be measured by a radioisotope dilution assay based on the principle that endogenous serum cobalamin will compete with radioactive cobalamin for binding to a limited amount of cobalamin-binding protein.[1014] The radioisotope dilution methods produce data indicating that the serum concentrations of B_{12} are substantially higher than those determined by microbiologic assays using *Lactobacillus leichmannii* or *Euglena gracilis.*[1015] Copper and Whitehead[1016] report that as many as ten percent of cobalamin-deficient patients may be overlooked if the serum concentration is measured by a radioisotope dilution with commercial reagents. Radioisotope dilution assays measure the extent to which the serum cobalamin competes with radioactively labelled cyanocobalamin for binding sites on a protein. The specificity of the binding protein used is crucial to the accuracy of the assay.[1017] Three distinct kinds of proteins have high B_{12} affinity. Intrinsic factor is remarkably specific. TC II is reasonably specific but also can bind at least a few cobalamin analogues. The so-called R proteins effectively bind cobalamin but also have high affinity for a wide variety of its analogues. Kolhouse, *et al.,*[1015] have provided evidence that biologically inactive analogues are present in human serum in concentrations sufficient to interfere with the radioisotope dilution assays for B_{12} when pure R proteins are used as binders in that assay. In considering these deficiencies of the radioisotope dilution assay, it must also be remembered that the more accurate microbiological assays do require sterile technique, take from one to seven days to perform, and can not be used if the subjects under study have been taking antibiotics or certain other drugs.

Herbert, *et al.*,[894] have shown that the addition of potassium cyanide (KCN) prior to the heating step in the B_{12} radioisotope assay will prevent ascorbic acid from destroying vitamin B_{12}. Failure to add KCN at the appropriate time had led to erroneously low assayable B_{12} concentrations in the serum and tissues of patients who had been taking two grams daily of ascorbic acid.

Cullen and Oace,[1018] in examining the effects of cellulose or pectin supplements on B_{12} metabolism in the rat, observed that the rate of fecal excretion of vitamin B_{12} was increased and that the urinary excretion of methylmalonic acid was increased nine- to 21-fold by the addition of celluose or pectin to the diets of the rats. The authors suggest that both fibers interfere with the recovery of biliary vitamin B_{12} by binding it to a residue which is metabolized little or none before it leaves behind the receptor sites of the ileum. Pectins proved far more damaging to B_{12} homeostasis in the rat than did cellulose, presumably because they may also serve as substrate promoting an excessive growth of B_{12}-requiring bacteria.

Many drugs interfere with the absorption of vitamin B_{12}. Among these are paraaminosalicylic acid (PAS), ethanol, neomycin, colchicine, various anticonvulsants and possibly L-dopa. Antibiotics such as clindamycin which may adversely influence the functions of the gastrointestinal tract also must be included among those medications adversely influencing B_{12} metabolism. Cholestyramine, a bile sequestrant, may interfere with B_{12}'s enterohepatic circulation.

Another major problem in the study of B_{12} nutritional status, particularly among ambulatory, outpatient populations, lies in the universal availability of B_{12} supplements and of foods fortified with B_{12}. The use not only of oral but also of parenteral B_{12} supplementation for extremely dubious indications is widely practiced. The total lack of known toxicity and the pleasing red color of B_{12} solutions make them ideal placebos. Widespread fortification of cereal products with vitamin B_{12} adds to the difficulty of establishing a known intake of B_{12} during the type of meticulous investigation required to quantify B_{12}'s role in biologic aging and the diseases which complement the aging process.

A sixth problem is that the diseases which adversely influence B_{12} absorption and metabolism are legion. In addition to Addisonian pernicious anemia, various lesions destroying the gastric mucosa and certain endocrine disorders may lead to an inadequate secretion of intrinsic factor. Obviously, total and proximal and distal subtotal gastrectomies do the same. Antibodies to intrinsic factor may influence its effectiveness as a transporter of B_{12}. Disorders of the ileum such as gluten-induced enteropathy, regional ileitis, Crohn's disease (regional enteritis), small bowel anastomoses, blind-loop syndromes, intestinal resections, and inadequate pancreatic exocrine secretions are but a few. Competition by intestinal parasites or bacteria for B_{12} occurs in the presence of *Diphyllobothrium latum*, a fish-vectored tapeworm, and in the above-mentioned blind-loop syndrome in which large numbers of B_{12}-utilizing bacteria rob the host of an adequate supply. Inadequate utilization of B_{12} is seen in the presence of B_{12} antagonists, in protein malnutrition, in specific congenital and acquired enzyme deficiencies and deletions, in the presence of abnormal B_{12}-binding proteins such as abnormal TC I and TC II seen in myeloproliferative disorders and liver disease, and in those conditions characterized by an insufficient quantity of B_{12}-binding proteins in the serum. The requirement for vitamin B_{12} may be increased in hyperthyroidism and rises in the presence of certain malignant tissues. The main cause for increased excretion is interference with the enterohepatic circulation *(v.s.)*.

Finally, food faddists, especially strict vegetarians, may have inordinately low serum vitamin B_{12} concentrations without corresponding signs or symptoms of vitamin B_{12} deficiency disease. Avowed strict vegetarians with normal serum B_{12} concentrations should be treated circumspectly, since such persons may not, as they claim, be rigid adherents to vegetarian regimens or may be supplementing their diets with oral or parenteral vitamin B_{12}.

These problems create special difficulties for investigators seeking more information in regard to the role of vitamin B_{12} in aging and the diseases which complement the aging process. They suggest the need for additional studies in animals where environmental conditions including nutrient intake can be rigidly controlled and also the need for the conduct of studies in clinical investigation settings where elderly persons may be carefully screened for the presence of disease and constantly monitored in regard to dietary intake.

The Interrelations of Folic Acid and Vitamin B_{12}: Vitamin B_{12} deficiency produces the signs and symptoms of folic acid deficiency. Vitamin B_{12} is necessary if folic acid is to play its role in the synthesis of DNA and therefore of protein. DNA synthesis depends on the conversion of deoxyuridylate to thymidylate, a conversion which requires a supply of $N^{5,10}$ methylene tetrahydrofolate derived from tetrahydrofolate. Tetrahydrofolate in turn is derived from N^5methyl tetrahydrofolate. In the absence of vitamin B_{12}, the diminished activity of the methyl transferase enzyme prevents conversion of N^5methyl tetrahydrofolate to tetrahydrofolate. As a result, N^5methyl tetrahydrofolate "piles up" while other folates decrease, the so-called "folate trap".[1019,1020] The resulting decrease in the availability of tetrahydrofolate and of $N^{5,10}$ tetrahydrofolate yields a reduction in the conversion of deoxyuridylate to thymidylate and therefore a diminution of DNA synthesis. This decrease in DNA synthesis leads to the arrest of cell replication in the S (synthesis) phase resulting in megaloblastosis.[991,991a]

In the complementary side of the same reaction, B_{12} is involved in the synthesis of methionine from its precursor homocysteine (methionine = methyl homocysteine). In the conversion of N^5methyl tetrahydrofolate to tetrahydrofolate, the B_{12}-dependent enzyme methyl transferase removes the methyl group from N^5methyl tetrahydrofolate and adds it to homocysteine to produce methionine.

These reactions explain how patients with pernicious anemia – a true deficiency of B_{12} – become sufficiently secondarily deficient in folic acid coenzyme activity that they will respond temporarily (hematologically only) to folic acid therapy alone.[1021,1022]

Other folic acid-vitamin B_{12} interactions involve the facts that formiminoglutamic acid (FIGLU), formate and aminoimidazolecarboxamide (AIC) excretions are elevated in both folic acid and B_{12} deficiency states. The abnormally high excretions are diminished when methionine — produced from homocysteine when B_{12} is present — is added to the diet. In addition, ^{14}C-formate incorporation into serine is decreased in lymphocytes obtained from animals deficient in either folic acid or vitamin B_{12}. The oxidation of serine's beta carbon to respiratory CO_2 is markedly reduced in both deficiencies. The influences of B_{12} and methionine on FIGLU, formate and AIC metabolism suggest that folate metabolism is impaired in B_{12} deficiency and that B_{12} may serve by its role in the synthesis of methionine from homocysteine.[1023]

-11-

Water

Water, the most essential of all nutrients, has been mentioned repeatedly in previous chapters and has been treated in considerable depth in those segments of Chapter 9 dealing with sodium. This chapter, therefore, is placed here to give emphasis to the fact that water is prime among all nutrients and must be so considered in all deliberations in regard to the nutrition-health-aging triad.

The primacy of water in the management of illnesses and accidents among the old deserves the greatest of deference. Altogether too many older persons arrive in emergency rooms near death not for lack of proper medications or even of nursing care at home but for lack of knowledge that proper hydration is an ever-present requirement of good health. Refusal by older persons to accept water and food when ill or injured must be countered by truly persuasive persistence by those assuming responsibility that water and food receive priority equivalent to that given other forms of medical and surgical therapy.

Orally administered hydration is usually possible unless some anatomic obstruction intervenes. Such hydration may be given in minuscule quantities — a few milliliters at a time — with great success if the frequency of administration is high.

In patients who are totally uncooperative, combative or comatose, but whose gastrointestinal tract is free from anatomic obstruction, hydration via nasogastric tube may be indicated. As previously mentioned (Chapter 9 page 131), great care must be exercised to incorporate sufficient water in nutrient mixtures administered by tube to obviate the ever-present danger of hypernatremia.[593,594]

In patients with anatomic obstructions of the gastrointestinal tract, with adynamic ileus from whatever cause, or with conditions like fistulous regional enteritis in which food by mouth or nutrients by nasogastric tube may be contraindicated, parenteral hydration and nutrition take precedence. If total parenteral nutrition utilizing hyperosmolar solutions administered via catheters extending into the central veins is used, the danger of overhydration can be minimized. However, if parenteral hydration using isotonic solutions delivered into peripheral veins is utilized, care must be taken to assure that overhydration particularly in older patients with cardiac, renal and hepatic pathology influencing water and electrolyte metabolism does not further complicate their problems. The re-approval after a ban of several years by the Food and Drug Administration of isotonic fat emulsions as sources of Calories as well as essential fatty acids[386e-g,386h] will afford once again the means of providing Calories in small volumes of fluid. Nonetheless, parenteral nutrition is a technique requiring the skills of a highly trained and experienced team backed up by a laboratory capable of providing prompt, accurate information on the composition of body fluids.

Since both nasogastric and parenteral nutrition represent far higher levels of complexity of management than do hydration and nutrition via the oral route, the need for prompt attention to these requirements among older persons who become ill or who are the victims of accidents is evident if the costs — both in humanitarian and fiscal terms — is to be minimized.

For older persons in good health, the issue of how much fluid to consume daily frequently arises. From an academic standpoint, the reduced discrete renal functions of older persons[182,183] would suggest the desirability of increasing the fluid intake above that indicated for younger mature adults. Assuming an insensible water loss of twelve milliliters per kilogram of body weight[1024], this would suggest the need for a total fluid intake of about 2.5 liters per day for an 80 kilogram man. Such quantities may be impractical from the point of view of patient compliance. In addition, especially in aged persons with prostatic and incontinence problems of the lower urinary tract, the added fluid requiring excretion may prove to be not only a nuisance but also a danger should it necessitate trips to toilet facilities in the dark of night. Hence, prescriptions for hydration of ambulatory elderly persons in relatively good health should be individualized to meet the particular needs of a given elder, not applied indiscriminately to the aged as a class.

-12-

Calories

A unit of heat used in the study of metabolism is the "large Calorie", the "kilocalorie" or the "Calorie", the last being the designation used throughout this book. The Calories important to human nutrition and health are derived from fat, carbohydrate and protein, with none being contributed by minerals and trace elements and negligible quantities being derived from vitamins. In scientific terms, a Calorie is the amount of heat required to raise the temperature of one kilogram of water from 15° to 16° C, at one atmospheric pressure. The heat of fat, carbohydrate and protein in pure form and in food may be measured precisely in a combustion ("bòmb") calorimeter. The average values in Calories per gram using such a technique are 9.5 for animal fat, 3.96 for glucose, 4.2 for starch, and 5.6 for animal proteins, with vegetable proteins having slightly lower values. In the human body, however, protein is not completely oxidized, some of its amino groups being converted to and excreted as urea and ammonia. Taking this and interindividual variations in caloric value of specific fats, carbohydrates and proteins into account, the physiologic heats of combustion are usually given as 9.3 Calories per gram for fat, 4.1 for carbohydrate and 4.1 for protein. These numbers themselves are usually rounded off to 9, 4 and 4 Calories per gram on the grounds that ingested foods are not completely assimilated.

Restriction of Calorie intake is generally regarded as the most efficient way of preventing excessive weight gain or of losing excessive weight which has already been acquired. The avoidance of gross obesity through exercise of Calorie restriction has long been associated with the prevention of morbidity and mortality from chronic illness.[260] Calorie restriction in fish and animals has resulted in greater longevity than has *ad libitum* feeding.[7,20,21,24,25,30-32,1025,1026] Although a half century has passed since McCay, *et al.*,[20] first reported the influence of Calorie undernutrition on longevity, no scientific mechanisms fully explaining the mode of action have been reported.[37]

During the decade of the seventies, Ross[33] has shown that the age at which Calorie restriction begins is an important determinant of longevity in the rat. Feeding the rats a restricted intake from 21 to 70 days only, increased longevity. A restricted intake imposed at 70 days of age only partially overcame the adverse effects of feeding *ad libitum* early in life. Ross also demonstrated that the most favorable degree of restriction in terms of enhancing longevity changed with age. The oldest at death were those rats restricted severely from 21 days of age throughout life. Length of life decreased when similar restriction was imposed at 300 days of age. However, when imposed at 365 days of age, longevity was decreased drastically, even below that of *ad libitum* fed controls. Contrariwise, when less severe degrees of restriction were imposed on older rats of similar age, the lengths of their lives were extended.

In view of the high cost in time and money of determining the optimum nutrition for rats of various ages, Ross, *et al.*[36,1027,1028] explored self-selection as a method of feeding. Post-weanling rats were offered three different purified isocaloric diets simultaneously. The percentages of protein were 10, 22, and 51, and of carbohydrate, 70.5, 58.5, and 29.5, respectively. Ross[1029] has summarized many details of these studies. From their data, he and his colleagues have developed a mathematical model best explaining variances in rat longevity. In the model, seven variables describe dietary behavior and associated growth responses.[1028,1029] These seven variables are: (1) absolute and (2) relative preferences for protein between the 43rd and the 49th day of life, (3) the feed efficiency (unit of weight gain per unit of food fed) between the 49th and the 98th day of life; (4) body weight at 119 and (5) 133 days; (6) the time required to double the body weight of 250 grams; and (7) the age of attaining a weight of 500 grams.

This model has led Ross, *et al.* to conclude that longevity is inversely related to feed efficiency and rates of growth in early life. Diminished longevity was associated with low protein, high carbohydrate intakes early in life and high protein, low carbohydrate intakes later in life. The dietary protein: carbohydrate ratios after 400 days of age did not influence longevity. The variable contributing most to variance in longevity was the number of days required to double the specified body weight. Their finding that maximum body weight during maturity was unrelated to length of life lends support to the concept that dietary habits and growth responses early in life are those most associated with life's duration.

When relating the findings of these studies in rats to human concerns, the observations of Ross and Bras[1027] that rats on self-selection regimens had from two to five times the incidence of neoplasias and of diseases of the heart, kidney and prostate found in rats fed each of the diets singly is of particular interest. It suggests that the incidence of diseases which complement the aging process and in turn limit life's duration is governed by individual specificity which determines dietary habits which sequentially influence growth responses. In a similar vein, Berg and Simms[1030] have reported that, with the exception of morbidity from radiculoneuritis,[1031] Calorie restriction afforded protection against almost every disease afflicting the rat.

The Calorie-related aspect of health which devours far more concern of Americans than does longevity is that of obesity. Publishers and electronic media provide an endless procession of diets and other gimmicks guaranteeing weight losses and circumference reductions requiring little effort. Nonetheless, obesity and its related pathology described half a century ago by Dublin and Marks[5] continue to be prevalent in American society. The 1972 data of the Health and Nutrition Examination Survey (HANES)[256] indicated that over one-quarter of all women and over one-eighth of all men aged 45-74 fell in the obese category. Except for black males, all groups with incomes below the poverty level had prevalence rates for obesity higher than did those with incomes above.

Interpretation of such data is controversial *(v.i.)*. However, there are consequences which may accompany the consumption of Calories in excess of those required for energy balance other than technical obesity. With aging, the composition of the body changes to comprise more fat and less lean body mass.[1032] Decreased tolerance for dietary carbohydrate is associated with overweightness and may be corrected by reduction in total Calorie and particularly fat Calorie intake.[367,370] In normal volunteers, high Calorie dietary regimens have been associated with lower mechanical efficiencies measured during work on a motorized treadmill than have lower Calorie regimens ingested by subjects with equal training.[1033] Among institutionalized disabled elderly persons who are grossly obese, their health care is made so difficult by their mass alone that it is frequently inferior to that afforded older persons with comparable infirmities who are of normal weight.

Calories are of concern not only when consumed in excessive quantities but even of more concern when their consumption is insufficient. Among the elderly, this is often a very difficult management problem. The pathogenesis of insufficient Calorie intake among the elderly has many roots. A majority of older persons have some chronic illness or disability physical or metabolic in nature which *per se* may depress appetite and/or the ability properly to absorb and metabolize ingested food. In addition, many of the chronically ill and disabled elderly take medications which further depress appetite and/or adversely influence Calorie absorption and metabolism. Furthermore, many more are depressed or afflicted with other emotional problems which lead to their inattention to adequate Calorie intake. Finally, many elderly, particularly in times of serious inflation, give nutrition — even Calorie nutrition — a low priority in their budgets. Nutrition — even Calorie nutrition — becomes the most compressible item in budgets, falling well behind housing, fuel, utilities, phone, transportation, clothing, health care and alcohol *(v.i.)*.

From a more scientific standpoint, Shock,[18] using an analysis of data from the Baltimore longitudinal study of aging, has reported intraindividual decrements in men in height beginning at age 25 and in weight beginning at age 55. These data confirm for the first time the trend initially resulting from the interpretation of numerous studies based on cross-sectional data. Cross-sectional data have always been suspect because the possibility has existed that the heavier, more obese persons in the population under study had died at younger ages, leaving only survivors to represent the older aged decades.[269] The data reported by Shock suggest that aging *per se* within groups of particular individuals studied over periods of time is associated with progressive loss of weight. Investigations of dietary intake conducted *pari passu* with the above studies suggest that the loss of weight is accompanied by a comparable reduction in Calorie intake.[266] While this reduction undoubtedly is multifactorial in etiology, part of the drop may be attributed to the lower Calorie expenditures of older persons and to the concomitant reduction in appetite.

Andres[1034] has reviewed six sets of data on weights among adults in late maturity and old age and has concluded that persons who are overweight up to no more that 130 per cent of standard weight for height have lower mortality rates than do persons with 100 per cent or less of standard weight. While Andres' argument is based on statistics which do not always reveal the presence or absence of disease in persons at the time they were weighed, his point that overweight is more desirable than underweight among elderly Americans deserves further examination.

He makes the fascinating suggestion that, while less than morbid obesity may do harm to specific subsets of the population *(e.g.,* those with predilections for hypertension, diabetes, coronary atherosclerosis and certain neoplasms), there may be counterbalancing benefits derived from moderately obese body composition which have not yet been examined by epidemiologists, clinical investigators and laboratory scientists. He concludes that research more sophisticated than that which has induced so much anxiety and frustration over the hazards of obesity should be able to shed light on the mechanisms that lead some to benefit and others to be injured by moderate amounts of overweight.

Health and welfare agency records and news media[1035] abound in case histories of emaciated, cachectic old persons whom outreach workers have found suffering from Calorie undernutrition caused by a large number of health-related and socioeconomic circumstances which have received inappropriate attention from relatives, friends and society until publicity has put them in the limelight. Often these persons are recluses who rarely are represented in statistics short of mortality tables. Such persons were supposed to be the prime targets of the original concept[90] of the Nutrition Program for Older Americans (NPOA) authorized by Title VII of the older Americans Act of 1965, as Amended[1036] and now authorized by Title IIIc.[1037] However, older persons in this category do not necessarily come only from lower income groups. This fact was recognized in the conceptualization of NPOA which has never closed the door to those who could afford to make voluntary contributions to the support of the program, even though top priority was given to elderly in the impoverished category. While NPOA has contributed much to the improvement of some elderly who fall in the emaciated, cachectic, Calorie-deficient category, many more are so physically and emotionally drained of endogenous resources that their recovery if feasible at all depends on their receiving optimum care in facilities with the personnel, supplies and equipment to monitor their health and nutritional status hour by hour. This situation reemphasizes the need to prevent such disability and mortality by identifying such persons long before they become headline statistics and to introduce them to appropriate health care and good nutrition through a fusion of primary care and nutrition services which were initially conceived as the mission of NPOA.

Calorie nutrition must be considered in two different ways when developing strategies for managing (a) mature adults not yet elderly and (b) mature adults who are already physiologically old.[1038] Among younger mature adults, lifelong avoidance of Calorie accretion achieved by judiciously combining good nutrition with reasonable amounts of physical work *(v.i.,* Chapter 13) may not only prevent obesity but in certain subsets defer the incidence of diseases now characterizing old age. For those already aged who have not pursued healthful life styles when younger and who have become victims of the diseases which complement old age, Calorie intake sufficient to maintain at least ideal weight for height in conjunction with regularly scheduled physical work[284,1039] may be the most rational regimen in the light of present knowledge.

The provision of social and economic incentives for maintaining regularly scheduled meal and physical activity patterns is a proven means of assuring older persons adequate dietary Calories.[2] When combined with the delivery of primary health care, education and personal counseling (see Figure 1, Chapter 15), such incentives also assure the maintenance of the best health status possible for each individual.[1040] For those already old, such optimum health maintenance, even though diseases and disabilities may be present, is a rational, plausible and attainable goal. Reaching that objective requires not only the consumption by the elderly of adequate Calories and other nutrients but also the application of the concept inherent in the nutrition-health-aging triad.

A source of Calories not previously mentioned but one of concern in the management of all living persons but particularly of the elderly is ethyl alcohol (ethanol). Ethanol provides approximately seven Calories per gram making it, next to fat, the most concentrated source among the sources of Calories. Alcohol *per se* provides only empty Calories, although some alcoholic beverages such as beer do contain other nutrients.[943,944,1040c] Alcoholic beverages when ingested in moderation have been reported to have some virtues.[349h,104d] However, they pose an insidious and everpresent danger which is made even more menacing among the elderly because of their social isolation, their income maintenance problems, their health status, and their consumption of drugs, many of which produce undesirable side-effects in the presence of ethanol.

Among compensated alcoholics *(i.e.,* those who consume large quantities of ethanol daily but who nonetheless still perform well enough to avoid being fired in a job paying well enough to support both the alcohol habit and a reasonable standard of living), retirement with its reduced income may result in extreme compression of the nutrition item in the family budget, since the alcohol habit must be satisfied and can not be eliminated without great pain and effort. The reduction in nutrient intake may lead to serious malnutrition and even to acute nutritional deficiency syndromes, not to mention the toxic effects of ethanol *per se.*

The place of alcoholic beverages in nutrition has been reviewed in depth by many experts.[1040c] The role — both positive and negative — of alcoholic beverages in gerontology has also been summarized.[1040d] The solution to alcohol-induced social, economic and health problems among the elderly requires first the identification of those older persons who have responded negatively to the challenge posed by alcoholic beverages. This identification entails organized outreach. Once identification has been made, resources are needed whereby the older person may receive proper treatment. While alcoholic beverages consumed in moderation have produced some positive social, psychologic and even physiologic health-related results, the legal, image-related and logistic problems associated with their use in institutions and in community-based programs such as NPOA do not hold out great promise for their widespread use as forms of therapy. As a Calorie source in parenteral nutrition, alcohol has been tried but has been superannuated by hypertonic solutions infused into central veins and by fat emulsions.[386,386a-386h]

-13-

Physical Work

Stated in oversimplified terms, body composition is the resultant of a balance between the intake of Calories from food, the output of Calories from basal metabolism, the specific dynamic action of food (SDA), and physical work. Certain nutrients are required in proportion to Calorie intake. Calorie intake in turn should be directly proportional to total Calorie expenditure, the readily controllable variable of which is physical work. The Calorie intake is inversely proportional to the nutrient density of foods needed to supply the minimum daily requirements (MDR's) or the recommended dietary allowances (RDA).[734,737] Lower nutrient density foods usually cost less. Meals meeting the RDA's standards are more easily planned when a broad spectrum of low nutrient density, low cost foods may be used. Physical work, by increasing energy expenditure, permits an increase in Calorie intake while maintaining constant body weight, thereby making possible the consumption of low nutrient density foods which in turn lower the cost of the food budget. In addition, physical work sufficient to raise the heart rate to 120 per minute or over, if maintained for substantial intervals of time, has been observed to improve physiological performance,[284] raise morale,[1041] increase collateral circulation in the heart,[283,1042,1043] serve as an anabolic stimulant,[1044,1045] reduce circulating lipid concentrations,[245] and improve glucose tolerance.[1046] Many devotees of strenuous daily physical work maintain that it diminishes appetite chronically and hence aids in the prevention of obesity. Some even report an addiction to strenuous physical work which results in withdrawal symptoms if daily workouts are terminated abruptly. Even among the well trained, physical work has produced sudden death.[1047,1048]

With these many attributes, physical work is a basic component of each third and of the entire integrated nutrition-health-aging triad. In order to focus the attention of every health professional coping with the triad, physical work should be considered as the "eighth nutrient group" in full partnership with protein, fat, carbohydrate, minerals and trace elements, vitamins, water and Calories.

Among the aged, vigorous physical work should be promoted cautiously especially among those whose daily occupation or avocation may not include it. Among those elderly accustomed to strenuous physical work daily, no differences in Calorie output compared to those of younger persons have been reported. Studies among Swiss farmers, for example, have revealed energy expenditures of equal Calorie value whether the farmer was aged or young.[1049] In many projects of the Nutrition Program for Older Americans (NPOA), physical work schedules have been introduced which are programmed to provide gradually increasing amounts of physical work regardless of the degree of disability of the participants.[133] Such deliberate efforts to promote physical work programs have been extremely popular among NPOA participants. Unfortunately, evaluations of impact using objective measures have not been carried out. Hence, research on the "eighth nutrient group" as it relates to the health and nutritional status of those already old is a field seeking investigators. The inclusion of regularly scheduled physical work among the life styles of persons of all ages may contribute importantly to improved health status.[1050]

The role of regularly scheduled physical work in the management of many diseases deserves far more attention than it has received. In adolescents with incurable neoplasms, preliminary studies produced evidence strongly suggesting that strenuous work daily *per se* could induce reductions in the physical size of unresectable neoplasms and in the values of parameters proportional to their activity.[1044] Studies in parabiotic animals strongly suggest that muscular work by one of the pairs produces a factor transmitted through the blood which is anabolic and improves carbohydrate tolerance in the other nonworking members of the pairs.[1051] Other studies have suggested that strenuous physical work daily must be accompanied by a diet high in protein if cardiac arrythmias occasioned by loss of potassium when work is performed by persons on low protein diets is to be avoided.[1033,1052] Physical work performed daily improves depressions.[1041] While it reduces the concentrations of certain plasma lipids, it also has the desirable effect of increasing concentrations of high density lipoproteins (HDL's). It will lower blood pressure and reduce pulse rate. However, it will not dissolve atheromata.[284] It will nonetheless improve the collateral circulation in diseased hearts.[283,1042,1043] If sudden death may be regarded as a disease, physical work even in trained persons has been associated with that ailment.[1047,1048]

For the elderly, the best approach to maximizing the advantages and minimizing the dangers of physical work is to begin increasing the daily work load slowly, eventually working up to the maximum tolerable level. Exercise testing among the elderly is probably a waste of time and money, since in the asymptomatic patient the number of false positives is high and in those who are symptomatic a very slowly increasing work regimen, if any, is the only one indicated.[1048,1053-1057] Physical work by elderly persons improves their psyche, reduces depressions, betters their affect and leads to often remarkable increases in their self-confidence. These internal changes enable the older person to do more, to go more places and to develop with greater ease an ever-expanding coterie of friends.

Little data is available regarding the non-Calorie nutrient requirements of persons of all ages performing strenuous physical work daily. Many opinions but few facts based on scientifically collected data pervade both popular and more authoratative views on this subject. Virtually no objective data describe the influence of work *per se* or the influence of variables in nutrient intake along with work among the elderly.

In conclusion, regularly scheduled physical work tailored to the capabilities of the particular person is an important component of any regimen designed to improve the physical and mental health of human beings. In view of the many mutual relations among physical work, nutrition and health, physical work must be incorporated in all considerations of the nutrition-health-aging triad.

Part III

PRESENT FEDERALLY-SPONSORED SERVICE PROGRAMS

PROLOGUE

In the ensuing chapter, resources derived by taxes received by and debts incurred by the Federal government are described. These resources never were conceived as complete answers to the problems of nutrition, health and aging among the elderly or any other group. They, however, do afford modest resources upon which to begin building more permanent systems which when applied will ultimately resolve the problems.

Ideally American society should be stimulated by these small Federal resources to devise answers which will enable the Federal funds to be shifted to the initiation of attacks on other priorities as answers to the previous problems are found. There is no justification for the institutionalization of demonstrations. No demonstration deserves to be started which does not include a planned mechanism for its own demise as more permanent mechanisms take over.

The activities described in this section should be viewed in that context. If they are so-viewed, changes in particular funding levels created by new administrations, new economic conditions or new international challenges need not create panic among older persons. Since most of these activities have been here for many years, substitutes for or complements to them should long ago have been developed. If they are not yet capable of sound performance, thorough investigations of these substitutes or complements are long overdue.

-14-

Federal Government Activities In Nutrition, Health And Aging

THE DEPARTMENT OF HEALTH AND HUMAN SERVICES (DHHS)

DHHS comprises more agencies dealing with nutrition than any other department or independent agency in the Federal Government.

The Secretary

The most important component of this vast department influencing Federal health, nutrition and aging activities is the Office of the Secretary (OS). The person of the Secretary has authority to establish priorities which are reflected in policy statements, organizational patterns, personnel allocations and budgetary allotments. Furthermore, the Secretary chooses the personnel who lead all agencies in the department. While such choices do require prior approval of the administration in power and advice and consent of the Senate, the Secretary, through the selection process, is able to appoint persons whose social, political and economic philosophies have major impact on the various bureaucracies under their control. Many Secretaries have definite concepts they wish to promote which influence programs of every agency in the Department. The political appointees in charge of the subordinate agencies have little opportunity for self-expression but are required under threat of dismissal to carry out policies promulgated by the Secretary.

The Office of the Assistant Secretary for Health (OASH) and the Surgeon General (SG)

OASH not only houses the Assistant Secretary, who may double as Surgeon-General of the United States, but also comprises other units which have direct and indirect effects on the Department's activities in the field of nutrition, health and aging.

One of these is the National Center for Health Statistics (NCHS) which is responsible for assembling the data bases on which technical decisions may be made and also for managing the Health and Nutrition Examination Surveys (HANES) conducted periodically on probability samples of the American population. HANES provide the only nationwide organized nutrition and health surveillance mechanism. Since the sampling unit is the household, HANES give cross-sectional evaluations of the nutritional status and health status of Americans of all ages.

OASH also is the locus for the National Center for Health Services Research (NCHSR). New concepts of the delivery of health services, including nutrition services, to persons of all ages including the elderly may arise from the Center's activities.

OASH contains in addition the Health Maintenance Organization (HMO) program. HMO's, in return for an annual fee, provide prepaid medical care covering practically all types of pathology. In concept, they also are supposed to provide sufficient health and nutrition education to warrant a high level of self-responsibility among their beneficiaries. Although a few HMO's such as those managed by Kaiser-Permanente in the western United States have been operating many years and have developed reputations for their results in health promotion, most HMO's are of recent origin and are still struggling with the problem of meeting the needs posed by presenting complaints of members. They have had little time, few personnel and limited resources to devote to health promotion. Nonetheless, the HMO concept affords a theoretically cost-effective method of resolving problems caused by diseases, accidents and inherited defects as well as those resulting from long-term practice of life styles inimical to health. In time, the HMO's may become vehicles for health promotion as well as curative medicine throughout the nation.

OASH, in its capacity as the Office of the Surgeon-General of the Public Health Service (PHS), serves as the locus for the Office of International Health (OIH). The OIH is the component of the department which extends overseas not only to assist in the management of health problems abroad but also to learn from the experiences of foreign governments in the management of problems dealing with nutrition, health and aging.

The Public Health Service (PHS)

By far the largest health-oriented consortium of agencies within DHHS is the PHS. The Surgeon-General in charge of the PHS may or may not be the Assistant Secretary for Health.

Included in the PHS is the Health Services Administration (HSA) which itself comprises the Indian Health Service (IHS), the Bureau of Medical Services (BMS) which controls Public Health Service Hospitals and Clinics, and the Bureau of Community Health Services (BCHS). All of these components have actual and potential roles to play in the management of nutrition, health and aging programs within the populations subject to their jurisdiction. For example, the IHS is responsible for the health and nutrition of all Native Americans and Alaskan natives who still maintain their tribal and historical identities. The BMS has a mandate to serve merchant seamen, personnel of the Coastguard, many other specifically entitled Federal government beneficiaries and those retirees from the Uniformed Services who choose to obtain their medical care at Public Health Service facilities. In addition, since the late seventies, the Public Health Service Hospitals have been working closely with the governments of the jurisdictions in which they operate in developing and elaborating health-oriented community based programs. The BCHS, which comprises urban health initiatives, rural health initiatives, migrant health initiatives, community health centers, and the National Health Service Corps (NHSC), to mention a few of its responsibilities, works with other Federal agencies *(v.i.)* to provide health and nutrition services to populations of all ages, including the elderly.

The PHS's Health Resources Administration (HRA) has many components which impact directly or indirectly on nutrition, health and aging. Important among these are the Health Systems Agencies (HSA's) which are responsible for the allocations of resources among health-oriented institutions in the specific geographic Health Service Areas of their responsibility.

Most prestigious and widely known among Public Health Service components are the National Institutes of Health (NIH). While only two of the National Institutes have a specific mandate to examine aging as a biologic process, *i.e.*, the National Institute for Child Health and Human Development (NICHD) and the National Institute of Aging (NIA), many of the other categorical Institutes have mandates in their respective categorical disease areas which give them reasonable arguments for relating their studies to biologic aging. Foremost among these are the National Heart, Lung and Blood Institute (NHLBI), the National Institute of Neurological and Communicative Disorders and Stroke (NINCDS), the National Cancer Institute (NCI) and the National Institute of Arthritis, Diabetes, Digestive and Kidney Diseases (NIADDKD). However, since all aspects of health have some component dealing with nutrition, every Institute within the National Institutes of Health is involved in nutrition one way or another. This has led to some controversy, since members of the Congress have not always agreed that the NIH-defined nutrition-related activities of NIH impact directly on the nutritional status of Americans.

Also a part of the Public Health Service are the Centers for Disease Control (CDC) located in Atlanta, Georgia. Since the CDC, formerly called the Communicable Disease Center, is now responsible for investigating diseases other than those characterized by acute or chronic infections, it is understandable that nutrition has become a component of CDC's national responsibility. A CDC laboratory is responsible for performance of a portion of the laboratory work of HANES. Also a part of the CDC is the Bureau of Health Education which has recently focused on studies of better methods of promoting nutrition education for the elderly.

Also in the Public Health Service, the Food and Drug Administration (FDA) plays a key role in the Federal government activities in the fields of health and nutrition and through them has an influence on aging. All new drugs must be approved by the FDA before they can be used in investigations or released for public sale. FDA laboratories monitor the hygienic properties of many food products. FDA writes regulations concerning the labelling of food. It has established the so-called USRDA (United States Recommended Dietary Allowances), distinct from the RDA,[92a] which assist in implementation of the food labelling regulations. In addition to the Bureau of Drugs and the Bureau of Foods, the FDA comprises the Bureau of Biologics, the Bureau of Radiologic Health, the Bureau of Veterinary Medicine and the Bureau of Medical Devices. All of these have direct and indirect impact on nutrition, health and aging.

Another component of the Public Health Service is the Alcohol, Drug Abuse and Mental Health Administration (ADAMHA). ADAMHA comprises the National Institute of Mental Health (NIMH), the National Institute on Alcohol Abuse and Alcoholism (NIAA) and the National Institute of Drug Abuse (NIDA). The influence of alcohol and drugs on the health and nutritional status of Americans is well understood. Somewhat less well known is the impact of emotional disorders on the physical health and nutritional status of persons afflicted with them. ADAMHA has major responsibility for Federal research and service programs dealing with these problems.

The Office of Human Development Services (OHDS)

That component of DHHS most directly concerned with the provision of nutrition services is OHDS whose Assistant Secretary is responsible for the activities of the Administration for Children, Youth and Families (ACYF), the Administration for Native Americans (ANA), the Administration on Aging (AoA) and the Administration for Public Services (APS).

ACYF has a major impact on the health and nutrition of children and youth through its components, the Head Start Bureau, the Children's Bureau and the Youth Development Bureau. ANA is an advocacy agency for Native Americans which has direct contact with the tribal councils which in turn assist in the policy making, resource allocation and program development of health and nutrition programs managed through other government agencies.

AoA, through the Nutrition Program for Older Americans (NPOA) *(v.i.)*, operates the largest activity in the world directed toward the provision of nutrition services to older people. Conceptually NPOA provides a means of making available to older Americans access to primary health care, to education and counselling on many topics and to a variety of so-called social services. The NPOA will be discussed in more detail in chapter 14 *(v.i.)*.

APS administers the Social Service Program for Individuals and Families authorized by Title XX of the Social Security Act, as Amended, enacted by P.L. 93-647 and signed into law by the President on October 1, 1975. Title XX in many jurisdictions plays an important role in complementing the resources of NPOA. Title XX will be discussed under Social Security Administration immediately below.

The Social Security Administration (SSA)

Another DHHS agency which plays an absolutely vital role in the health and nutrition of Americans is the Social Security Administration (SSA). By providing financial assistance to families and children in need, to disabled persons of all ages and to older Americans who have retired, SSA makes the difference between mere subsistence and a plausible standard of living for millions of Americans. A component of SSA, the Bureau of Supplemental Security Income (SSI), provides from general revenue (not from SSA's own trust fund) in cooperation with State welfare agencies a guaranteed minimum income for the old (65 years of age and over), the blind and the permanently disabled regardless of their eligibility for other SSA-paid benefits.

Title XX of the Social Security Act (administered by APS of OHDS) *(v.s.)* mandates that certain essential social services be provided by the collaborating jurisdiction (State or the District of Columbia). Federal Financial Participation (FFP) is available for 75 per cent of the service costs and for personnel training and retraining directly related to the provision of services under the jurisdiction's plan for services.

Title XX requires that the jurisdictional plan for services be directed at the following goals and objectives: (a) achieving or maintaining economic self-support to prevent, reduce or eliminate dependency; (b) achieving or maintaining self-sufficiency, including reduction or prevention of dependency; (c) preventing or remedying neglect, abuse or exploitation of children and adults unable to protect their own interests, or preserving, rehabilitating or reuniting families; (d) preventing or reducing inappropriate institutional care by providing for community-based care, home-based care or other forms of less intensive care; or (e) securing referral or admission for institutional care when other forms of care are not appropriate, or providing services to individuals in institutions.

Eligibility for such services is restricted to the poor and near-poor. By Federal regulations, 50 per cent of the funds in any jurisdiction must be used to serve persons on welfare. Almost all of the remainder must be used to serve people whose family income is 65 per cent or less of the jurisdiction's average. Members of families with incomes as high as 115 per cent of the jurisdiction's average may receive services but must pay a fee to receive them. The relation of Title XX to NPOA will be discussed in Chapter 14 *(v.i.)*.

The Health Care Financing Administration (HCFA)

Operating symbiotically with SSA in DHHS is HCFA. This agency is responsible for the Medicare and Medicaid programs which finance the provisions of health care to the elderly and to low income persons of all ages. In addition to funding the provision of these health services, HCFA also cooperates with State health departments and the U.S. Public Health Service in assuring quality control in the provision of health care.

The Office of Education (OE)

DHHS's OE, which became the independent Department of Education under the provisions of P.L. 96-88, signed into law by the President on October 17, 1979, was party to an interagency agreement with AoA which committed the Commissioner of Education to utilize the resources at OE's disposal to improve the education, including the health and nutrition education, of older Americans. The intent of this agreement foundered because of the various reorganizations which preceded P.L. 96-88 and must be renegotiated to comply with the new interdepartmental format, should the new Department indeed survive.

THE UNITED STATES DEPARTMENT OF AGRICULTURE (USDA)

The USDA comprises many agencies which play impressive roles in feeding persons of all ages. In addition, it comprises agencies which perform and subsidize research in food production, others which are devoted to research in animal and human metabolism of nutrients and others which are the major bastions of education in food production, in food safety and in nutrition in the Federal establishment.

In recent years, Congress has authorized and funded four new USDA Human Nutrition Research Centers and has continued support of the Nutrition Institute at Beltsville, Maryland. Reporting through Regional Offices of the Agricultural Research Service *(v.i.),* these Centers and the Institute have obscured the once clear dividing line between DHHS and USDA responsibilities in the field of human nutrition as it relates to health and aging. It is no secret that USDA, through the moves of its own political leaders and bureaucrats and their allies — the staff members of Senate and House Agriculture Committees — is moving deliberately in directions which will make USDA more influential than DHHS in all aspects of human nutrition with the exception of those rigidly associated with categorical diseases. A review of major USDA components which influence the nutrition-health-aging triad follows.

The Secretary

USDA's presidentially appointed political leader serves a constituency represented in Congress by Senators and Representatives whose seniority places them in position to support effectively programs proposed by the Secretary. Lobbyists for agribusiness provide additional leverage to assist in promotion, authorization and funding of USDA proposals. The Secretary is in a position to move ahead in developing new programs and in expanding existing programs with great impact on the components of and on the entire nutrition-health-aging triad.

The Assistant Secretary for Food and Consumer Services (ASFCS)

This Assistant Secretary is responsible for three agencies which have great influence on the nutrition of millions of Americans.

The Food and Nutrition Service (FNS): FNS operates on the principle that a better diet means better health for millions of Americans, particularly those with low incomes, whom it serves. Through its various programs, FNS makes available the indispensable ingredients of that better diet, *viz.,* access to wholesome foods and knowledge of the relationship between nutrition and health. In conducting this crucial operation, FNS comprises several programs.

The Food Stamp Program — Whether measured in millions of people served or by billions of dollars invested therein, the Food Stamp Program is the largest enterprise in the USDA. Its *raison d'etre* is to assist low income households purchase the foods they need for good health.

The Food Stamp Act of 1977 which authorized the Food Stamp Program's operation through 1981 is an example of a series of Federal food assistance programs going back to the Great Depression of the early 1930's. At that time, unsold farm surpluses combined with thousands of people in breadlines induced the Federal establishment to begin distributing surplus foods to the hungry. Food stamps *per se* were first used in the late 1930's in Rochester, New York, and subsequently in 1700 counties and 88 cities. This plan at its zenith served three million people monthly. Households purchased stamps equal in value to cash paid, with which to purchase food at retail outlets but also received as a bonus additional stamps with which designated surplus foods could be purchased at retail stores. Elimination of surplus foods by World War II terminated the program.

In 1961, USDA established a pilot food stamp program which was reaching 350,000 people in 43 areas by 1964. The Food Stamp Act of 1964 made the program permanent and authorized its expansion to all States. During the next five years national concern over hunger in the United States led to augmentation of direct food distribution or food stamp programs.

Stimulated by the activities of the 1969 White House Conference on Food, Nutrition and Health,[89] the Congress in 1971 established national standards of eligibility and required States to inform low income people about food stamp availability. It was not until 1974, however, that the Food Stamp Program under court order became truly national in scope when States were required to offer food stamps to the poor in all intra-State jurisdictions. Since 1974 the Food Stamp Program has mushroomed, reaching a peak of 19.5 million participants during the recession of 1975. Since then participation has fluctuated with economic conditions.

Under the regulations issued to implement the Food Stamp Act of 1977,[1058] purchase requirements were completely eliminated. Under the old law, most households had to purchase food stamps with cash in order to receive bonus stamps issued in proportion to their need. Now they get only the bonus stamps. This change has been of particular benefit to low income elderly who frequently did not participate because of lack of cash to buy the stamps.

A survey in 1976 indicated that 54.8 per cent of the people participating in the Food Stamp Program were under age 18. This suggests that older Americans even though eligible have not been taking full advantage of the Food Stamp Program. While the reforms of 1977 may have led to more participation, many older Americans are still deterred by pride and the stigma of welfare from enrolling in the program. To combat this problem, the 1977 Act included provisions for outreach. It requires States to inform low-income people — including all on public assistance, unemployment compensation and SSI — about the availability of food stamps. Nonetheless, the elderly still may not participate without specific assistance from local agencies like NPOA in overcoming not only considerations of pride but also the not inconsiderable bureaucratic maze leading to certificaton which, in spite of many simplifications, still is difficult to traverse unaided. Getting the stamps and later getting food with the stamps is sometimes physically and emotionally impossible for many elderly unless they receive the assistance of relatives, friends, neighbors or volunteers from the community.

Since March 1, 1979, States have been required by Federal regulations to have more flexible certification procedures for elderly and handicapped persons. These may include home visits and telephone interviews. SSI recipients are able to apply for food stamps at Social Security Offices when they apply for SSI. The information collected for SSI is used to determine food stamp eligibility. (SSI recipients are ineligible for food stamps in the two "cashout" States — California and Massachusetts — where SSI recipients receive a larger SSI payment instead of food stamps).

As with most Federally-initiated programs, the Food Stamp Program must be applied at the grass roots level if it is to be successful in meeting the needs of Americans of all ages. When applied properly at the community level, the Food Stamp Program assures that no American need be hungry. The challenge facing society is to make certain that all Americans are familiar with the program and know the mechanisms through which they may be benefited by it.

The Food Distribution Program — This Program donates food to certified outlets, *e.g.*, schools, charitable institutions, the NPOA, summer camps, disaster relief agencies and programs for needy families on some Indian reservations. While logistic problems in distribution of foods *per se* led to cashout by NPOA projects in many States, other States have continued to use donated foods. Some States use cashout in certain regions, donated foods in others.

The use of surplus commodities (usually available in limited variety) in NPOA was authorized in NPOA's initial legislation (P.L. 92-258). However, in the 1974 Amendments to the Older Americans Act (P.L. 93-351), the Secretary of Agriculture was required to maintain a specific level of assistance (expressed in cents) per meal served by NPOA. This amount has risen by Congressional action and also because it is adjusted to reflect changes in the series for food away from home of the Consumer Price Index published by the Bureau of Labor Statistics of the Department of Labor. In contrast to the initial Act (P.L. 92-258), the 1974 Amendments made available to NPOA the wide variety of foods being distributed to the School Lunch Program. Hence, by virtue of the Donated Food Program, USDA became a major contributor to the resources of NPOA.

Other FNS Programs — Since aging begins no later than conception, the Special Supplemental Food Program for Women, Infants and Children (WIC) plays an important role by providing specific nutritious foods to pregnant and breast feeding women and to children up to five years of age. Eligibility requires that the health of the mothers and children be threatened by low income and poor nutrition. The specific foods are prescribed at WIC centers. Vouchers are given to participants who may exchange them for prescribed foods at retail stores.

The National School Lunch Program and School Breakfast Program make nutritious, low-cost lunches and breakfasts available daily to children attending participating schools and institutions. Needy children receive meals free or at reduced prices.

The Special Milk Program allows all children attending participating schools or institutions to buy milk at a reduced price or, if they are needy, to receive it free.

The Child Care Food Program runs year-round in non-residential institutions. In daycare centers, Head Start Centers and family day care homes, participating children receive breakfasts, lunches, suppers and snacks. The extension of this program to encompass comparable facilities involved in the care of dependent and disabled elderly would not be unreasonable.

The Summer Food Service Program for Children provides meals for children from low-income areas during extended vacations when schools are closed. Children enrolled in eligible summer camps and similar institutions get the meals free. An extension of this program logically could assist comparable summer camps and similar institutions serving low-income elderly.

The Nutrition Education and Training Program (NET), authorized by P.L. 95-166, is designed to reinforce the Federal, State and local alliances already addressing the mutual relations of food and nutrition, health and aging among school-age populations and those other persons associated with them. It is a prototype of a program which could be developed to reinforce the relatively feeble alliances now attempting to disseminate knowledge of the mutual relations among nutrition, health and aging within NPOA.

NET is a Federal to State grant program based on a formula of n¢ per year child (50¢, in the initial legislation) enrolled in public and private schools, residential child care institutions and day care centers. States must use these funds to disseminate effectively nutrition information to children and to provide inservice training to foodservice and teaching personnel. A State Coordinator for Nutrition Education and Training is appointed in each jurisdiction. This person must conduct a needs assessment and develop a State Plan. The law also requires a State Advisory Council composed of teachers, foodservice personnel, health professionals, food and nutrition professionals and paraprofessionals, administrators, consumer groups and parents. In many States, the Cooperative Extensions Service *(v.i.)* based in land-grant universities have played significant roles in implementing NET.

The Human Nutrition Information Service (HNIS): This agency reporting to the ASFCS came into being in 1981 and provides the public and the media with access to facts and figures about nutrition in general and the USDA's roles in human nutrition in particular. Also under the ASFCS is a Food and Nutrition Information Service which is centered in the National Agricultural Library which is a function of the Director of Science and Education *(v.i.)*.

The Office of the Consumer Advisor (OCA): This Office also began operating in 1981. Its function is to provide consumers with reliable information about food quality and pricing and about the nutritional values of various food products.

The Under Secretary for International Affairs and Commodity Programs (USIACP)

The Agricultural Stabilization and Conservation Service (ASCS): This Under Secretary's importance to older persons arises primarily from the control exercised over the Agricultural Stabilization and Conservation Service (ASCS). This service has great potential for playing a major role in meeting the nutritional requirements of many older Americans. ASCS administers specified commodity and related land-use programs designed for voluntary production adjustment, resource protection and price, market and farm income stabilization. ASCS administers commodity stabilization programs for a number of food products including wheat, corn, peanuts, rice, milk and the products of milk, barley, oats, sorghum, soybeans, dried edible beans and honey. In the case of milk and milk products, prices are stabilized through ASCS purchases of processed dairy products.

The Secretary of Agriculture has authority to authorize ASCS purchases of dairy-based products for donation to organizations like NPOA serving needy elderly. Using this authority, ASCS made available to 6,000 NPOA participants distributed among 20 projects in all ten DHEW Federal regions a dairy-based product designated Limited Use Supplemental Food (LUSF) which had been formulated by DHEW's AoA and USDA's Agricultural Research Service (ARS).[732a-732c] In this demonstration program, ASCS contracted with a corporation capable of mixing nonfat dry milk solids with vitamins, trace elements and enough corn syrup solids to bring the Calorie content to 150 per serving. The product was packaged to insure long shelf life and to be available in emergencies when NPOA participants, because of weather, illness or failure of their NPOA site to operate, had no access to other sources of nutrition. It also served as a supplemental food for those whose daily regimen included only a major meal at an NPOA site and who frequently were without nutrition when their NPOA site was closed on weekends. The demonstration program indicated a better than 90 per cent acceptability of the product. Projections suggested that distribution of LUSF throughout the NPOA network would within one year result in the consumption of and therefore the disposition of 40 million kg of nonfat dry milk solids annually. The LUSF project suggested the potential of ASCS to serve millions of elderly people through a mechanism which also would have the power to dispose of truly enormous amounts of a commodity which at the time of the LUSF acceptability trial comprised a 700 million kg glut on the world market.

The Assistant Secretary for Marketing and Inspection Services (ASMIS)

In 1981, this Assistant Secretary became responsible for the newly named Food Safety and Inspection Service (FSIS) which previously had been under the jurisdiction of the ASFCA under the name Food Safety and Quality Service (FSQS).

The Food Safety and Inspection Service (FSIS): FSIS provides assurance to the consumer that foods are safe, wholesome and nutritious, that they are of good quality and that they are informatively and honestly labelled. It also provides assistance to the marketing system through purchase of surplus food commodities and those needed in the National Food Assistance Programs. The Service is responsible for promulgating the regulations dealing with various aspects of the food chain from livestock health, veterinary medicine and pest control through meat and poultry processing and standards for dairy products, fruits and vegetables. In these many roles, it represents the interests of the American consumer and may, when indicated serve as an advocate for those consumers. In its exercise of responsibility, FSIS must work closely with the Animal and Plant Health Inspection Service (APHIS) which also reports directly to the ASMIS and is responsible for implementing at the processing level the regulations promulgated by FSIS. As the USDA's voice in guaranteeing the safety and quality of the American food supply, FSIS shares with DHHS's FDA Federal government authority in assuring the American public freedom from risk or injury from the food supply and in guaranteeing also a high degree of excellence in the character of that food supply.

The Director of Science and Education (DSE)

In a 1981 reorganization, the DSE was given purview of the Agricultural Research Service (ARS), the Cooperative State Research Service (CSRS), the Extension Service (ES), the National Agricultural Library (NAL) and the Science and Education Management Staff (SEMF).

In cooperation with Federal departments and agencies, State agricultural experiment stations, colleges and universities and consumer groups, these agencies conduct and support research, extension and teaching programs in the food and agricultural sciences responsive to local, State, regional, national and worldwide needs in the fields of human nutrition, home economics, consumer services, family life, rural and community development, agricultural energy, agricultural economics, environmental quality, natural and human resources, forestry, range management, animal and plant production and protection, aquaculture, and the processing, distribution and utilization of food and agriculture products.

From their numerous missions, it is obvious that the agencies reporting to the DSE play major roles in nutrition, health and aging and in the mutual relations of these in the integrated nutrition-health-aging triad.

Through its Regional Offices, the ARS oversees the Nutrition Institute and the Consumer and Food Economics Institute located in Beltsville, Maryland and four Human Nutrition Research Centers located in Grand Forks, Boston, Houston and San Francisco. The Consumer and Food Economics Institute is responsible for conduct of the decennial Household Food Consumption Surveys. The Nutrition Institute conducts research in many fields of nutrition science and also is responsible for USDA's Food Analysis Laboratory. The Human Nutrition Research Centers have in-house programs with special areas of emphasis. The Grand Forks center focuses on studies of trace elements. The Boston Center investigates nutrition and aging. The Houston center is concerned with nutritional considerations of neonatology and pediatrics. The San Francisco center, formerly the U.S. Army's Medical Research and Nutrition Laboratory, is engaged in research covering a broad spectrum of nutritional physiology and biochemistry.

The Human Nutrition Research Centers may engage in collaborative ventures with investigators throughout the nation. In its own community, each center is affiliated with a specific university *e.g.*, the University of North Dakota at Grand Forks. The centers represent a major USDA thrust in the field of human nutrition.

ARS comprises units dealing with soil, water and air sciences; livestock and veterinary sciences; plant and entomological sciences; and marketing, nutrition and engineering sciences. The four Regional Research Laboratories of the Department and special laboratories such as the Metabolism and Radiation Laboratory in Fargo, North Dakota fall under its jurisdiction.

ARS comprises units dealing with natural resources and forestry; animal sciences; plant sciences; and human nutrition, food and social sciences. Very importantly it also includes the Competitive Research Grants Office (CRGO) which receives applications for research support from universities and other research oriented organizations throughout the United States and subjects them to peer review processes similar to those used by NIH. The "Cooperative" in the CSRS title signifies long-standing cooperation between the Federal and State governments mediated through the land grant colleges and universities in each jurisdiction.

ES is composed of six divisions: agriculture, natural resources, food and nutriton, family education, rural development and 4-H youth. The agriculture, natural resources and rural development divisions focus on economic aspects of farm life. The food and nutrition, family education and 4-H youth divisions are more people oriented. Through them, not only rural but also metropolitan area households are afforded the opportunity to learn more about the interrelations of nutrition, health and aging.

Gerontology has become a major component of extension programs in many States. An example of this is the Generations Alliance Program started in 1974 by a 4-H Club and a chapter of the American Association of Retired Persons (AARP) in northern Cook County, Illinois. It is now a nation-wide Program of the AARP with a Washington Office and has been extended to include cooperation with other youth organizations such as the Girl Scouts, Student Nurses, the Red Cross, the Key Club and the Campfire Girls. In Arkansas, one of the first States to appoint an extension specialist in gerontology, the 4-H Adopt a Grandparent Program is another example of how the Extension Service is seeking to serve the elderly and to bridge the generation gaps. In Connecticut, the Extension Service has worked closely with the Department of Aging to bring more effective health and nutrition education into NPOA projects. In Utah, the Extension Family Life Programs based at Utah State University have assisted elderly residents of southern counties of the State in establishing the Senior Nutrition Aid Program (SNAP) through which small groups of elderly persons join together in food production projects, in meal preparation and consumption in individual homes and in education projects for increasing their self-responsibility for personal health.

Throughout the nation practically all Cooperative Extension Services cooperate directly with State Agencies on Aging and involve many of their personnel in the activities of the State Councils and Advisory Committees on Aging. Well over one-third of State Extension Services have projects in the field of nutrition funded by their State Agencies on Aging. All States, through their Extension Home Economists or Expanded Food and Nutrition Education Program (EFNEP) aides conduct nutrition education exercises for older Americans at NPOA sites or at Senior Centers. Over two-thirds of the State Extension Services have developed special materials suitable for nutrition education among the elderly. Extension Service personnel have made extensive use of publications of other USDA agencies such as *Cooking for Two*[1059] prepared by the Nutrition and Technical Service Staff of the FNS and the Consumer and Food Economics Institute.

The Extension Service and the EFNEP Program have personnel

and resources in all U.S. jurisdictions which have long histories of contact with households in rural and, more recently, in metropolitan areas. In the past decade, the growing interest in older members of households has complemented the traditional emphasis on children and youth. The Extension Service now is a major resource available for promoting concepts inherent in the nutrition-health-aging triad.

OTHER FEDERAL DEPARTMENTS AND AGENCIES

While DHHS and USDA represent the largest of the departments and agencies concerned with the nutrition-health-aging triad, other departments and independent agencies may make significant contributions to specific persons and groups.

The Department of Defense (DOD)

For career Armed Forces personnel and their families and for all enlisted and officer personnel and their families on active duty, DOD provides medical services at its own installations or through contract health care providers. The opportunities to employ periods of military service for education of military personnel in considerations of the nutritition-health-aging triad are far greater than have been utilized to the present time. Considering the fact that many 20 and 30 year veterans of military service continue to be DOD responsibilities in their retirement years, the opportunity to reach large numbers of mature and elderly Americans is also present.

The Department of Housing and Urban Development (HUD)

HUD, through its ability to provide safe and suitable housing for many low-income households and particularly for the elderly and the handicapped, contributes greatly to the maintenance of the health and nutrition of those individuals so housed. Many HUD-sponsored facilities serve as project sites for NPOA.

The Veterans Administration (VA)

The Veterans Administration, through its VA Medical Centers, provides medical care for those veterans with service-connected disabilities and for those needy veterans who are unable to obtain health care elsewhere. Very important to all veterans, regardless of their economic status, the VA provides appropriate care when catastrophic illness or accident disrupts the income-producing capability of a wage earner. Within the walls of VA Medical Centers, Dietetic Services supervise nutrition services and provide excellent professional advice in regard to the interrelations of health and nutrition. However, since nutrition is regarded by the VA as a subsistence item, not a medical benefit, nutrition advice and consultation and the provision of adequate nutrition in the form of meals outside VA Medical Centers is currently impossible. While medication and prostheses are regarded as medical benefits, the provision of nutrients in any format outside VA Medical Centers is held to be the responsibility of the individual veteran, to be paid for from his own resources or VA subsistence payments.

The Department of Commerce (DOC)

DOC plays a direct role in nutrition through its control of the National Oceanic and Atmospheric Administration (NOAA) which incorporates in its domain the National Marine Fisheries Service (NMFS). NMFS not only analyzes the economic aspects of fisheries operations with an eye to improving man's ability to conserve and protect these resources but also conducts research designed to improve the quality of and reduce the cost of edible marine food to the consuming public.

EPILOGUE

This chapter has cited the major agencies in the Federal government which have played in the past and will play in the future major roles in the provision of services and the performance of research and development in realms pertinent to the nutrition-health-aging triad. The large number of mysterious acronyms attached to various departmental agencies and independent agencies suggests the confusion prevalent in the minds of many citizens unschooled in the sometimes Byzantine machinations of the Federal establishment.

In order to assist in directing older American citizens to Federal programs which might be of assistance, Congress established, through the Older Americans Act, as Amended, the Administration on Aging and mandated its functioning via State-level Agencies on Aging which in turn function through regional Area Agencies on Aging within the States. Every American has easy access to such an Area Agency on Aging by telephone if not by personal visit. In addition, the Nutrition Program for Older Americans operates over 12,000 project sites through State Agencies on Aging and Area Agencies on Aging. The Area Agencies on Aging also coordinate the activities of other Federal, State and local agencies for the benefit of older Americans. Because of its very significant role in guiding older Americans through the maze of programs by which they may be aided in time of need, the next chapter will be devoted to an in-depth look at the organization and operations of the Administration on Aging and its various components at the State and intra-State level.

Part IV

PUTTING IT ALL TOGETHER

PROLOGUE

The Administration on Aging (AoA) has the responsibility for and the potential for integrating the social, political, economic and physical sciences, the arts of medicine and the conceptual goals of public health into an agglomerate capable of providing effective and cost-effective approaches to the revolution in thought and process which is now demanded to resolve the problems associated with biologic aging at the end of the twentieth century.

Responsibility and potential without authority delegated by society generate frustration, since they are able to sweep back but a few drops of the onrushing tide of problems. Nonetheless, by building on AoA's structure, personnel, resources and particularly experience, American society has a means of granting to AoA the authority needed to press forward toward solutions. As related in the next chapter, AoA's conceptualization has never changed. Throughout its history, the approaches toward implementing the conceptualization have been altered from time to time by the persons who have held the reins of power.

Given the right of every American to participate in the activities of AoA, the manpower needed by AoA to fulfill the needs of older persons is surely available if it can be mobilized. Given the ample fiscal resources and the needs to which AoA can respond of well over half of older persons in the United States, a blending of their resources with AoA's need-fulfilling talents could resolve financial pressures on AoA programs and give them the authority needed to fulfill their responsibility and potential.

AoA represents opportunity to demonstrate that older persons have the clout to overcome huge problems. In helping the older less fortunate, the older more fortunate can perform miracles for many others but certainly also can derive benefits which will improve dramatically the quality of their own lives. AoA's network is designed to put the sciences, medicine and public health to work by using present knowledge of nutrition, health and aging to work producing lives for older Americans that are happier and more productive. All Americans are welcome to use the AoA network in developing more and better ways of meeting the challenges of growing old.

-15-

The Administration on Aging

Among all Federal departments and independent agencies, one — the Administration on Aging (AoA) — has a Congressionally authorized mandate to implement service programs designed to assist those who are already old. AoA is also mandated to serve as a center for information and for coordination of resources — Federal, State, county, community, nonprofit and private — which may in any way be of benefit to older Americans.

By far the largest Federally funded program administered by AoA (measured either in terms of dollars expended or persons reached) is the Nutrition Program initially authorized by Title VII of the Older Americans Act of 1965, as Amended (P.L. 92-258) and presently comprising the major service function of the newly authorized Title III (P.L. 95-478). The Nutrition Program for Older Americans (NPOA) not only serves meals at over 12,000 sites but also is mandated by its own legislation and regulations and through cooperation with the Area Agencies on Aging initially authorized by Title III of the Older Americans Act (P.L. 93-29) to coordinate delivery of a host of supportive services with the provision of meal services to elderly participants (Figure 1).

Heading the list of supportive services, both in the initial legislation and in the 1978 amendments (which consolidated Titles III, V and VII), is outreach through which those elderly persons most in need of assistance are identified, advised about available services and, when necessary, persuaded to take advantage of the services offered. As needed, escort and transportation services are provided to enable disabled persons and those without accessible personal or public transportation to reach their destinations, be they meal service sites, health

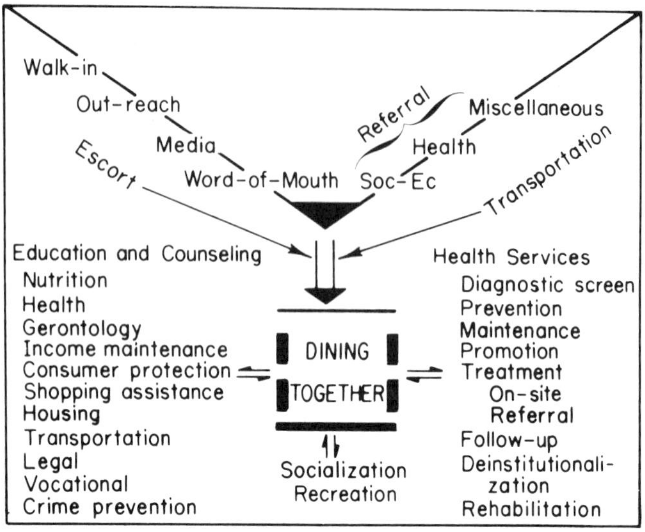

Figure 1: Alpha through omega conceptualization of the Nutrition Program for Older Americans (NPOA) authorized by Title VII (now by Title IIIc) of the Older Americans Act of 1965, as Amended. Reproduced with permission from *Fermented Food Beverages in Nutrition*, edited by C.F. Gastineau, W.J. Darby, and T.B. Turner, a publication of The Nutrition Foundation's Monograph Series, Academic Press, New York, 1979.

care sites, shopping centers, senior citizen centers, etc. NPOA sites serve as centers of gravity drawing participants to locations where meals and the other supportive services may be provided.

Foremost among these services is the delivery of primary health care. This includes diagnostic screening, treatment within the scope of primary care, monitoring of compliance with treatment regimens, health promotion, disease and accident prevention, referral for more sophisticated diagnostic measures as needed, referral for indicated treatment beyond the scope of primary care, referral for any indicated institutional care, provision of community-based services for the care of deinstitutionalized elderly persons and the provision of rehabilitation services when these are indicated and can be provided in a noninstitutional setting. Additional services essential to independent living may be arranged as indicated. These include housekeeping assistance, performance of chores such as shopping and home maintenance and the maintenance of daily contact in person or by telephone with the elderly participant, even when he or she does not attend the meal service site.

The origins of NPOA may be traced back to 1966 when the first meal service site where elderly persons congregated to eat, to socialize and to receive the supportive services then available was implemented in Miami, Florida.[87] The success of this venture was so great that in 1968 Congress authorized the Administration on Aging to set up a nationwide demonstration program comprising over thirty meal service projects.[88] These projects were operated under a variety of environmental, climatic and demographic conditions with the intent of finding out if the Florida experience could be duplicated elsewhere and, if so, what organizational patterns would be most effective and cost-effective. This demonstration program continued through 1971. At that time, the success of almost all of the demonstration projects was so great that the demand for their continuation until they could be absorbed into a larger program of national scope led to annual refunding in 1972 and 1973. The very popularity of these demonstration projects left moot the question of the most effective organizational patterns. In other words, no analysis of the effectiveness or cost-effectiveness of the various methods of administration and management was ever undertaken.

Conceptualization of the present NPOA took shape during the deliberations of the Panel on Aging at the White House Conference on Food, Nutrition and Health from July through December of 1969. Recommendations of the Panel[89] led to the gathering under the sponsorship of the Administration on Aging of a group of experts who, in the summer of 1970, elaborated on the Panel's recommendations.[90] Within a few months legislation was introduced in the House of Representatives by Claude Pepper and in the Senate by Edward Kennedy proposing a national nutrition program for older Americans. After appropriate hearings, committee actions and floor debate, NPOA was authorized by a new Title VII added by the 1972 Amendments to the Older Americans Act. The 1972 Amendments (P.L. 92-258) became law on March 22, 1972 with the signature of the President.

Unfortunately, the appropriation bill funding NPOA failed to pass during the 92nd Congress. In 1973, the Senate of the 93rd Congress attempted to halt the bombing of Cambodia by attaching a rider to the NPOA appropriation. This was not acceptable to the White House. A compromise regarding cessation of the Cambodian bombing was reached and the appropriation bill eventually passed in July, 1973. By the time the funds had been distributed to the States and the Program actually began to function nationwide, September, 1973 had arrived.

The long delay between the authorization in March, 1972 and implementation of the Nutrition Program in September, 1973 proved unfortunate. In that interval, P.L. 93-29, the 1973 Amendments to the Older Americans Act, became law and funds to support it were appropriated, enabling the then new Title III program to be implemented simultaneously with the implementation of the Nutrition Program. This temporal coincidence led to conflicts in priorities at the Central Office of AoA, at the ten DHEW Regional Offices and at the State Offices on Aging. Under the terms of the then new Title III, the State Agencies were directed to divide their States into Planning and Service Areas, to determine for which tasks an area plan would be developed and to designate an Area Agency on Aging to draft, implement and administer a plan for each task. Since such chores were less scientifically complicated than establishing the Nutrition Program, many State agencies put limited resources which should have gone into the employment of trained personnel to implement NPOA into the employment of numbers of generalists whose skills were adequate for implementation of the Title III laws and regulations.

The prolonged delay between authorization and funding of NPOA created an unusual situation best described as an abomination of riches. The FY '73 appropriation and the FY '74 appropriation, each in the amount of $100,000,000, become available simultaneously. Suddenly, AoA was confronted with more funds to implement the Program than could possibly be utilized in a single year by a Program which for lack of prior funding had never gotten off the ground. To resolve this conundrum, a decision was reached by the DHEW Comptroller's Office to put NPOA on what was called forward funding. In other words, the FY '73 appropriation would be used to fund the Program during 1974 and the FY '74 appropriation would be used to fund the Program in 1975. This decision led to considerable confusion at all Program levels in subsequent funding of the NPOA during FY's '76, '77 and '78.

Another part of the fallout from the long interval between authorization and appropriation was the decision in September, 1973 to expand the meal service component of NPOA as rapidly as possible regardless of the readiness of other components. The first evidence of this decision was the issuance of regulations placing a moratorium on the development of supportive services for a period of six months. This meant that outreach, which had originally been planned to bring into NPOA those elderly persons who were in greatest need, whether because of physical or emotional disease or disability or because of economic circumstances, was temporarily suspended. NPOA was opened wide to any persons age 60 or over who might choose to attend meal service sites. Weekly records of the meals served and estimates of the number of minority persons and those in the so-called poverty level were phoned in from projects to State Agencies to Regional Offices and then to the AoA Central Office in Washington. Stress was placed on getting the most possible meals on the table at each of the project sites.

While this method did succeed in producing data showing a rapid expansion of NPOA toward AoA-established objectives in terms of meals served, it also resulted in bringing into NPOA large numbers of persons who were affable, gregarious, well-socialized, healthy, relatively affluent and well-transported. As these individuals gained control of the project site councils and project councils, all of which were required to have participant majorities, subtle devices quickly evolved which tended to keep new recruits to the project sites confined to the same socio-economic strata from which were derived the original participants. With no outreach and no other supportive services mandated during the first six months, the impression spread rapidly that these were not elements of consequence in NPOA. Hence, although the moratorium lasted technically only six months, it lasted in effect for many years.

In spite of this unfortunate beginning, NPOA did expand, did receive sufficient popular support to encourage the Congress to increase the appropriation level each succeeding Fiscal Year, did receive considerable support from State legislatures and from communities in which projects and project sites were located and, finally, did receive from the participants themselves reasonable though small voluntary contributions in cash or food stamps as encouraged by the law and regulations.

Beginning with the 1974 Amendments to the Older Americans Act (P.L. 93-351), the Secretary of Agriculture was required to maintain an annually programmed level of assistance indexed to meals served which began at 10 cents per meal in FY '74. This amount per meal was increased in the 1975 Amendments (P.L. 94-135) to 15 cents during FY '76 and 25 cents during FY '77. The Amendments also provided that the amount per meal should be adjusted annually each Fiscal Year to reflect changes in the series for food away from home of the Consumer Price Index published by the Bureau of Labor Statistics of the Department of Labor. The Amendments also required that the Secretary give special emphasis among the commodities delivered under this subsection of the Act to high protein foods, meat and meat alternatives.

Since the assistance from USDA originally was in the form of food acquired at economy-of-scale-no-middleman prices identical to those paid for food acquired for the School Lunch Program, the true value of the donated food to NPOA projects was appreciably more than the prices of comparable foods purchased on the retail market. Nonetheless, logistic problems in ordering, shipping, receiving and storing the donated foods led many NPOA projects and many State Agencies to demand the cashout of the amount specified by law instead of the delivery of donated foods. Since some States had great success in managing the donated foods, a controversy arose among those favoring cashout and those wishing to continue to receive donated foods. A compromise finally established the system under which a State may determine whether to receive food or cash from USDA and may in fact even receive both cash and food depending on intra-State logistics in regard to delivery and storage of the donated foods.

By 1978, the resources of NPOA had exceeded half a billion dollars. In spite of this remarkable achievement in the short space of 5 years, estimates of need suggested that five times this amount would be required to satisfy the legitimate demands of only those categorized as being in desperate need.

Neither law nor regulations stipulated that NPOA Federal allocations to States be used only to subsidize meals served to elderly congregated at projects sites. However, AoA, after finding Congressional intent in the legislative history of the various Amendments to the Older Americans Act, strongly suggested to States that projects devoting more than 15 per cent of their annual Federally derived allotment to home-delivered meals be investigated to establish clearly whether such home delivery truly was justified. This Congressionally backed AoA policy was based on experiences in the 1966-1973 demonstration programs which revealed greater benefits for elderly persons when they could join their peers for meals, on the availability of funds within project budgets for outreach, escort and transport services to assure that disabled persons could reach meal service sites, and on the extreme cost of providing meal service and other supportive services mandated by the Older Americans Act to elderly persons confined to their own places of residence.

In spite of the logic involved, the demand for a legislatively authorized home-delivered meal phase of NPOA, expressed through lobbyists for already existing but not Federally subsidized home-delivered meal programs, grew rapidly. In the 1978 Amendments to the Older Americans Act (P.L. 95-478), a home-delivered meal phase of NPOA was authorized.

The Comprehensive Older Americans Act Amendments of 1978 (P.L. 95-478) consolidated under an amended Title III the Nutrition (Title VII), Multipurpose Center (Title V) and Social Services (Title III) Programs. Many NPOA project leaders were opposed to this consolidation on the grounds that it put them at the mercy of politically appointed directors of Area Agencies on Aging who might not have an appreciation of the tremendous contributions NPOA had made to the welfare of older Americans. Their arguments were insufficient to overcome the underlying consideration as expressed by a House Committee, *viz.*, to eliminate duplicative and overlapping functions such as outreach, advocacy, needs assessment, planning, staff training and various administrative tasks.[1060] The same House Committee also noted that the consolidation would increase the visibility, political strength and significance of Area Agencies on Aging in the community and would provide for more effective coordination of community resources for the elderly. The Senate Committee on the 1978 Amendments,[1060] in recognition of the opposition to the consolidation, took pains to indicate that in many instances throughout the country NPOA sites and multipurpose senior centers have served effectively as focal points within the community for the delivery of a full range of supportive services. The Senate Committee report urged that each Area Agency in carrying out its plan should take these facts into account and should assure that nutrition services and supportive services are fully integrated. The 1978 Amendments provided a transition period of two years (and necessary waivers permitting longer transition intervals in the event that such were necessary) to allow State and Area Agencies to come into full compliance with the new requirements of the Act.

Also included in the 1978 Amendments was a new Title VI providing for a program of direct grants from AoA's Commissioner to Indian Tribal Organizations. Even though regulations for the Title III and Title VI programs were issued separately, the two programs are closely related. Any eligible Indian Tribal Organization may apply for Federal funding under Title VI but also may continue, if it so desires, to seek funding under Title III. Title III provides that Indian Tribal Organizations may be designated as Area Agencies and gives any Indian Tribal Organization the right of appeal to AoA's Commissioner if its reservation is denied funding in service area status by the State Agency. Any Indian Tribal Organization designated as an Area Agency on Aging receives Older Americans Act Title III funds directly from the Administration on Aging through the State Agency on Aging. Organizations funded under Title VI would function as Area Agencies receiving direct grants from the Federal government. In such a case the State allotment would be reduced based on the number of older Indians funded under Title VI.

In anticipation of the 1978 Amendments, AoA was internally reorganized to reflect the intent of the law and also the desires of a new Commissioner. The reorganization is reflected in Figure 2. While NPOA has disappeared from this table of organization, it has by no means been eliminated from its major role in serving the old and in providing major visibility to AoA. From a conceptual standpoint, the 1978 Amendments afford a means of bringing the performance of NPOA nationally into compliance with the conceptualization originally envisioned by the Panel on Aging of the White House Conference on Food, Nutrition and Health in 1969. That conceptualization is illustrated in Figure 1.

AoA as now structured[1061] provides an appropriate vehicle for the delivery to all older Americans of the health, nutrition and social ser-

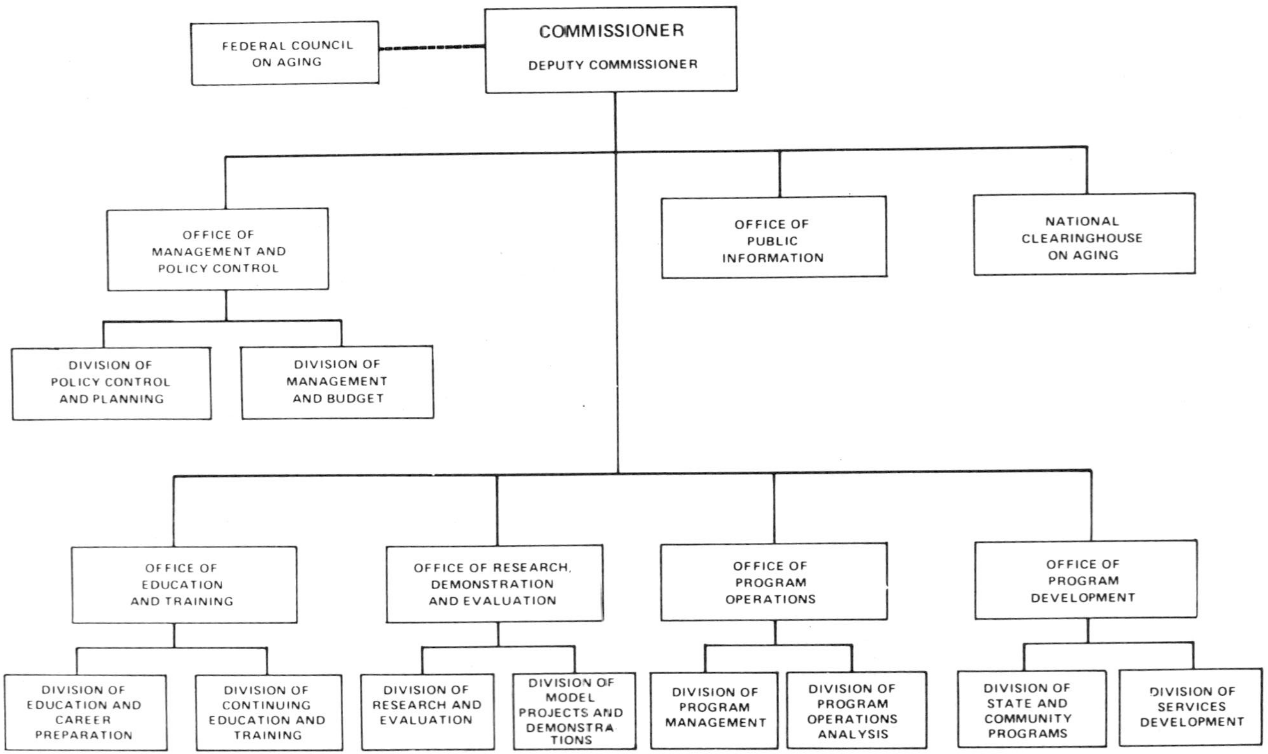

Figure 2: Table of Organization of the Administration on Aging, Office of Human Development Services, Department of Health, Education and Welfare (now Department of Health and Human Services), following the President's signing into law the Comprehensive Older Americans Act Amendments of 1978, P.L. 95-478.

vices of a supportive nature which they may from time to time or on a long-term basis require. Through the present Title III, the conceptualization of NPOA (Figure 1) has become reality in many communities and should be the objective of every community in the nation.[732b] While AoA policy now focuses resources on the impoverished elderly, this is solely because resources are in short supply. All elderly persons may, if they so desire, take advantage of the programs of the AoA national network. Those who can afford to do so should make voluntary contributions to support their local programs. While far from perfect at its present stage of maturation, the AoA network does provide one key by which elderly persons may open the doors leading to healthier, more prosperous and happier lives.[1062]

–Appendix–

Recommended Dietary Allowances (RDAs)

Revised 1980, by the Food and Nutrition Board, Division of Biological Sciences, National Research Council, National Academy of Sciences, Washington, D.C. Reproduced from: *Recommended Dietary Allowances, Ninth Edition* (1980), with the permission of the National Academy of Sciences, Washington, D.C.

FOOD AND NUTRITION BOARD, NATIONAL ACADEMY OF SCIENCES–NATIONAL RESEARCH COUNCIL
RECOMMENDED DAILY DIETARY ALLOWANCES,[a] Revised 1980

Designed for the maintenance of good nutrition of practically all healthy people in the U.S.A.

	Age (years)	Weight (kg)	Weight (lb)	Height (cm)	Height (in)	Protein (g)	Fat-Soluble Vitamins: Vitamin A (μg RE)[b]	Vitamin D (μg)[c]	Vitamin E (mg α-TE)[d]	Water-Soluble Vitamins: Vitamin C (mg)	Thiamin (mg)	Riboflavin (mg)	Niacin (mg NE)[e]	Vitamin B-6 (mg)	Folacin[f] (μg)	Vitamin B-12 (μg)	Minerals: Calcium (mg)	Phosphorus (mg)	Magnesium (mg)	Iron (mg)	Zinc (mg)	Iodine (μg)
Infants	0.0–0.5	6	13	60	24	kg × 2.2	420	10	3	35	0.3	0.4	6	0.3	30	0.5[g]	360	240	50	10	3	40
	0.5–1.0	9	20	71	28	kg × 2.0	400	10	4	35	0.5	0.6	8	0.6	45	1.5	540	360	70	15	5	50
Children	1–3	13	29	90	35	23	400	10	5	45	0.7	0.8	9	0.9	100	2.0	800	800	150	15	10	70
	4–6	20	44	112	44	30	500	10	6	45	0.9	1.0	11	1.3	200	2.5	800	800	200	10	10	90
	7–10	28	62	132	52	34	700	10	7	45	1.2	1.4	16	1.6	300	3.0	800	800	250	10	10	120
Males	11–14	45	99	157	62	45	1000	10	8	50	1.4	1.6	18	1.8	400	3.0	1200	1200	350	18	15	150
	15–18	66	145	176	69	56	1000	10	10	60	1.4	1.7	18	2.0	400	3.0	1200	1200	400	18	15	150
	19–22	70	154	177	70	56	1000	7.5	10	60	1.5	1.7	19	2.2	400	3.0	800	800	350	10	15	150
	23–50	70	154	178	70	56	1000	5	10	60	1.4	1.6	18	2.2	400	3.0	800	800	350	10	15	150
	51 +	70	154	178	70	56	1000	5	10	60	1.2	1.4	16	2.2	400	3.0	800	800	350	10	15	150
Females	11–14	46	101	157	62	46	800	10	8	50	1.1	1.3	15	1.8	400	3.0	1200	1200	300	18	15	150
	15–18	55	120	163	64	46	800	10	8	60	1.1	1.3	14	2.0	400	3.0	1200	1200	300	18	15	150
	19–22	55	120	163	64	44	800	7.5	8	60	1.1	1.3	14	2.0	400	3.0	800	800	300	18	15	150
	23–50	55	120	163	64	44	800	5	8	60	1.0	1.2	13	2.0	400	3.0	800	800	300	18	15	150
	51 +	55	120	163	64	44	800	5	8	60	1.0	1.2	13	2.0	400	3.0	800	800	300	10	15	150
Pregnant						+30	+200	+5	+2	+20	+0.4	+0.3	+2	+0.6	+400	+1.0	+400	+400	+150	*h*	+5	+25
Lactating						+20	+400	+5	+3	+40	+0.5	+0.5	+5	+0.5	+100	+1.0	+400	+400	+150	*h*	+10	+50

[a] The allowances are intended to provide for individual variations among most normal persons as they live in the United States under usual environmental stresses. Diets should be based on a variety of common foods in order to provide other nutrients for which human requirements have been less well defined.

[b] Retinol equivalents. 1 retinol equivalent = 1 μg retinol or 6 μg β carotene.

[c] As cholecalciferol. 10 μg cholecalciferol = 400 IU of vitamin D.

[d] α-tocopherol equivalents. 1 mg d-α-tocopherol = 1 α-TE.

[e] 1 NE (niacin equivalent) is equal to 1 mg of niacin or 60 mg of dietary tryptophan.

[f] The folacin allowances refer to dietary sources as determined by *Lactobacillus casei* assay after treatment with enzymes (conjugases) to make polyglutamyl forms of the vitamin available to the test organism.

[g] The recommended dietary allowance for vitamin B-12 in infants is based on average concentration of the vitamin in human milk. The allowances after weaning are based on energy intake (as recommended by the American Academy of Pediatrics) and consideration of other factors, such as intestinal absorption.

[h] The increased requirement during pregnancy cannot be met by the iron content of habitual American diets nor by the existing iron stores of many women; therefore the use of 30–60 mg of supplemental iron is recommended. Iron needs during lactation are not substantially different from those of nonpregnant women but continued supplementation of the mother for 2–3 months after parturition is advisable in order to replenish stores depleted by pregnancy.

Bibliography

1. World Health Organizaton (1946): Constitution of WHO. Preamble. World Health Organization Geneva, p. 3.
2. Watkin, D.M. (1977): Nutrition and aging. The Nutrition Program for Older Americans: a successful application of current knowledge in nutrition and gerontology. *World Review of Nutrition and Dietetics.* 26:26-40.
3. Genesis V: 21-27 (1859): *The Holy Bible*, Eighth Edition, The American Bible Society, New York.
4. Shaw, G.B. (1947): *Back to Methuselah*, Rev. Ed. Oxford University Press, New York.
5. Dublin, L.I., and Marks, H. (1930): Influence of weight on certain causes of death. *Human. Biol.* 2:159-184.
6. McCay, C.M. (1952): Chemical aspects of aging and the effect of diet upon aging. In: *Cowdry's Problems of Aging*, Third Edition, edited by A.I. Lansing. Williams and Wilkins, Baltimore. pp. 139-202.
7. Ross, M.H. (1969): Aging, nutrition and hepatic enzyme activity patterns in the rat. *J. Nutr.* 97: Suppl. 1:565-601.
8. Bierman, E.L. (1976): Obesity, carbohydrate, and lipid interactions in the elderly. In: *Nutrition and Aging*, edited by M. Winick. John Wiley & Sons, New York. pp. 171-176.
9. Stunkard, A.J. (1976): Nutrition, aging and obesity. In: *Nutrition, Longevity and Aging*, edited by M. Rockstein and M.L. Sussman. The Academic Press, New York. pp. 253-284.
10. Keys, A. (1970): Diets of middle-aged farmers in Japan. *Amer. J. Clin. Nutrition* 23:212-223.
11. Burkitt, D.P. (1973): Some diseases characteristic of modern Western civilization. *Brit. Med. J.* 1:274-278.
12. Leaf, A. (1973): Observations of a peripatetic gerontologist. *Nutr. Today* 8:4-12.
14. Dawber, T.R., Kannel, W.B., and Lyell, L.P. (1963): An approach to longitudinal studies in a community: the Framingham study. *Ann. N.Y. Acad. Sci.* 107:539-556.
15. Murphy, E.A., Thomas, C.B., and Bolling, D.R. (1967): The precursors of hypertension and coronary disease: statistical considerations of distributions in a population of medical students. II. Blood pressure. *Johns Hopkins Med. J.* 120:1-120.
16. Epstein, F.H., Francis, T., Jr., Hayner, N.S., Johnson, B.C., Kjelsberg, M.O., Napier, J.A., Ostrander, L.D., Jr., Payne, M.W., and Dodge, H.J. (1965): Prev-

alence of chronic diseases and distribution of selected physiologic variables in a total community, Tecumseh, Michigan. *Am. J. Epidemiol.* 681:307-322.
17. Bell, B.C., Rose, C.L., and Damon, A. (1972): The normative aging study: an interdisciplinary and longitudinal study of health and aging. *Aging and Human Develop.* 3:5-17.
18. Shock, N.W. (1972): Energy metabolism, Calorie intake and physical activity of the aging. In: *Nutrition in Old Age*, edited by L.A. Carlson. Almquist & Wiksell, Uppsala. pp. 12-23.
19. Panorama de Iberoamerica (1971): Diario las Américas. Miami, Florida. August 6. p. 2.
20. McCay, C.M., Dilley, W.E., and Crowell, T.F. (1929): Growth rates of brook trout reared upon purified rations, upon dry skim milk diets, and upon feed combinations of cereal grains. *J. Nutr.* 1:233-246.
21. McCay, C.M., Crowell, M.F., and Maynard, L.A. (1935): Effect of retarded growth upon length of life span and upon ultimate body size. *J. Nutr.* 10:63-79.
22. McCay, C.M., Maynard, L.A., Sperling, G., and Barnes, L.L. (1939): Retarded growth, life span, ultimate body size and age changes in albino rats after feeding diets restricted in calories. *J. Nutr.* 18:1-13.
23. McCay, C.M., Maynard, L.A., Sperling, G., and Osgood, H.S. (1941): Nutritional requirements during latter half of life. *J. Nutr.* 21:45-60.
24. McCay, C.M., Sperling, G., and Barnes, L.L. (1943): Growth, aging, chronic diseases, and life span in rats. *Arch. Biochem.* 2:469-479.
25. McCay, C.M. (1947): Effect of restricted feeding upon aging and chronic diseases in rats and dogs. *Am. J. Pub. Health* 37:521-528.
26. Widdowson, E.M., and McCance, R.A. (1960): Some effects of accelerating growth. I. General somatic devlopment. *Proc. Roy. Soc. B.* 152:188-206.
27. Berg, B.N., and Simms, H.S. (1960): Nutrition and longevity in the rat. II. Longevity and onset of diseases with different levels of food intake. *J. Nutr.* 71:255-263.
28. Simms, H.S., and Berg, B.N. (1962): Interrelation between longevity, mortality, and the onset of disease. In: *Biological Aspects of Aging*, edited by N.W. Shock. Columbia University Press, New York. pp. 30-34.
29. Berg, B.N., and Simms, H.S. (1962): Relation of nutrition to longevity and onset of disease in rats. In: *Biological Aspects of Aging*, edited by N.W. Shock. Columbia University Press, New York. pp. 35-37.
30. Ross, M.H. (1959): Protein, Calories and life expectancy. *Fed. Proc.* 18:1190-1207.
31. Ross, M.H. (1961): Length of life and nutrition in the rat. *J. Nutr.* 75:197-210.
32. Ross, M.H. (1964): Nutrition, disease and length of life. In: *Diet and Bodily Constitution*, edited by G.E.W. Wolstenholme, and M. O'Conner, J. & A. Churchill, London. pp. 90-107.
33. Ross, M.H. (1972): Length of life and Caloric intake. In: *Symposium on Nutrition and Aging* — Part I, edited by D.M. Watkin. *Am. J. Clin. Nutr.* 25:834-838.
34. Ross, M.H., and Bras, G. (1965): Tumor incidence patterns and nutrition in the rat. *J. Nutr.* 87:245-260.
35. Ross, M.H., and Bras, G. (1973): Influence of protein under- and overnutrition on spontaneous tumor prevalence in the rat. *J. Nutr.* 103:944-963.
36. Ross, M.H., and Bras, G. (1975): Food preference and length of life. *Science* 190:165-167.
37. Watkin, D.M. (1976): Biochemical impact of nutrition on the aging process. In: *Nutrition, Longevity, and Aging*, edited by M. Rockstein and M.L. Sussman. The Academic Press, New York. pp. 47-66.
38. Lutwak, L. (1964): Osteoporosis — a mineral deficiency disease? *J. Am. Diet. Assoc.* 44:173-175.
39. Watkin, D.M., Froeb, H.F., Hatch, F.T., and Gutman, A.B. (1950): Effects of diet in essential hypertension: I. Baseline study: effects in 86 cases of prolonged hospitalization on regular hospital diet. *Amer. J. Med.* 9:428-440.
40. Watkin, D.M., Froeb, H.F., Hatch, F.T., and Gutman, A.B. (1950): Effects of diet in essential hypertension: II. Results with unmodified Kempner rice diet in 50 hospitalized patients. *Amer. J. Med.* 9:441-493.

41. Hatch, F.T., Wertheim, A.R., Eurman, G.H., Froeb, H.F., and Watkin, D.M. (1954): Effects of diet in essental hypertension: III. Alterations in sodium chloride, protein and fat intake. *Amer. J. Med. 17:499-513.*
42. Council on Foods and Nutrition, American Medical Association, Committee on Dietary Fat Levels, Hand, D.B., Chairman (1962): The regulation of dietary fat. *J. Amer. Med. Assoc.* 181:411-429.
43. National Diet Heart Study Research Group with the approval of the Executive Committee on Diet and Heart Disease (1968): The National Diet and Heart Study Final Report. American Heart Association Monograph Number Eighteen. *Circulation* 37: No. 3, supplement No. I, pp. I-1 - I-428.
44. Diet-Heart Panel of the National Heart Institute, E.H. Ahrens, Jr., Chairman (1969): Mass Field Trials and the Diet-Heart Question: their significance, timeliness, feasibility, and applicability. American Heart Association Monograph Number 28. American Heart Association, Inc., New York.
45. Dayton, S., Pearce, M.L., Hashimoto, S., Dixon, W.J., and Tomiyosu, U. (1969): A controlled clinical trial of a diet high in unsaturated fat in preventing complication of atherosclerosis. *Circulation* 40:Supplement II, 1-69.
46. Dayton, S., Chapman, J.M., Pearce, M.L., and Papjak, G.J. (1970): Cholesterol, atherosclerosis, ischemic heart disease, and stroke. *Ann. Int. Med.* 72:97-109.
47. Pearce, M.L., and Dayton, S. (1971): Incidence of cancer in men on a diet high in polyunsaturated fat. *Lancet* 1:464 -467.
48. Goodman, D.S., and Smith, F.R. (1976): Hyperlipidemia, arteriosclerosis, and ischemic heart disease. In: *Nutrition and Aging*, edited by M. Winick. John Wiley & Sons, New York. pp. 177-189.
49. Hazzard, W.R. (1976): Aging and atherosclerosis: Interactions with diet, heredity, and associated risk factors. In: *Nutrition, Longevity, and Aging*, edited by M. Rockstein and M.L. Sussman. Academic Press, New York. pp. 143-195.
50. National Institutes of Health (1977): Nutrition Plan. Office of the Director. National Institutes of Health, Bethesda, Maryland.
51. Wynder, E.L., Lemon, F.R., and Bross, I.J. (1959): Cancer and coronary artery disease among Seventh-day Adventists. *Cancer* 12:1016-1028.
52. Dungal, N. (1961): The special problem of stomach cancer in Iceland with particular reference to dietary factors. *J.A.M.A.* 178:789-798.
53. Doll, R. (1967): Worldwide distribution of gastro-intestinal cancer. In: *Tumors of the Alimentary Tract in Africans.* National Cancer Institute Monograph Number 25. U.S. Government Printing Office, Washington, D.C., pp. 173-190.
54. Wynder, E.L., Kajitani, T., Ishikawa, S., Dodo, H., and Takano, A. (1969): Environmental factors of cancer of the colon and rectum. II. Japanese epidemiological data. *Cancer* 23:1210-1220.
55. Haenszel, W., Berg, J.W., Segi, M., Kurichara, M., and Locke, F.B. (1973): Large-bowel cancer in Hawaiian Japanese. *J. Natl. Cancer Inst.* 51:1765-1779.
56. Breslow, N.E., and Enstrom, J.E. (1974): Geographic correlations between cancer mortality rates and alcohol-tobacco consumption in the United States. *J. Natl. Cancer Inst.* 53:631-639.
57. Burkitt, D.P. (1975): Editorial: Large-bowel cancer; an epidemiologic jigsaw puzzle. *J. Natl. Cancer Inst.* 54:3-6.
58. Lyon, J.L., Klauber, M.R., Gardner, J.W., and Smart, C.P. (1976): Cancer incidence in Mormons and non-Mormons: Utah 1966-1970. *New Eng. J. Med.* 294:129-133.
59. Rhoads, C.P., Castle, W.B., Payne, G.C., and Lawson, H.A. (1934): Observations on the etiology and treatment of anemia associated with hookworm infection in Puerto Rico. *Medicine* 13:317-375.
60. Herbert, V. (1968): Folic acid deficiency in man. In: *Vitamins and Hormones*, Vol. 26. Academic Press, New York. pp. 525-538.
61. Herbert, V. (1973): Section J. Folic acid and vitamin B_{12}. In: *Modern Nutrition in Health and Disease*, Fifth Edition, edited by R.S. Goodhart and M.E. Shils. Lea & Febiger, Philadelphia. pp. 221-244.
62. Horwitt, M.K., Harvey, C.C., Duncan, G.D., and Wilson, W.C. (1956): Symposium on role of some newer vitamins in human metabolism and nutrition; effects of limited tocopherol intake in man with relationships to erythrocyte hemolysis and lipid oxidations. *Am. J. Clin. Nutr.* 4:408-419.

63. Majaj, A.S., Dinning, J.S., Azzam, S.A., and Darby, W.J. (1963): Vitamin E responsive megaloblastic anemia in infants with protein-calorie malnutrition. *Am. J. Clin. Nutr.* 12:374-379.
64. Horrigan, D.L, and Harris, G.W. (1968): Pyridoxine-responsive anemias in man. In: *Vitamins and Hormones*, Vol. 26. Academic Press, New York. pp. 549-571.
65. Lane, M., and Alfrey, C.P. (1965): The anemia of human riboflavin deficiency. *Blood* 25:432-442.
66. Schnegg, A., and Kirchgessner, M. (1976): Zur interaktion von nickel mit eisen, kupfer und zink. *Arch. Tierernaehr* 26:543-549.
67. Hopkins, L.L. Jr., and Mohr, H.E. (1974): Vanadium as an essential nutrient. *Federation Proc.* 33:1773-1775.
68. Wintrobe, M.M. (1967): The erythrocyte. In: *Clinical Hematology*, Sixth Edition. Lea & Febiger, Philadelphia. p. 127.
69. Nielson, F.H., Myron, D.R., Givand, S.H., and Allerick, D.A. (1975): Nickel deficiency and nickel-rhodium interaction in chicks. *J. Nutr.* 105:1607-1619.
70. Drabkin, D.L. (1951): Metabolism of hemin chromoproteins. *Physiol. Rev.* 31:345-431.
71. Victor, M., and Adams, R.D. (1961): On the etiology of the alcoholic neurologic diseases: with special reference to the role of nutrition. *Am. J. Clin. Nutr.* 9:379-397.
72. Victor, M., Adams, R.D., and Collins, G.H. (1971): *The Wernicke-Korsakoff Syndrome.* F.A. Davis Co., Philadelphia. pp. 1-206.
73. Farmer, T.W. (1974): Neurologic complications of vitamin and mineral disorders. In: *Clinical Neurology*, Vol. 3, edited by A.B. Baker, and L.H. Baker. Harper & Row, New York. Chap. 42:1-25.
74. Murphy, F., Srivastava, P.C., Varadi, S., *et al.* (1969): Screening of psychiatric patients for hypovitaminosis B_{12} *Brit. Med. J.* 3:559-560.
75. Batata, M., Sproy, G.H., Bolton, F.G., Higgins, G., and Wollner, L. (1967): Blood and bone marrow changes in elderly patients, with special reference to folic acid, vitamin B_{12}, iron, and ascorbic acid. *Brit. Med. J.* 2:667-669.
76. Elvehjem, C.A. (1940): Relation of nicotinic acid to pellagra. *Physiol. Rev.* 20:249-271.
77. Hartles, R.L. (1967): Carbohydrate consumption and dental caries. *Am. J. Clin. Nutr.* 20:152-156.
78. Zamcheck, N., and Broitman, S.A. (1973): Section B. Nutrition in diseases of the intestine. In: *Modern Nutrition in Health and Disease*, Fifth Edition, edited by R.S. Goodhart and M.E. Shils. Lea & Febiger, Philadelphia. pp. 789-798.
79. Holt, P.R. (1971): Medium chain triglycerides. DM Jun 1-30.
80. Kopple, J.D., Sorensen, M.K., Coburn, J.W., Gordon, S., and Rubini, M.E. (1968): Controlled comparison of 20-g and 40-g protein diets in the treatment of chronic uremia. In: Proceedings of the Conference on the Nutritional Aspects of Uremia, guest editors E.J. Lewis, and J.W. Magill. *Amer. J. Clin. Nutr.* 21:553-564.
81. Watkin, D.M. (1972): Practical solutions to malnutrition in spinal cord dysfunction. *Proceedings of the Eighteenth Veterans Administration Spinal Cord Injury Conference, 1971.* U.S. Government Printing Office. Washington, D.C. pp. 231-233.
82. Yu, T.F., and Gutman, A.B. (1967): Uric acid nephrolithiosis in gout: predisposing factors. *Ann. Intern. Med.* 67:1133-1148.
83. Dayton, S., Chapman, J.M., Pearce, M.L., and Popjak (1970): Cholesterol, atherosclerosis, ischemic heart disease, and stroke. *Ann. Intern. Med.* 72:97-109.
84. Dayton, S., and Pearce, M.L. (1969): Prevention of coronary heart disease and other complications of arteriosclerosis by modified diet. *Amer. J. Med.* 46:751-762.
85. Christakis, G., Rinzler, S.H., Archer, M. and Kraus, A. (1966): Effect of the Anti-Coronary Club program on coronary heart disease. Risk factor status. *J.A.M.A.* 198:597-604.
86. National Council on the Aging (1965): Home-delivered meals for the ill, the handicapped and the elderly. *Amer. J. Pub. Health* 55:May supplement. pp. 1-86.

87. McKibben, G.B. (1966): Dept. HEW/SRS R&D Grant AA-4014 (66-3). National Technical Information Service, Springfield, Virginia.

88. Bechill, W.D., and Wolgamot, I. (1973): Nutrition for the Elderly. Program Highlights of Research and Development Nutrition Projects funded under Title IV of the Older Americans Act of 1965. June 1968 to June 1971. DHEW Publication No. (SRS) 73-20236. U.S. Department of Health, Education and Welfare, Washington, D.C.

89. White House Conference on Food, Nutrition and Health. Final Report and Addendum: (1970): U.S. Government Printing Office, Washington, D.C. pp. 62-64 plus Addendum pp 1-5.

90. Watkin, D.M. (1970): A year of developments in nutrition and aging. *Med. Clin. North Amer.* 54:1589-1597.

91. Reifenstein, E.C., Jr., Albright, F., and Wells, S.L. (1945): Accumulation, interpretation and presentation of data pertaining to metabolic balances, notably those of calcium, phosphorus and nitrogen. *J. Clin. Endocrinology* 5:367-395; correcton 6:232, 1946.

92. Food and Nutrition Board (1974): Recommended Dietary Allowances, Eighth Edition. National Academy of Sciences, Washington, D.C.

92a. Food and Nutrition Board (1980): Recommended Dietary Allowances, Ninth Edition. National Academy of Sciences, Washington, D.C.

93. Lintz, L.P. (1976): Weber County Health Screening Project: Senior Citizens Health Screening Report. Weber County Department on Aging. Ogden, Utah. pp. 49.

94. Watkin, D.M., Katz, M., Shock, N.W., Todhunter, N., and Wilcox, J. (1973): Nutritional assessment of the elderly. In: *Nutritional Assessment in Health Programs*, edited by G. Christakis. *Amer. J. Public Health* 63: November Supplement. pp. 68-75.

95. Roe, D.A. (1976): *Drug-induced Nutritional Deficiencies.* A.V.I. Publishing Company, Westport, Connecticut. pp. 272.

96. Dudrick, S.J. (1972): Parenteral hyperalimentation. *Ann. Surg.* 176:259-264.

97. Eagleton, T.F., and Hathaway, W.D., Cochairmen (1976): Alcohol and Drug Abuse Among the Elderly, Joint Hearings before the Subcommittee on Aging and the Subcommittee on Alcoholism and Narcotics of the Committee on Labor and Public Welfare, United States Senate, June 7. U.S. Government Printing Office, Washington, D.C.

98. Bosse, R., Costa, P., Cohen, M., and Podolsky, S. (1975): Age, smoking inhalation, and pulmonary function. *Arch. Environ. Health* 30:495-498.

99. U.S. Department of Health, Education and Welfare (1972): Ten State Nutrition Survey, 1968-1970. V-Dietary. DHEW Publication No. (HSM) 72-8133. Center for Disease Contol, Atlanta, GA. pp. V1-V-340.

100. McWhirter, N. (1980): *The Guinness Book of World Records*, Bantam Books, New York. pp. 25-29.

101. Watkin, D.M. (1973): Nutrition for the aging and the aged. In: *Modern Nutrition in Health and Disease, Fifth Edition*, edited by R.S. Goodhart and M.E. Shils. Lea & Febiger, Philadelphia. p. 681.

101a. Levy, R.I. (1977): Statement of Robert I. Levy, M.D., Director, National Heart, Lung and Blood Institute. In: Diet Related to Killer Diseases. II. Hearings before the Select Committee on Nutrition and Human Needs of the United States Senate, G. McGovern, Chairman. Committee Print No. 83-693 O, U.S. Government Printing Office, Washington, D.C.

101b. Havlik, R.J., and Feinlieb, M. Editors. (1979): *Proceedings of the Conference on the Decline of Coronary Heart Disease Mortality.* U.S. Department of Health, Education and Welfare, Washington, D.C.

101c. Stallones, R.A. (1980): The rise and fall of ischemic heart disease. *Sci. Amer.* 243:53-59.

101d. Moment, G.B. (1978): The Ponce de Leon trail today. In: *The Biology of Aging*, edited by J.A. Behnke, C.E. Finch and G.B. Moment. Plenum Press, New York. pp. 1-17.

101e. Watkin, D.M. (1982): The physiology of aging. *Amer. J. Clin. Nutrition* 36:750-758.

101f. Watkin, D.M. (1983): Aging, nutrition and health. *Resident & Staff Physician* (In preparation).

101g. Linn, M.W., Linn, B.S., and Gurel, L. (1967): Physical resistance of the aged. *Geriatrics* 22:134-138.

101h. Linn, B.S., Linn, M.W., and Gurel, L. (1968): Cumulative illness rating scale. *J. Amer. Geriatrics Soc.* 16:622-626.

101i. Linn, B.S. (1968) Viewpoint: a personal opinion on progress in care of the aged. Elite physical resistance seen as key to longevity. *Geriatrics* 23 (4):48, 55, 58.

101j. Linn, B.S., Linn, M.W., and Gurel, L. (1969): Physical resistance and longevity. *Gerontol. Clin. (Basel)* 11:362-370.

101k. Belloc, N.B. and Breslow, L. (1972): Relationship of physical health status and health practices. *Preventive Med.* 1:409-421.

101l. Gompertz, B. (1825): On the nature of the function expressive of the law of human mortality. *Phil. Trans.* A 115:513-585.

101m. Upton, A.C. (1977): Pathobiology. In: *Handbok of the Biology of Aging*, edited by C.E. Finch and L. Hayflick. Van Nostrand Reinhold Company, New York. pp. 513-535.

101n. Belloc, N.B. (1973): Relationship of health practices and mortality. *Preventive Med.* 2:67-81.

102. Medvedev, Zh. A. (1974): Caucasus and Altay longevity: a biological or social problem? *Gerontologist* 14:381-387.

103. Hayflick, L. (1965): The limited *in vitro* life time of human diploid cell strains. *Exp. Cell. Res.* 25:285-621.

104. Hayflick, L. and Moorhead, P.S. (1961): The serial cultivation of human diploid cell strains. *Exp. Cell. Res.* 25:585-621.

105. Martin, G.M., Sprague, C.A., and Epstein, C.J. (1970): Replicative life span of cultivated human cells. Effects of donor's age, tissue, and genotype. *Lab. Invest.* 23:36-92.

106. Cristofolo, V.J. (1976): A model system approach to the biology of aging. In: *Nutrition and Aging,* edited by M. Winick. John Wiley & Sons, New York. pp. 3-22.

107. Medvedev, Zh. A. (1962): Aging at the molecular level and some speculations concerning maintaining the functioning of systems for replicating specific macromolecules. In: *Biologic Aspects of Aging,* edited by N.W. Shock. Columbia University Press, New York. pp. 255-266.

108. Brooks, A.L., Mead, D.K., and Peters, R.F. (1973): Effect of aging on the frequency of metaphase chromosome aberrations in the liver of Chinese hamsters. *J. Gerontology* 28:452-454.

109. Harman, D. (1968): Free radical theory of aging: effect of free radical reaction inhibitors on the mortality rate of male LAF mice. *J. Gerontology* 23:476-482.

110. Pocher, L., Deamer, D.W., and Heath, R.L. (1967): Regulation and deterioration of structure in membranes. In: *Advances in Gerontological Research*, Volume 2, edited by B.L Strehler. Academic Press, New York. pp. 77-120.

111. Gordon, P. (1974): Free radicals and the aging process. In: *Theoretical Aspects of Aging,* edited by M. Rockstein. Academic Press, New York. pp. 61-81.

112. José. D.G., and Good, R.A. (1973): Quantitative effects of nutritional essential amino acid deficiency upon immune responses to tumors in mice. *J. Exptl. Med.* 137:1-9.

113. Walford, R.L., Liu, R.K., Gerbase-DeLima, M., Methies, M., and Smith, G.S. (1973-74): Long-term dietary restriction and immune function in mice; response to sheep red blood cells and to mitogenic agents. *Mechan. Aging & Develop.* 2:447-454.

114. Teller, M.N. (1972): Interrelationships among aging, immunity and cancer. In: *Tolerance, Autoimmunity and Aging,* edited by M.M. Segel and R.A. Good. Charles C. Thomas, Springfield, Illinois. pp. 18-32.

115. Adelman, R.C. (1976): Age-dependent hormonal regulation of mammalian gene expression. In: *Hypothalamus, Pituitary and Aging,* edited by A.V. Everitt and J.A. Burgess. Charles C. Thomas, Springfield, Illinois. pp. 668-675.

116. Liu, R.K., and Walford, R.L. (1975): Mid-life temperature-transfer effects on lifespan of annual fish. *J. Gerontology* 30:129-131.

117. Schmeck, H.M., Jr. (1977): Scientists fear bid to regulate genetic studies. *New York Times, February 20. p. 30.*
118. Verzar, F. (1963): The aging of collagen. *Sci. Amer.* 208:104-114.
119. Takacs, I., and Verzar, F. (1968): Macromolecular aging of collagen. I. Experiments *in vivo* and *in vitro* with different animal races. *Gerontologia* 14:15-34.
120. Hrůza, Z., Fábry, P., Chvapil, M., and Holecková, E. (1962): Adaptation to undernutrition and trauma and influence of undernutrition on biological age. In: *Medical and Clinical Aspects of Aging,* edited by H.T. Blumenthal. Columbia University Press, New York. pp. 45-52.
121. Holecková, E., Chytil, F., and Chvapil, M. (1961): (Effect of domestication on the biological age of rats). *Cas Lek. Ces.* 100:612-616.
122. Chvapil, M., and Holecková, E. (1962): Lowered structural stability of collagenous fibers induced by intermittent feeding and fasting in the rat. *Physiol. Bohemoslov.* 11:505-509.
123. Bjorksten, J. (1968): The crosslinkage theory of aging. *J. Amer. Geriat. Soc.* 16:408-427.
124. Piez, K.A. (1969): Chemistry of collagen and elastin and biosynthesis of covalent cross links. In: *Aging of Connective and Skeletal Tissue,* edited by Engel, A., and Larsson, T. Nordiska Bokhandelns Förlag, Stockholm. pp. 15-32.
125. Verzar, F. (1968): Intrinsic and extrinsic factors of molecular aging. *Exp. Gerontol.* 3:69-75.
126. Piez, K.A. (1968): Cross-linking of collagen and elastin. *Ann. Rev. Biochem.* 37:547-570.
127. Von Hahn, H.P., and Fritz, E. (1966): Age-related alterations in the structure of DNA. III. Thermal stability of rat liver DNA, related to age, histone content and ionic strength. *Gerontologia* 12:237-250.
128. Harman, D. (1972): Free radical theory of aging: dietary implications. In: *Symposium on Nutrition and Aging. Part I.,* edited by D.M. Watkin, *Amer. J. Clin. Nutrition* 25:839-843.
129. Couch, R.B., Watkin, D.M., Smith, R.R., Rosenberg, L.E., Winitz, M., Birnbaum, S.M., Otey, M.C., and Greenstein, J.P. (1960): Clinical trials of water-soluble chemically defined diets. *Federation Proc.* 19:13 (abstract).
130. Schwarz, K. (1970): An agent promoting growth of rats fed amino acid diets (Factor G). *J. Nutrition* 100:1487-1500.
131. Spiller, G.A., and Amen, R.G. (Editors) (1976): *Fiber in Human Nutrition.* Plenum Press, New York.
132. FAO/WHO (Food and Agriculture Organization/World Health Organization). (1973): Energy and protein requirements. Report of a joint FAO/WHO *ad hoc* Expert Committee. WHO Tech. Rept. Ser. No. 522; FAO Nutrition Meetings Report Series 52. WHO, Geneva. pp. 1-118.
133. National Association for Human Development (1976): Final evaluation report: health education and fitness activity program for older persons. Administration on Aging, DHEW. Washington, D.C., pp. 1-22.
134. Astrand, I., Astrand, P., Hallbock, I., and Kilhom, A. (1973): Reduction in maximal oxygen uptake with age. *J. Applied Physiol.* 35:649-654.
135. Drinkwater, B.L., Horvath, S.M., and Wells, C.L. (1975): Aerobic power of females, ages 10 to 68. *J. Gerontol.* 30:385-394.
136. Kountz, W.B., Hofstatter, L., and Ackerman, P.G. (1947): Nitrogen balance studies in elderly people. *Geriatrics* 2:173-182.
137. Kountz, W.B., Hofstatter, L., and Ackerman, P.G. (1948): Nitrogen balance studies under prolonged high nitrogen intake levels in elderly individuals. *Geriatrics* 3:171-184.
138. Kountz, W.B., Hofstatter, L., and Ackermann, P.G. (1951): Nitrogen balance studies in four elderly men. *J. Gerontology* 6:20-33.
139. Kountz, W.B., Ackermann, P.G., Kheim, T., and Toro, G. (1953): Effects of increased protein intake in older people. *Geriatrics* 8:63-69.
140. Schulze, W. (1954): Untersuchungen uber den Eiweiss-Stoffwechsel im Alter. *Altersforsch.* 8:65-75.
141. Schulze, W. (1955): Protein metabolism and requirement in old age. In: *Old Age in the Modern World,* 3rd Congr. Internat. Assoc. Gerontol., London, 1954. E & S Livingstone, Ltd., London. pp. 122-127.

142. Watkin, D.M., Froeb, H.F., Hatch, F.T., and Gutman, A.B. (1950): Effects of diet in essential hypertension: results with unmodified Kempner rice diet in 50 hospitalized patients. *Am. J. Med.* 9:485-486.
143. Bogdonoff, M.D., Shock, N.W., and Nichols, M.P. (1953): Calcium, phosphorus, nitrogen and potassium balance studies in the aged male. *J. Gerontology* 8:272-288.
144. Horwitt, M. (1953): Dietary requirements of the aged. *J. Am. Dietet. Assoc.* 29:443-448.
145. Watkin, D.M. (1964): Protein metabolism and requirements in the elderly. In: *Mammalian Protein Metabolism,* Volume II, edited by H.N. Munro and J.B. Allison. Academic Press, New York. pp. 248-249.
146. Watkin, D.M. (1966): The impact of nutrition on the biochemistry of aging in man. Eighth Annual Ciba Foundation Lecture on Research on Aging, Glasgow, 1964. *World Rev. Nutrition and Dietetics,* 6:124-164. S. Karger, New York. pp. 137-139.
147. Watkin, D.M. (1966): Nutrition and aging. In: *Nutrition: a Comprehensive Treatise,* Volume III, edited by G.H. Beaton and E.W. McHenry. Academic Press, New York. pp. 160-162.
148. Watkin, D.M. (1973): Nutrition for the aging and the aged. In: *Modern Nutrition in Health and Disease, Fifth Edition,* edited by R.S. Goodhart and M.E. Shils. Lea & Febiger, Philadelphia. pp. 689-691.
149. McCoy, R.H., Meyer, C.E., and Rose, W.C. (1935). Feeding experiments with mixtures of highly purified amino acids; isolation and identification of a new essential amino acid. *J. Biol. Chem.* 112:283-302.
150. Rose, W.C., Oesterling, M.J., and Womack, M. (1948). Comparative growth on diets containing ten and 19 amino acids, with further observations upon the role of glutamic and aspartic acids. *J. Biol. Chem.* 176:753-762.
151. Rose, W.C., Smith, L.C., Womack, M., and Shane, M. (1949). Utilization of nitrogen of ammonium salts, urea, and certain other compounds in synthesis of nonessential amino acids *in vivo. J. Biol. Chem.* 181:307-316.
152. Rose, W.C. (1949). Amino acid requirements of man. *Federation Proc.* 5:546-552.
153. Rose, W.C. (1957). The amino acid requirements of adult man. *Nutr. Abstr. Rev.* 27:631-647.
154. Leverton, R.M. (1959). Amino acid requirements of young adults. In: *Protein and Amino Acid Nutrition,* edited by A.A. Albanese. Academic Press, New York, pp. 477-505.
155. Holt, L.E., Jr., and Snyderman, S.E. (1956): *Some Aspects of Amino Acid Supplementation.* Rutgers University Press, New Brunswick, New Jersey.
156. Mertz, E.T., Baxter, E.J., Jackson, L.E., Roderick, C.E., and Weis, A. (1952): Essential amino acids in self-selected diets of older women. *J. Nutrition* 46:313-322.
157. Albanese, A.A., Higgons, R.A., Orto, L.A., and Zavattaro, D.N. (1957): Protein and amino acid needs of the aged in health and convalescence. *Geriatrics* 12:465-475.
158. Tuttle, S.G., Swendseid, M.E., Mulcare, D., Griffith, W.H., and Bassett, S.H. (1957): Study of the essential amino acid requirements of men over fifty. *Metabolism* 6:564-573.
159. Watts, J.H., Mann, A.N., Bradley, L., and Thompson, (1964): Nitrogen balances of men over 65 fed the FAO and milk patterns of essential amino acids. *J. Gerontology* 19:370-374.
160. Tuttle, S.G., Swendseid, M.E., and Bassett, S.H. (1960): Methionine requirements of men over sixty. *Federation Proc.* 19:11 (abstract).
161. Tuttle, S.G. Swendseid, M.E., Mulcare, D., Griffith, W.H., and Bassett, S.H. (1959): Essential amino acid requirements of older men in relation to total nitrogen intake. *Metabolism* 8:61-72.
162. Swendseid, M.E., Feeley, R.J., Harris, C.L., and Tuttle, S.G. (1959): Egg protein as a source of the essential amino acids: requirement for nitrogen balance in young adults studied at two levels of nitrogen intake. *J. Nutrition* 68:203-211.
163. Tuttle, S.G., Bassett, S.H., Griffith, W.H., Mulcare, D., and Swendseid, M.E. (1965): Further observations on the amino acid requirements of older men. I.

Effects of nonessential nitrogen supplements fed with different amounts of essential amino acids. *Am. J. Clin. Nutr.* 16:225-228.

164. Swendseid, M.E., and Tuttle, S.G. (1961): In: *Progress in Meeting Protein Needs of Infants and Preschool Children.* Publ. No. 843, National Acad. Sci., National Research Council, Washington, D.C. p. 323.
165. Tuttle, S.G., Bassett, S.H., Griffith, W.H., Mulcare, D., and Swendseid, M.E. (1965): Further observations on the amino acid requirements of older men. II. Methionine and lysine. *Am. J. Clin. Nutr.* 16:229-231.
166. Reynolds, M.S., Steel, D.L., Jones, E.M., and Baumann, C.A. (1958): Nitrogen balances of women maintained on various levels of methionine and cystine. *J. Nutrition* 64:99-111.
167. Tontisirin, K., Young, V.R., Miller, M., and Scrimshaw, N.S. (1973): Plasma tryptophan response curve and tryptophan requirements of elderly people. *J. Nutrition* 103:1220-1228.
168. Young, V.R., Hussein, M.A. Murray, E., and Scrimshaw, N.S. (1971): Plasma tryptophan response curve and its relation to tryptophan requirements in young adult men. *J. Nutrition* 101:45-59.
169. Tontisirin, K., Young, V.R., Rand, W.M., and Scrimshaw, N.S. (1974): Plasma threonine response curve and threonine requirements of young men and elderly women. *J. Nutrition* 104:495-505.
170. Young, V.R., Perera, W.D., Winterer, J.C., and Scrimshaw, N.S. (1976): Protein and amino acid requirements of the elderly. In: *Nutrition and Aging,* edited by M. Winick. John Wiley and Sons, New York. pp. 77-118.
171. Young, V.R. (1976): Protein metabolism and needs in elderly people. In: *Nutrition, Longevity and Aging,* edited by M. Rockstein and M.L. Sussman. Academic Press, New York. pp. 67-102.
172. Scrimshaw, N.S., and Young, V.R. (1976): The requirements of human nutrition. *Scientific American* 235:50-64.
173. Watkin, D.M., Parsons, J.M., Yiengst, M.J., and Shock, N.W. (1955): Metabolism in the aged: the effect of stanolone on the retention of nitrogen, potassium, phosphorus, and calcium and on the urinary excretion of 17-keto, 11-oxy, and 17-hydroxy steroids in eight elderly men on high and low protein diets. *J. Gerontology* 10:268-287.
174. Watkin, D.M. (1958): The assessment of protein nutrition in aged man, *Ann. N.Y. Acad. Sci.* 69:902-913.
175. Watkin, D.M., Silverstone, F.A., and Shock, N.W. (1965): The effect of abrupt changes in dietary protein on metabolic and renal parameters in old and middle-aged men. *Federation Proc.* 24:629 (abstract).
176. Watkin, D.M. (1973): Nutrition for the aging and the aged. In: *Modern Nutrition in Health and Disease,* Fifth Edition, edited by R.S. Goodhart and M.E. Shils. Lea & Febiger, Philadelphia. p. 690.
177. Couch, R.B., Watkin, D.M., Smith, R.R., Rosenberg, L.E., Winitz, M., Birnbaum, S.M., Otey, M.C., and Greenstein, J.P. (1960): Clinical trials of water-soluble, chemically defined diets. *Federation Proc.* 19:13 (abstract).
178. Watkin, D.M. (1961): Nitrogen balance as affected by neoplastic disease and its therapy. *Am. J. Clin. Nutr.* 9:446-460.
179. Shaffer, P.A., and Coleman, W. (1909): Protein metabolism in typhoid fever. *A.M.A. Arch. Int. Med.* 4:538-600.
180. Coleman, W., and DuBois, E.F. (1914): The influence of the high calorie diet on the respiratory exchanges in typhoid fever. *Arch. Int. Med.* 14:168-209.
181. DuBois, E.F. (1922): Metabolism in fever and in certain infections. In: *Endocrinology and Metabolism,* Vol. 4, edited by L.F. Barker. Appleton, New York.
182. Davies, D.F., and Shock, N.W. (1950): Age changes in glomerular filtration rate, effective renal plasma flow, and tubular excretory capacity in adult males. *J. Clin. Invest.* 29:496-507.
183. Watkin, D.M., and Shock, N.W. (1955): Agewise standard value for C_{IN}, C_{PAH}, and TM_{PAH} in adult males. *J. Clin. Invest.* 34:969 (abstract).
184. Giovanetti, S., and Maggione, O. (1964): A low-nitrogen diet with proteins of high biological value for severe chronic uremia. *The Lancet* 1:1000-1003.
185. Senior, J.R., Van Itallie, T.B., and Greenberger, N.J. Editors (1968): *Medium Chain Triglycerides,* University of Pennsylvania Press, Philadelphia.

186. Greenberger, N.J., and Skillman, T. (1969): Medium chain triglycerides. *New Engl. J. Med.* 280:1045-1058.
187. Sinclair, H.M. (1964): Carbohydrates and fats. In: *Nutrition: A Comprehensive Treatise, Volume I,* edited by G.H. Beaton and E.W. McHenry. Academic Press, New York, pp. 96-105.
188. Karlson, P. (1963): Nutrition and vitamins. In: *Introduction to Modern Biochemistry,* Academic Press, New York, pp. 377-378.
189. Feeley, R.M., Criner, P.E., and Watt, B.K. (1972): Cholesterol content of foods. *J. Amer. Diet. Assoc.* 61:131-149.
190. Coburn, A.F. (1963): The pathogenesis of rheumatic fever — a concept. *Perspectives in Biology and Medicine* 6:493-511.
191. Rubner, M. (1902): *Die Gesetze des Energieverbrauchs bei der Ernahrung.* Deutiche. Leipzig.
192. Forbes, E.B., and Swift, R.W. (1944): Associative dynamic effects of protein, carbohydrate and fat. *J. Nutrition* 27:453-468.
193. Forbes, E.B., Swift, R.W., Elliott, R.F., and James, W.H. (1946): Relation of fat to economy of food utilization by growing albino rat. *J. Nutrition* 31:203-212.
194. Forbes, E.B., Swift, R.W., Thacker, E.J., Smith, V.F., and French, C.E. (1946): Further experiments of relation of fat to economy of food utilization by the growing albino rat. *J. Nutrition* 32:387-396.
195. Forbes, E.B., Swift, R.W., Thacker, E.J., Smith, V.F., and French, C.E. (1946): Further experiments of relation of fat to economy of food untilization by mature albino rat. *J. Nutrition* 32:397-403.
196. Burr, G.O., and Burr, M.M. (1929): New deficiency disease produced by rigid exclusion of fat from diet. *J. Biol. Chem.* 82:345-367.
197. Sinclair, H.M. (1958): Essential fatty acids and the skin. *Brit. Med. Bull.* 14:258-262.
198. Norby, J.G. (1965): Effects of giving a fat-free diet for up to 10 weeks on the male weanling rat. *Brit. J. Nutr.* 19:209-224.
199. Hansen, A.E., Wiese, H.F., Boelsche, A.N., Haggard, M.E., Adam, D.J.D., and Davis, H. (1963): Role of linoleic acid in infant nutrition. *Pediatrics* 31:171-192.
200. Ramalingaswami, V., and Sinclair, H.M. (1953): Relation of deficiencies of vitamin A and of essential fatty acids to follicular hyperkeratosis in the rat. *Brit. J. Dermatol.* 65:1-22.
201. Bagchi, K., Halder, K., and Chowdbury, S.R. (1959): The etiology of phrynoderma; histologic evidence. *Am. J. Clin. Nutr.* 7:251-258.
202. Kinsell, L.W., Patridge, J., Boling, L., Margen, S., and Michaels, G. (1952): Dietary modification of serum-cholesterol and phospho-lipid levels. *J. Clin. Endocrinol.* 12:909-913.
203. Alfin-Slater, R.B., Aftergood, L., Wells, A.F., and Devel, H.J. Jr. (1954): The effect of essential fatty acid deficiency on the distribution of endogenous cholesterol in the plasma and liver of the rat. *Arch. Biochem. Biophysics* 52:180-185.
204. Van Dorp, D.A., Beerthuis, R.K., Nugteren, D.H., and Vonkeman, H. (1964): The biosynthesis of prostaglandins. *Biochim. Biophys. Acta* 90:204-207.
205. Bergstrom, S., Danielsson, H., and Samuelsson, B. (1964): The enzymatic formation of prostaglandin E_2 from arachidonic acid. *Biochim. Biophys. Acta* 90:207-210.
206. Van Dorp, D.A., Beerthuis, R.K., Nugteren, D.H., and Vonkeman, H. (1964): Enzymatic conversion of all-cis-polyunsaturated fatty acids into prostaglandins. *Nature* 203:839-841.
207. Alfin-Slater, R.B., and Aftergood, L. (1973): Fats and other lipids. In: *Modern Nutrition in Health and Disease,* edited by R.S. Goodhart and M.E. Shils. Lea and Febiger, Philadelphia, pp. 136-137.
208. Patel, N. (1970): Prostaglandins: newest of the hormones? (editorial). *Ann. Internal Med.* 73:483-485.
209. Hertelendy, F., Todd, H., Ehrhart, K., and Blute, R. (1972): Studies on growth hormone secretion: IV. In vivo effects of prostaglandin E_1. *Prostaglandins* 2:79-91.

210. Dukes, P.P., Shore, N.A., Hammond, D., Ortega, J.A., and Datta, M.C. (1973): Enhancement of erythropoiesis by prostaglandins. *J. Lab. Clin. Med.* 82:704-712.
211. Sylven, C., and Borgstrom, B. (1969): Intestinal absorption and lymphatic transport of cholesterol in the rat: influence of the fatty acid chain length of the carrier triglyceride. *J. Lipid Res.* 10:351-355.
212. Swell, L., Flick, D.F., Field, H. Jr., and Treadwell, C.R. (1955): Role of fat and fatty acid in absorption of dietary cholesterol. *Am. J. Physiol.* 180:124-128.
213. Ivy, A.C., Karvinen, E., Lin, T.M., and Ivy, E.K. (1957): Some parameters of sterol metabolism in man on a sterol-free and fat-free diet. *J. Appl. Physiol.* 11:1-7.
214. Wilson, J.D., and Lindsey, C.A. (1965): Studies on the influence of dietary cholesterol on cholesterol metabolism in the isotopic steady state in man. *J. Clin. Invest.* 44:1805-1814.
215. Borgström, B. (1967): Comments on a paper by J. Wilson, "The influence of dietary cholesterol on cholesterol metabolism," In: *Proceedings of the 1967 Deuel Conference on Lipids,* edited by G.R. Cowgill and L.W. Kinsell. U.S. Government Printing Office, Washington, D.C. p. 63-66.
216. Keys, A. (1965): Diet and Coronary Heart Disease. In: *World Trends in Cardiology: Cardiovascular Epidemiology,* Vol., 1, edited by A. Keys and P.D. White. Harper & Row, New York p. 135.
217. Cantorow, A., and Schepartz, B. (1962): Metabolism of lipids. In: *Biochemistry, Third Edition.* W.B. Saunders Company, Philadelphia. pp. 489-492.
218. Siperstein, M.D., and Fagan, V.M., (1966): Feedback control of mevalonate synthesis by dietary cholesterol. *J. Biol. Chem.* 241:602-609.
219. Bhattathiry, E.P., and Siperstein, M.D. (1963): Feedback control of cholesterol synthesis in man. *J. Clin. Invest.* 42:1613-8.
220. Fujiwara, T., Hirono, H., and Arakawa, T. (1965): Idiopathic hypercholesterolemia: demonstration of an impaired feedback control of cholesterol synthesis *in vivo. Tohoku J. Expotl. Med.* 87:155-67.
221. Miettinen, T.A. (1970): Detection of changes in human cholesterol metabolism. *Ann. Clin. Res.* 2:300-20.
222. Nestel, P.J. (1970): Cholesterol turnover in man. *Adv. Lipid Res.* 8:1-39.
223. Mann, G.V., and Spoerry, A. (1974): Studies of a surfactant and cholesteremia in the Massai. *Amer. J. Clin. Nutrition* 27:464-2169.
224. Mann, G.V., Geyer, R.P., Watkin, D.M., and Stare, F.J. (1949): Parenteral Nutrition IX, Fat emulsion for intravenous nutrition in man. *J. Lab. & Clin. Med.* 34:699-712.
225. Patek, A.J., Jr., and Post, J. (1941): Treatment of cirrhosis of liver by nutritious diet and supplements rich in Vitamin B complex. *J. Clin. Invest.* 20:481-505.
226. Davidson, C.S. (1973): Section D, Diseases of the liver. In: Chapter 28, Nutrition in diseases of the gastrointestinal tract. In: *Modern Nutrition in Health and Disease,* edited by R.S. Goodhart and M.E. Shils. Lea and Febiger, Philadelphia. p. 838.
227. DuVigneaud, V. (1942-1943): The significance of labile methyl groups in the diet and their relation to trans-methylation. *Harvey Lecture* 38:39-62.
228. Artom, C., and Swanson, M.A. (1948): On absorption of phospholipides. *J. Biol. Chem.* 175:871-881.
229. Blomstrand, R. (1955): Intestinal absorption of phospholipids in rat. *Acta. Physiol. Scandanav.* 34:147-157.
230. Stein, Y., and Stein, O. (1966): Metabolism of labeled lysolecithin, lysophosphatidyl ethanolamine and lecithin in the rat. *Biochim. Biophys. Acta.* 116:95-107.
231. Select Committee on Nutrition and Human Needs of the United States Senate (1977): *Dietary Goals for the United States. Second Edition.* U.S. Government Printing Office, Washington, D.C. Stock No. 052-070-04376-8.
232. Friend, B. (1974): *Changes in Nutrients in the U.S. Diet Caused by Alterations in Food Intake Patterns.* Agricultural Research Service, U.S. Department of Agriculture, Washington, D.C.
233. Friend, B. (1967): Nutrients in United States food supply. Review of trends, 1909-13 to 1965. *Amer. J. Clin. Nutrition* 20:907-914.

234. Rizek, R.L., Friend, B., Page, L. (1974): Agricultural Research Service, Consumer & Food Economics Institute, Hyattsville. Fat in today's food supply level of use and sources. *J. Amer. Oil Chemist's Soc.* 41(6): 244-250.
235. Morgan, D. (1977): The hamburger society and America's love affair with beef. *Washington Post,* February 2, p. A12.
236. Morgan, D. (1977): Cattle feedlots in economic pincer. *Washington Post,* January 31, p. A1.
237. Vergroesen, A.J. (1976): Physiologic effects of dietary linoleic acid. Hearing on nutrition information in food advertising. Federal Trade Commission, Washington, D.C.
238. Harper, J.M., Jansen, G.R., Shigetomi, C.T., Frey, A.L., and Fallis, L.K. (1975): *Nutrient Standard Method (NSM): Menu Planning and Menu Monitoring.* Administration on Aging, DHEW, Washington, D.C. pp. 1-128.
239. Connor, W.F., and Conner, S.L. (1972): The key role of nutritional factors in the prevention of coronary heart disease. *Prev. Med.* 1:49-83.
240. Armstrong, B., and Doll, R. (1975): Environmental factors and cancer incidence and mortality in different countries, with special reference to dietary practices. *Int. J. Cancer* 15:617-631.
241. Wynder, E.L., and Reddy, B.S. (1975): Dietary fat and colon cancer. *J. Natl. Cancer Inst.* 54:7-10.
242. Brown, J., Bourke, G.J., Gearty, G.F., Finnegan, A., Hill, M., Heffeman-Fox, F.C., Fitzgerald, D.E., Kennedy, J., Childers, R.W., Jessop, W.J.E., Trulson, M.F., Latham, M.C., Cronin, S., McCann, M.B., Clancy, R.E., Gore, I., Stoudt, H.W., Hegsted, D.M., and Stare, F.J. (1970): Nutritional and epidemiologic factors related to heart disease. *World Rev. Nutr. Diet.* 12:1-42.
243. Kato, H., Tillotson, J., Nichaman, M.Z., Rhoads, G., and Hamilton, H. (1973): Epidemiologic studies of coronary heart disease and stroke in Japanese men living in Japan, Hawaii and California. *Am. J. Epidemiol.* 97:372.
244. Insull, W., Oiso, T., and Tsuchiya, K. (1968): Diet and nutritional status of Japanese. *Am. J. Clin. Nutrition* 21:753-777.
245. Nikkila, E.A., and Konttinen, A. (1962): Effect of physical activity on postprandial levels of fats in serum. *Lancet* 1:1151-54.
246. Watkin, D.M. (1973): Nutrition and aging in technically underdeveloped societies. In: *Food, Nutrition, and Health.* Rechcigl, M., Editor. *World Rev. Nutr. Dietet.* 16:46-58.
247. Reid, T.J. (1974): Energy metabolism in the whole animal. In: *The Control of Metabolism.* The Pennsylvania State University Press, p. 133-134.
248. Reid, T.J. (1975): Comparative efficiency of animals in the conversion of feedstuffs to human foods. *Proceedings of the Cornell Nutrition Conference,* 1975. Cornell University Press, Ithaca, pp. 16-24.
249. Watkin, D.M. (1973): Nutrition for the aging and the aged. In: *Modern Nutrition in Health and Disease,* Fifth Edition, edited by R.S. Goodhart and M.E. Shils. Lea & Febiger, Philadelphia. p. 683.
250. Manoff, R. (1975): "Toward a New American Mentality" — Commentary. *J. Nutr. Ed.* 7(8):139-140.
251. McLuhan, M. (1965): *Understanding Media: The Extension of Man.* McGraw-Hill Book Company, New York, pp. 7-21.
252. U.S. Bureau of the Census (1977): Current Population Reports. Series P-25, No. 643. "Estimates of the Population of the United States, by Age, Sex, and Race: July 1, 1974 to 1976". U.S. Government Printing Office, Washington, D.C.
253. Select Committee on Nutrition and Human Needs of the United States Senate (1976): *Title VII Survey.* U.S. Government Printing Office, Washington, D.C. pp. 1-338.
253a. Watkin, D.M. (1978): Logical bases for action in nutrition and aging. *J. Amer. Geriatrics Soc.* 36:193-202.
254. Administration on Aging, DHEW (1976): National nutrition program for older Americans. Fact Sheet. DHEW Publication No. (OHD) 76-20230. Washington, D.C. pp. 1-3.

254a. Bureau of Health Education, Center for Disease Control, U.S. Department of Health, Education and Welfare (1980): Nutrition Education for the Elderly, by Westinghouse Public Applied Systems. Contract No. HEW 200-79-0923. Center for Disease Control, Atlanta, Georgia.

254b. U.S. Department of Agriculture and U.S. Department of Health, Education and Welfare (1980): *Nutrition and Your Health: Dietary Guidelines for Americans.* U.S. Government Printing Office, Washington, D.C.

254c. Rifkin, B.M. Chief, Program Office (1979): The Coronary Primary Prevention Trial: design and implementation. The Lipid Research Clinics Program. *J. Chronic Dis.* 32:609-631.

254d. Food and Nutrition Board, Task Force on Guidelines Toward Healthful Diets, R.E. Olson, Chairman (1980): *Toward Healthful Diets.* National Research Council. National Academy of Sciences, Washington, D.C.

254e. Department of National Health and Welfare (1977): Recommendations for prevention programs in relation to nutrition and cardiovascular disease. Bureau of Nutritional Sciences, Health Protection Branch, Ottawa, Canada.

254f. MacNeil, R., Lehrer, J., Goodman, D., Calloway, W., and Olson, R. (1980): The cholesterol question. The MacNeil/Lehrer Report, May 28, 1980, library #1218, show #5238. Journal Graphics, Inc. New York.

255. Read, P.P. (1974): *Alive: The Story of the Andes Survivors.* J.B. Lippincott Co., New York.

256. Abraham, S., Lowenstein, F.W., and O'Connell, M.A. (1975): Preliminary findings of the first health and nutrition examination survey, United States. 1971-1972: Anthropometric and clinical findings. DHEW Publication No. (HRA) 75-1229. U.S. Government Printing Office, Washington, D.C. Stock Number 017-021-00026-5.

257. Kannel, W.B., Pearson, G., and McNamara, P.M. (1969): Obesity as a force of morbidity and mortality. In: *Adolescent Nutrition and Growth,* edited by F.P. Heald. Appleton-Century-Crofts, New York.

258. Watkin, D.M. (1968): La epidemiologia de la obesidad en América Latina. *Transacciones del I Congress de la Sociedad Latinoamericana de Nutrición y III Jornaclas Venezolanas de Nutrición,* Instituto de Nutrición, Caracas.

259. U.S. Department of Health, Education and Welfare (1972): Ten State Nutrition Survey, 1968-1970. III. Clinical. Anthropometry. Dental. DHEW Publication No. (HSM) 72-8131. Center for Disease Control, Atlanta, Georgia.

259a. Andres, R. (1980): Influence of obesity on longevity in the aged. In: *Aging, Cancer and Cell Membranes. Volume VII, Advances in Cancer Biology Series,* edited by C. Borek. Stratton Intercontinental Medical Book Corporation, New York.

259b. Metropolitan Life Insurance Company (1959): New weight standards for men and women. *Statistical Bull.* 40:1-4.

259c. Sorlic, P., Gordon, T., and Kannel, W.B. (1980): Body build and mortality. The Framingham Study. *J. Amer. Med. Assoc.* 243:1828-1831.

260. Armstrong, D., Dublin, L.I., Wheatley, G.M., and Marks, J.H. (1951): Obesity and its relation to health and disease. *J.A.M.A.* 147:1007-1014.

261. Dublin, L.I. (1953): Relation of obesity to longevity. *N. Engl. J. Med.* 243:971-974.

262. Kannel, W.B., LeBauer, E.J., Dawber, T.F., and McNamara, P.M. (1967): Relation of body weight to the development of coronary heart disease: The Framingham Study. *Circulation* 35:734-744.

263. Keys, A., Aravanis, C., Blackburn, H., vanBuchem, F.S.P., Buzina, R., Djordjevic, B.S., Fidanza, F., Karvanen, M.J., Menotti, A., Puddu, V., and Taylor, H.L. (1972): Probability of middle-aged men developing coronary heart disease in five years. *Circulation* 45:815-828.

264. Select Committee on Nutrition and Human Needs. U.S. Senate (1977): *Diet and Killer Diseases with Press Reaction and Additional Information.* U.S. Government Printing Office, Washington, D.C.

265. Select Committee on Nutrition and Human Needs. United States Senate (1977): *Dietary Goals for the United States,* Second Edition. U.S. Government Printing Office, Washington, D.C. Stock No. 052-070-04376-8.

266. McGandy, R.B., Barrows, C.H., Jr., Spanias, A., Meredith, A., Stone, J.L., and Norris, A.H. (1966): Nutrient intake and energy expenditure in men of different ages. *J. Gerontol.* 21:581-587.
267. Shock, N.W. (1972): Energy metabolism, caloric intake and physical activity of the aging. In: *Nutrition in Old Age,* edited by L.A. Carlson. Alquist & Wiksell. Uppsala. pp. 16-17.
268. McGandy, R.B., Barrows, C.H., Jr., Spanias, A., Meredith, A., Stone, J.L., and Norris, A.H. (1966): Nutrient intakes and energy expenditures in men of different ages. *J. Gerontol.* 21:581-587.
269. Watkin, D.M. (1968): Nutritional problems today in the elderly in the United States. In: *Vitamins in the Elderly,* edited by A.N. Exton-Smith and D.L. Scott. John Wright & Sons, Ltd. Bristol, U.K., pp. 73-75.
270. Stone, J.L., and Norris, A.H. (1966): Activities and attitudes of participants in the Baltimore longitudinal study. *J. Gerontol.* 21:575-580.
271. McFarland, R.A., and O'Doherty. Work and occupational skills. In: *Handbook of Aging and the Individual,* edited by J.E. Birren, pp. 452-500.
272. Pincus, A. (1976): The village elders. Potomac Magazine. pp. 14-19. *The Washington Post,* August 15.
273. American Heart Association (1968): The National Diet Heart Study: Final Report. American Heart Association Monograph Number Eighteen. New York.
274. Atkins, R.D. (1972): *Dr. Atkins' Diet Revolution: The High Calorie Way to Stay Thin Forever.* David McKay, Inc., New York.
275. Mann, G.V. (1977): Diet and Obesity (Editorial). *N. England J. Med.* 296:812.
276. Council on Foods and Nutrition. American Medical Association (1973): A critique of low-carbohydrate ketogenic weight reduction regimens: A review of Dr. Atkins' Diet Revolution. *J. Am. Med. Assoc.* 224:1414-1419.
277. Harvey, W. (1872): *On Corpulence in Relation to Disease.* Henry Renshaw, London. pp. 109, 122.
278. Banting, W. (1863): *Letter on Corpulence, Addressed to the Public.* (London, 1863), Edition Two. Harrison, London. p. 22.
279. Lewis, S.B., Vallin, J.D., Kane, J.P., and Gerich, J.E. (1977): Effect of diet composition on metabolic adaptations to hypocaloric nutrition: comparison of high carbohydrate and high fat isocaloric diets. *Amer. J. Clin. Nutrition* 30:160-170.
279a. Linn, R., and Stuart, S. (1976): *The Last Chance Diet.* Lyle Stuart, Inc. Secaucus, N.J.
279b. Food and Drug Administration, HEW. (1978): Protein diets. *FDA Drug Bulletin* 8:(1) 2-4.
279c. Center for Disease Control, HEW. (1977): Deaths associated with liquid protein diets. *Morb. Mortal. Wkly. Rep.* 26:(46) 383; 26:(52) 443.
280. Watkin, D.M., Shock, N.W., Todhunter, E.N., Wilcox, J., and Katz, M. (1973): Nutritional assessment of the elderly. In: Nutritional Assessment in Health Programs, edited by Christakis, G., *Amer. J. Public Health* 63: November, Suppl. pp. 68-75.
281. Sickroom Service (1977): *Exercises While You Watch T.V.* Sickroom Services, Inc., Milwaukee, pp. 1-32.
282. Yoshimura, H. (1961): Adult protein requirements. *Federation Proc.* 20: Suppl. No. 7, pp. 103-110.
283. Borer, J.S., Bacharach, S.L., Green, M.V., Kent, K.M., Epstein, S.E., and Johnston, G.S. (1977): Real-time radionucleotide cineangiography in the noninvasive evaluation of global and regional left ventricular function at rest and during exercise in patients with coronary-artery disease. *New England J. Med.* 296:839-844.
284. Conner, J.F., LaCerva, F., Jr., Swanick, E.J., Oldham, M.J., Holzaepfel, D.W., and Lyczkowskyj, O. (1976): Effects of exercise on coronary collateralization — angiographic studies in six patients in a supervised exercise program. *Medicine and Science in Sports* 8:145-151.
285. Nikkilä, E.A., and Konttinen, A. (1962): Effect of physical activity on postprandial levels of fats in serum. *Lancet* 1:1151-1154.
286. Keys, A. (1956): The Diet and the Development of Coronary Heart Disease. *J. Chron. Dis.* 4:364-380.

287. Schlierf, G. (1975): Polyunsaturated fats and atherosclerosis. *American Oil Chemists Society Journal* 42: Supp. p. 433A.

288. Wilmot, V.A., and Swank, R.L. (1952): The influence of low-fat diet on blood lipid levels in health and in multiple sclerosis. *Amer. J. Med. Sci.* 223:25-34.

289. Starke, H. (1950). Effect of rice diet on serum cholesterol fractions of 154 patients with hypertensive vascular disease. *Amer. J. Med.* 9:494-499.

290. Hildreth, F.A., Mellinkoff, S.M., Blair, G.W., and Hildreth, D.M. (1951): An experimental study of practical diets to reduce the human serum cholesterol. *J. Clin. Invest.* 30:649.

291. Keys, A. (1950): Relation in man between cholesterol levels in diet and in blood. *Science* 112:79-81.

292. Keys, A., Brozek, J., Henschel, A., Mickelsen, O., and Taylor, H.L. (1950): *The Biology of Human Starvation.* The University of Minnesota Press. Minneapolis, pp. 488-498.

293. Hatch, F.T., Abell, L.L., and Kendall, F.E. (1955): Effects of restriction of dietary fat and cholesterol on serum lipids and lipoproteins in patients with hypertension., *Am. J. Med.* 19:48-60.

294. Zarkovic, G., Levi, M., Radovanovic, M., and Plecas, T. (1955): Effects of dietary fat habits on serum cholesterol and blood pressure in group of Bosnian villages. *Acta. Med. Jugoslav.* 9:129-137.

295. Keys, A., Anderśon, J.T., Fidanza, F., Keys, M.H., and Swahn, B. (1955): Effects of diet on blood lipids in man, particularly cholesterol and lipoproteins. *Clin. Chem.* 1:34-52.

296. Keys, A. (1956): Diet and the development of coronary heart disease. *J. Chronic Dis.* 4:364-380.

297. Keys, A., Anderson, J.T., Aresu, M., Biörck, G., Brock, J.F., Bronte-Stewart, B., Fidanza, F., Keys, M.H., Malmros, H., Poppi, A., Posteli, T., Swahn, B., and del Vecchio, A. (1956): Physical activity and diet in populations differing in serum cholesterol. *J. Clin. Invest.* 25:1173-1181.

298. Sacko, F.M., Castelli, W.P., Donner, A., and Kass, E.H. (1975): Plasma lipids and lipoproteins in vegetarians and controls. *New Eng. J. Med.* 292:1148-1150.

299. Yudkin, J. (1957): Diet and coronary thrombosis: hypothesis and fact. *Lancet* 2:155-162.

300. Goldbloom, A.A., Eiber, H.B., and Boyd, L.G. (1954): Clinical studies in blood lipid metabolism: IX. Effect of lipotropic agents on serum lipid partitions in 50 patients with generalized atherosclerosis; three year study. *Am. J. Digest. Dis.* 21:152-157.

301. Mayer, G.A., Connell, W.F., DeWolfe, M.S., and Beveridge, J.M.R. (1954): Diet and plasma cholesterol. *Amer. J. Clin. Nutr.* 2:316-322.

302. Wilkerson, C.F., Jr., Boyle, E., Jackson, R.S., and Benjamin, M.R. (1955): Effects of varying the intake of dietary fat and the ingestion of sitosterol on lipid and lipoprotein fractions of human serum. *Metabolism* 4:302-309.

303. Horlick, L., and Craig, B.M. (1957): Effect of longchain polyunsaturated and saturated fatty acids on serum lipids in man. *Lancet* 2:566-569.

304. American Heart Association, Committee on Nutrition (1973): *Diet and Coronary Heart Disease.* New York.

305. Lees, R.S., and Wilson, D.E. (1971): The treatment of hyperlipidemia. *New Eng. J. Med.* 284:186-95.

306. Wilson, W.S., Hulley, S.B., Burrows, M.I., and Nichaman, M.Z. (1971): Serial lipid and lipoprotein responses to American Heart Association fat-controlled diet. *Am. J. Med.* 51:491-503.

307. Hall, Y., Stamler, J., Cohen, D.B., Majonnier, L., Epstein, M.B., Berkson, D.M., Whipple, I.T., and Catchings, S. Effectiveness of a low saturated fat, low cholesterol, weight-reducing diet for the control of hypertriglyceridemia. *Atherosclerosis* 16:389-403.

308. Mann, G.V., and Andrus, S.B. (1956): Xanthomatosis and atherosclerosis produced by diet in adult rhesus monkey. *J. Lab. & Clin. Med.* 48:533-550.

309. Portman, O.W., Hegsted, D.M., Stare, F.J., Bruno, D., Murphy, R., and Sinisterra, L. (1956): Effect of the level and type of dietary fat on the metabolism of

cholesterol and beta lipotroteins in the cebus monkey. *J. Exper. Med.* 104:817-828.
310. Moore, N.S., Young, C.M., and Maynard, L.A. (1954): Blood lipid levels as influenced by weight. *Am. J. Med.* 17:348-354.
311. Schroeder, H.A. (1956): Practical method for reduction of plasma cholesterol in man. *J. Chronic Dis.* 4:461-468.
312. Connor, W.E., Stone, D.B., and Hodges, R.E. (1964): The interrelated effects of dietary cholesterol and fat upon human serum lipid levels. *J. Clin. Invest.* 43:1691-96.
313. Connor, W.E., and Connor, S.L. (1972): The key role of nutritional factors in the prevention of coronary heart disease. *Prev. Med.* 1:49-83.
314. Cox, G.E., Taylor, C.B., Cox, L.G., and Counts, M.A. (1958): Atherosclerosis in rhesus monkeys: I. Hypercholesterolemia induced by dietary fat and cholesterol. *A.M.A. Arch. Path.* 66:32-52.
315. Nichols, A.B., Ravenscroft, C., Lamphiear, D.E., and Ostrander, L.D., Jr. (1976): Daily nutritional intake and serum lipid levels. The Tecumseh study. *Amer. J. Clin. Nutrition* 29:1384-1392.
316. Nichols, A.B., Ravenscroft, D., Lamphiear, D.E., and Ostrander, L.D., Jr. (1976): Independence of serum lipid levels and dietary habits. *J. Am. Med. Assoc.* 236:1948-1953.
317. Kannel, W., and Gordon, T. (1970): The Framingham Study. An epidemiologic investigation of cardiovascular diseases. Section 24: The Framingham diet study: Diet and the regulation of serum cholesterol. U.S. Government Printing Office, Washington, D.C.
318. Kahn, H., Medalie, J., Neufeld, H., Riss, E., Balogh, M., and Groen, J. (1969) Serum cholesterol: its distribution and association with dietary and other variables in a survey of 10,000 men. *Israel J. Med. Sci.* 5:1117-27.
319. Stulb, S.C., McDonough, J.R., Greenberg, B.S., and Hames, C.G. (1965): The relationship of nutrient intake and exercise to serum cholesterol levels in white males in Evans County, Georgia. *Am. J. Clin. Nutr.* 16:238-242.
320. Keys, A., (1970): Coronary heart disease in seven countries. *Circulation* 1970, Vol. 41, Suppl. #1, pp. I1-I211.
321. Ashley, F., and Kannel, W. (1974): Relation of weight changes to changes in atherogenic traits: The Framingham Study. *J. Chronic Dis.* 27:103-14.
322. Ostrander, L.D., Jr., and Lamphiear, D.E. (1976): Coronary risk factors in a community. Findings in Tecumseh, Michigan. *Circulation* 53:152-56.
323. Bleiler, R.E., Yearick, E.S., Schnur, S.S., Singson, I.L., and Ohlson, M.A. (1963): Seasonal variations in cholesterol in serum of men and women. *Amer. J. Clin. Nutr.* 12:12-16.
324. Thomas, C.B., Halljes, H.W.D., and Eisenberg, F.F. (1961): Observations on seasonal variations in serum cholesterol level among healthy prisoners. *Ann. Internal Med.* 54:413-430.
325. Keys, A., Mickelsen, O., Miller, E.B., Hayes, E.W., and Todd, R. (1950): The concentration of cholesterol in the blood serum of normal man and its relation to age. *J. Clin. Invest.* 29:1347-1353.
326. Mann, G.V., Teel, K., Hayes, O.B., McNally, A., and Bruno, D. (1955): Exercise in the disposition of dietary Calories: regulation of serum lipoprotein and cholesterol levels in human subjects. *New Eng. J. Med.* 253:349-355.
327. Trowell, H. (1975): Coronary heart disease and dietary fiber. *Am. J. Clin. Nutr.* 28:798-800.
328. Heaton, K.W., and Pomare, E.W. (1974): The effect of bran on blood lipids and calcium. *Lancet* 1:49-50.
329. Connell, A.M., Smith, C.L., and Somsell, M. (1975): Absence of effect of bran on blood lipids. *Lancet* 1:496-497.
330. Truswell, A.S., and Kay, R.M. (1975): Absence of effect of bran on blood lipids. *Lancet* 1:922-923.
331. Wilson, D.E., Schreibman, P.H., Brewster, A.C., and Arky, R. (1970): The enhancement of alimentary lipemia by ethanol in man. *J. Lab. Clin. Med.*75:264-74.

332. Kudzma, D., and Schonfeld, G. (1974): Alcoholic hyperlipidemia: Induction by alcohol but not carbohydrate. *J. Lab. Clin. Med.* 77:384-95.
333. Ostrander, L.D., Jr., Lamphiear, D.E., Block, W.D., Johnson, B., Ravenscroft, C., and Epstein, F.H. (1974): Relationship of serum lipid concentrations to alcohol consumption. *Arch. Internal Med.* 134:451-56.
334. Fredrickson, D.S., Levy, R.I., and Lees, R.S. (1967): Fat transport in lipoproteins. An integrated approach to mechanisms and disorders. *N. Eng. J. Med.* 276:34-42, 94-103, 148-56, 215-25, and 273-81.
335. Levy, R.I., Fredrickson, D.S., Shulman, R., Bilheimer, D.W., Breslow, J.L., Stone, N.J., Lux, S.E., Sloan, H.R., Krauss, R.M., and Herbert, P.N. (1972): Dietary and drug treatment of primary hyperlipoproteinemia. *Ann. Int. Med.* 77:267-294.
336. American Medical Association. Council on Foods and Nutrition, Committee on Dietary Fat Levels, Hand, D.B., Chairman. (1962): The regulation of dietary fat. *J. Amer. Med. Assoc.* 181:411.
337. Ahrens, E.H., Jr. (1976): The management of hyperlipidemia: Whether, rather than how. *Ann. Internal Med.* 85:87-93.
338. Rose, G.A., Thompson, W.B., and Williams, R.T. (1965): Corn oil in the treatment of ischaemic heart disease. *Br. Med. J.* 1:1531-1533.
339. Christakis, S., Rinzler, S.H., Archer, M., Winslow, G., Jampel, S., Stephenson, J., Friedman, G., Fein, H., Draus, A., and James, G. (1966): The Anti-Coronary Club: a dietary approach to the prevention of coronary heart disease — a 7-year report. *Amer. J. Public Health* 56:299-314.
340. Leren, P. (1966): Effect of plasma cholesterol-lowering diet in male survivors of myocardial infarction: a controlled clinical trial. *Acta. Med. Scandinav.* Supp. 466.
341. Bierenbaum, M.L., Fleischman, A.I., Raichelson, R.I., Hayton, T., and Watson, P.B. (1973): Ten-year experience with modified fat diets on younger men with coronary heart disease. *Lancet* 1:1404-1407.
342. Medical Research Council (1968): Controlled trial of soya-bean oil in myocardial infarction. *Lancet* 2:693-700.
343. Turpeinen, O., Miettinen, M., Karvonen, M.J., Roine, P., Pekkarinen, M., Lehtosuo, E.J., and Alivirta, P. (1968): Dietary prevention of coronary heart disease; long-term experiment: I. Observations on male subjects. *Am. J. Clin. Nutrition* 21:255-276.
344. Miettinen, M., Turpeinen, O., Karvanen, M.J., Elosuo, R., and Paavilainen, E. (1972): Effect of cholesterol-lowering diet on mortality from coronary heart disease and other causes. 12-year clinical trial in men and women. *Lancet* 2:835-838.
345. Dewar, H.A. (1971): Trial of clofibrate in the treatment of ischaemic heart disease. Five-year study by a group of physicians in the Newcastle-upon-Tyne region. *Br. Med. J.* 4:767-775.
346. Oliver, M.F. (1971): Ischaemic heart disease: a secondary prevention trial using clofibrate. Report by a research committee of the Scottish Society of Physicians. *Br. Med. J.* 4:775-784.
347. Stamler, J. (1975): The Coronary Drug Project. Clofibrate and niacin in coronary heart disease. *J. Amer. Med. Assoc.* 231:360-381.
348. Whyte, H.M. (1975): Potential effect on coronary-heart disease morbidity of lowering blood cholesterol. *Lancet* 1:906-910.
349. Gordon, T., and Kannel, W.B. (1972): Predisposition to atherosclerosis in the head, heart, and legs. *J. Amer. Med. Assoc.* 221:661-664.
349a. Mann, G.V. (1977): Current concepts: Diet-heart: End of an era. *New England J. Med.* 297:644-650.
349b. Barr, D.P., Russ, E.M, and Eder, H.A. (1951): Protein lipid relationships in human plasma. II. In atherosclerosis and related conditions. *Amer. J. Med.* 11:480-493.
349c. Rhoads, G.G., Gulbrandsen, C.L., and Kagan, A. (1977): Serum lipoproteins and coronary heart disease. *New England J. Med.* 294:293-298.
349d. Miller, N.E., Fórde, O.H., and Thelle, D.S. (1977): The Troms Heart Study: High

density lipoprotein and coronary heart disease: A prospective case control study. *Lancet* 1:965-967.

349e. Gordon, T., Castelli, W.P., Hjortland, M.C., Kannel, W.B., and Dawber, T.R. (1977): High density lipoprotein as a protective factor against coronary heart disease. *Amer. J. Med.* 62:707-714.

349f. Kannel, W.B., and Gordon, T. (1977): Cardiovascular risk factors in the aged: The Framingham Study. In *Proceedings of a Conference on the Epidemiology of Aging.* National Institute on Aging. Bethesda, Maryland.

349g. Glueck, C.J., Fallat, R.W., Spadafora, M., and Gartside, P. (1975): Longevity syndromes. *Circulation* 52:II-272.

349h. Yano, K., Rhoads, G.R., and Kagan, A. (1977): Coffee, alcohol, and risk of coronary heart disease in Japanese-Americans. *New England J. Med.* 297:405-409.

349i. Bondjers, G., and Bjorkerud, S. (1975): HDL-dependent elimination of cholesterol from human arterial tissues. *Proc. Europ. Soc. Clin. Invest.* 9:51-52.

349j. Miller, G.J., and Miller, N.E. (1975): Plasma-high-density lipoprotein concentration and development of ischaemic heart disease. *Lancet* 1:16-19.

349k. Carew, T.E., Kaschinsky, T., Hayes, S.B., and Steinberg, D. (1976): A mechanism by which high-density lipoproteins may slow the atherogenic process. *Lancet* 1:1315-1317.

350. Sansum, W.D., Blatherwick, N.R., and Bowden, R. (1926): The use of high carbohydrate diets in the treatment of diabetes mellitus. *J. Amer. Med. Assoc.* 86:178-181.

351. Himsworth, H.P. (1935): The dietetic factor determining the glucose tolerance and sensitivity to insulin of healthy man. *Clin. Sci.* 2:67-94.

352. Himsworth, H.P. (1939): Mechanism of diabetes mellitus. (Goulstonian Lecture). *Lancet* 2:1-6, 65-68, 118-122, and 171-175.

353. Kempner, W., Peschel, R.L., and Schlayer, C. (1958): Effects of rice diet on diabetes mellitus associated with vascular disease. *Postgrad. Med.* 24:359-371.

354. Brunzell, J.D., Lerner, R.L., Hazzard, W.R., Porte, D. Jr., and Bierman, E.L. (1971): Improved glucose tolerance with high carbohydrate feeding in mild diabetes. *N. Engl. J. Med.* 284:521-524.

355. Weinsier, R.L., Seeman, A., Herrera, M.G., Assal, J.P., Soeldner, J.S., and Gleason, R.E. (1974): High and low carbohydrate diets in diabetes mellitus. Study of the effects on diabetic control, insulin secretion, and blood lipids. *Ann. Internal Med.* 80:332-341.

356. Anderson, J.W., Herman, R.H., and Zakim, D. (1973): Effect of high glucose and high sucrose diets on glucose tolerance in normal man. *Am. J. Clin. Nutr.* 26:600-607.

357. Kiehm, T.G., Anderson, J.W., and Ward, K. (1976): Beneficial effects of a high carbohydrate, high fiber diet on hyperglycemic diabetic men. *Am. J. Clin. Nutr.* 29:895-899.

358. Dwyer, J.T., and Molitch, M.E. (1976): Clinical nutrition 1976: Where are we going? *Ann. Internal Med.* 84:329-331. (Editorial)

359. Bondy, P.K. (1972): Editorial Comment. *Year Book of Medicine.* Year Book Medical Publishers, Inc., Chicago. p. 546.

360. O'Sullivan, J.B., and Mahan, C.M. (1971): Evaluation of age-adjusted criteria for potential diabetes. *Diabetes* 20:811-15.

361. Smith, L.E., and Shock, N.W. (1949): Intravenous glucose tolerance tests in aged males. *J. Gerontol.* 4:27-33.

362. Silverstone, F.A., Brandfonbrener, M., Shock, N.W., and Yiengst, M. (1957): Age differences in the intravenous glucose tolerance tests and the response to insulin. *J. Clin. Invest.* 36:504-14.

363. Swerdloff, R.S., Pozefsky, T., Tobin, J.D., and Andres, R. (1967): Influence of age on the intravenous tolbutamide response test. *Diabetes* 16:161-170.

364. Andres, R., and Tobin, J.D. (1972): Aging, carbohydrate metabolism, and diabetes. *Proc. 9th International Congress of Gerontology, Kiev.* Vol. 1. pp. 276-280.

365. Andres, R. (1967): Aging, glucose tolerance, and diabetes — a proposal. In: *Endocrines and Aging,* edited by L. Gitman. Charles C. Thomas, Springfield, Illinois. pp. 200-207.

366. Andres, R. (1967): Diabetes and aging. *Hosp. Pract.* 2:63-67.
367. Andres, R. (1971): Aging and diabetes. *Med. Clin. North America* 55:835-846.
368. Bierman, E.L., Albrink, M.J., Arky, W.E., Dayton, S., Spritz, N., and Steinberg, D. (1971): Principles of nutrition and dietary recommendations for patients with diabetes mellitus. *Diabetes* 20:633-634.
369. Christakis, G., and Miridjanian, A. (1970): The nutritional aspects of diabetes. In: *Diabetes Mellitus: Theory and Practice*, edited by M. Ellenberg., and H. Rifkin. McGraw-Hill Book Co., Inc. New York. pp. 594-623.
370. Albrink, M.J., and Davidson, P.C. (1971): Dietary therapy and prophylaxis of vascular disease in diabetics. *Med. Clin. North Am.* 55:877-887.
371. West, K.M. (1973): Diet therapy in diabetes: An analysis of failure. *Ann. Int. Med.* 79:425-434.
372. West, K.M. (1975): Prevention and therapy of diabetes mellitus. *Nutrition Rev.* 33:193-198.
373. American Diabetes Association, Inc., and the American Dietetic Association (1976): Exchange Lists for Meal Planning. American Diabetes Association, Inc., New York, and the American Dietetic Association, Chicago, pp. 1-24.
374. Food and Drug Administration. (1976): Using nutrition labels with food exchange lists. HEW Publication No. (FDA) 77-2072. Public Health Service, Rockville, Md.
375. Tschudy, D.P., Bacchus, H., Weissman, S., Watkin, D.M., Eubanks, M., and White, J. (1959): Studies of the effects of dietary protein and caloric levels on the kinetics of nitrogen metabolism using N^{15} L-aspartic acid. *J. Clin Invest.* 38:892-901.
376. Watkin, D.M. (1959): Increased fat utilization in the hypermetabolism of active neoplastic disease. *ACTA Unio Internationalis Contra Cancrum.* 15:907-917.
377. Levenson, S.M., and Watkin, D.M. (1959): Protein requirements in injury and certain acute and chronic diseases. *Federation Proc.* 18:1155-1190.
378. Mueller, P.S., and Watkin, D.M. (1961): Plasma unesterified fatty acid (UFA) concentrations in neoplastic disease. *J. Lab. & Clin. Med.* 57:95-108.
379. Watkin, D.M. (1961): Nitrogen balance as affected by neoplastic disease and its therapy. *Am. J. Clin. Nutr.* 9:446-460.
380. Watkin, D.M. (1962): Nutritional care in advanced cancer. In: *The Physician and the Total Care of the Cancer Patient. A Symposium Presented at the 1961 Scientific Session.* The American Cancer Society, Inc. New York. pp. 120-123.
381. Shils, M.E. (1973): Nutrition and neoplasia. In: *Modern Nutrition in Health and Disease, Fifth Edition*, edited by R.S. Goodhart and M.E. Shils. Lea & Febiger, Philadelphia. pp. 981-996.
382. Watkin, D.M. (1957): Clinical, chemical, hematologic and anatomic changes accompanying repeated administration of fat emulsion to man. *Metabolism* 6:785-806.
383. Watkin, D.M., and Steinfeld, J.L. (1965): Nutrient and energy metabolism in patients with and without cancer during hyperalimentation with fat administered intravenously. *Amer. J. Clin. Nutrition* 16:182-212.
384. Watkin, D.M. (1965): Fecal excretion of lipids before, during and after hyperalimentation with fat administered intravenously. *Amer. J. Clin. Nutrition* 16:213-223.
385. Mueller, J.F., and Canham, J.E., Editors. (1965): Symposium on intravenous fat emulsions: preface. *Amer. J. Clin. Nutrition* 16:1-3.
386. Schwartz, G.F., Green, H.L., Bendon, M.L., Graham, W.P., III, and Blakemore, W.S. (1971): Combined parenteral hyperalimentation and chemotherapy in the treatment of disseminated solid tumors. *Amer. J. Surg.* 121:169-173.
386a. Copeland, E.M., MacFadyen, B.V., Jr., and Dudrick, S.J. (1974): Intravenous hyperalimentation in cancer patients. *J. Surg. Research* 16:241-247.
386b. Copeland, E.M., III, MacFadyen, B.V., Jr., Lanzotti, V.J., and Dudrick, S.J. (1975): Intravenous hyperalimentation as an adjunct to cancer chemotherapy. *Amer. J. Surg.* 129:167-173.
386c. Copeland, E.M., III, MacFadyen, B.V., Jr., Rapp, M.A., and Dudrick, S.J. (1975): Hyperalimentation and immune competence in cancer. *Surg. Forum* 26:138-140.

386d. Fleming, C.R., McGill, D.B., Hoffman, H.N., II, and Nelson, R.A. (1976): Total parenteral nutrition. *Mayo Clinic Proc.* 51:187-199.
386e. Moghissi, K., Hornshaw, J., Teasdale, P.R. and Dawes, E.A. (1977): Parenteral nutrition in carcinoma of the oesophagus treated by surgery: Nitrogen balance and clinical studies. *Brit. J. Surg.* 64:125-128.
386f. Solassol, C., and Joyeux, H. (1978): Artificial gut with nutritive mixtures as a major adjuvant in gastrointestinal cancer treatment. *J. Parenteral Enteral Nutrition* 2: Abstract 91.
386g. Dietel, M., Vasic, V., and Alexander, M. (1979): Specialized nutritional support and cancer. *J. Parenteral Enteral Nutrition* 2:671-675.
386h. Barlow, A.L., Editor (1979): *Liposyn®Research Conference Proceedings.* Abbott Laboratories, North Chicago, IL. pp. 1-112.
387. Greenberger, N.J., Ruppert, R.D., and Tzagournis, M.T. (1967): The use of medium chain triglycerides in malabsorption. *Ann. Internal Med.* 66: 727-734.
388. Senior, J.B., Editor (1968): *Medium Chain Triglycerides.* University of Pennsylvania Press, Philadelphia.
389. Bochenek, W., Rogers, J.B., Jr., and Balint, J.A. (1970): The effect of changes of dietary lipids on intestinal fluid loss in the short bowel syndrome. *Ann. Internal Med.* 72:205-213.
390. American Association for Cancer Research (1975): Symposium: Nutrition in the causation of cancer. *Cancer Research* 35:3231-3550.
391. Carroll, K.K., and Khor, H.T. (1975): Dietary fat in relation to tumorigenesis. In: *Progress in Biochemical Pharmacology: Lipids and Tumors,* Vol. 10. edited by K.K. Carroll, S. Karger, New York. pp. 308-373.
392. Wynder, E.L. (1977): Testimony and prepared statement for hearings on Diet Related to Killer Diseases. In: *Diet and Killer Diseases with Press Reaction and Additional Information.* Select Committee on Nutrition and Human Needs, United States Senate. U.S. Government Printing Office, Washington, D.C. pp. 192-207.
393. Gori, G.B. (1977): Testimony and prepared statement for hearings on Diet Related to Killer Diseases. In: *Diet and Killer Diseases with Press Reaction and Additional Information.* Select Committee on Nutrition and Human Needs, United States Senate. U.S. Government Printing Office, Washington, D.C. pp. 164-191.
394. Segi, M., and Kurchara, M. (1972): *Cancer Mortality for Selected Sites in 24 Countries.* Japan Cancer Society. Nagaya.
395. Oiso, T. (1975): Incidence of stomach cancer and its relation to dietary habits and nutrition in Japan between 1900 and 1975. *Cancer Research* 35:3254-3258.
396. Haenszel, W., and Kurichara, M. (1968): Studies in Japanese Migrants. I. Mortality from cancer and other diseases among Japanese in the United States. *J. Nat'l. Cancer Institute* 40:43-68.
397. Dunn, J.E., Jr. (1975): Cancer epidemiology in populations of the United States — with special emphasis on Hawaii and California — and Japan. *Cancer Research* 35:3240-3245.
398. Philips, R.L. (1975): Role of lifestyle and dietary habits in risk of cancer among Seventh-Day Adventists. *Cancer Research* 35:3513-3522.
399. Martinez, I., Torres, R., and Frias, Z. (1975): Cancer incidence in the United States and Puerto Rico. *Cancer Research* 35:3265-3271.
400. Fernandez, H.A. (1975): Nutrition in Puerto Rico. *Cancer Research* 35:3272-3291.
401. Hill, P., Chan, P.C., Cohen, L.A., Wynder, E.L., Helman, P., Kuno, K., and Rona, G. (1977): Diet and endocrine related cancer. *Cancer* 30:1820-1826.
402. Chan, P.C., and Cohen, L.A. (1975): Dietary fat and growth promotion of rat mammary tumors. *Cancer Research* 35:3384-3386.
403. Chan, P.C., and Cohen, L.A. (1974): Effect of dietary fat antiestrogen and antiprolactin on the development of mammary tumors in rats. *J. Nat'l. Cancer Inst.* 52:25-30.
404. DeWaard, F., and Baanders-von Halewyn, E.A. (1974): A prospective study in general practice on breast cancer risk in postmenopausal women. *Int. J. Cancer* 14:153-160.

405. Wynder, E.L. (1976): Nutrition and cancer. *Federation Proc.* 35:1309-1315.
406. Hegsted, D.M. (1977): Testimony and prepared statement for hearings on Diet Related to Killer Diseases. In: *Diet and Killer Diseases with Press Reaction and Additional Information.* Select Committee on Nutrition and Human Needs, United States Senate. U.S. Government Printing Office, Washington, D.C. pp. 208-211.
407. Benditt, E.P. (1977): The origin of atherosclerosis. *Scientific American* 236:(2), 74-85.
408. Benditt, E.P., and Benditt, J.M. (1973): Evidence for a monoclonal origin of human atherosclerotic plagues. *Proc. Nat'l. Acad. Sci. U.S.A.* 70:1753-1756.
409. Benditt, E.P. (1976): Implications of the monoclonal character of human atherosclerotic plagues. *Beiträge zur Pathologie* 158:405-416.
410. Ross, R., and Glomset, J. (1974): Atherosclerosis. *University of Washington Medicine* 1:(2) 3-9.
411. Daoud, A.S., Jarmolych, J., Fritz, K.E., and Augustyn, J.M. (1975): Serum factor influencing peripheral growth in the medial explant — relation to DNA synthesis. *Artery* 1:495-506.
412. Fritz, K.E., Augustyn, J.M., Peters, T., Jr., Jarmolych, J., and Daoud, A.S. (1976): Protein synthesis and its relation to DNA synthesis in aortic medial explants. *Atherosclerosis* 23:177-190.
413. Daoud, A.S. Personal communication.
414. Cohn, P.F., Gabbay, S.I., and Weglicki, W.B. (1976): Serum lipid levels in angiographically defined coronary artery disease. *Ann. Internal Med.* 84:241-245.
415. Miller, D.S., and Mumford, P. (1967): Gluttony. 1. An experimental study of overeating low or high-protein diets. *Am. J. Clin. Nutr.* 20:1212-1222.
416. Miller, D.S. Mumford, P., and Stock, M.J. (1967): Gluttony. 2. Thermogenesis in overeating man. *Am. J. Clin. Nutr.* 20:1223-1229.
417. Kasper, H., Thiel, H., and Ehl, M. (1973): Response of body weight to a low carbohydrate, high fat diet in normal and obese subjects. *Am. J. Clin. Nutr.* 26:197-204.
418. Hampers, C.L., Soeldner, T.S., Doak, P.B., and Merrill, T.P. (1966): Effect of chronic renal failure and hemodialysis on carbohydrate metabolism. *J. Clin. Invest.* 45:1719-31.
419. Bilbrey, G.L., Faloona, G.R., White, M.G., Atkins, C., Hill, A.R., and Knochel, J.P. (1975): Hyperglucagonemia in uremia: Reversal by renal transplantation. *Ann. Intern. Med.* 82:525-528.
420. Bilbrey, G.L., Faloona, G.R., White, M.G. and Knochel, J.P. (1974): Hyperglucagonemia of renal failure. *J. Clin. Invest.* 53:841-847.
421. Salter, J.M., Ezrin, C., Laidlaw, J.C., Gornall, A.G. (1960): Metabolic effects of glucagon in human subjects. *Metabolism* 9:753-768.
422. Unger, R.H., Aguilar-Parada, E., Muller, W.A., and Eisentraut, A.M. (1970): Studies of the pancreatic alpha cell function in normal and diabetic subjects. *J. Clin. Invest.* 49:837-848.
423. Murase, T., Cattran, D.C., Rubenstein, B., Steiner, G. (1975): Inhibition of lipoprotein lipase by uremic plasma; a possible cause of hypertriglyceridemia. *Metabolism* 24:1279-1286.
424. Cattran, D.C., Fenton, S.S.A., Wilson, D.R., and Steiner, G. (1976): Defective triglyceride removal in lipemia associated with peritoneal dialysis and haemodialysis. *Ann. Intern. Med.* 85:29-33.
425. Cattran, D.C., Fenton, S.S.A., Wilson, D.R., and Steiner, G. (1976): Dialysis and triglycerides (In comment on a comment). *Ann. Intern. Med.* 85:680.
426. Information Canada. Bureau of Nutritional Sciences. Department of National Health and Welfare. *Dietary Standards for Canada.* Ottawa. 1975.
427. DeFronzo, R.A., Andres, R., Edgar, P., and Walker, W.G. (1973): Carbohydrate metabolism in uremia: a review. *Medicine (Baltimore)* 52:469-481.
428. Burton, B.T. (1974): Current concepts of nutrition and diet in diseases of the kidney. I. General principles of dietary management. II. Dietary regimen for specific kidney disorders. *J. Am. Dietetic Assoc.* 65:623-633.
429. Walser, M. (1975): Treatment of renal failure with ketoacids. *Hosp. Prac.* 9:59-66.
430. Watkin, D.M. (1957): Clinical, chemical, hematological and anatomic changes

accompanying repeated intravenous administration of fat emulsion to man. *Metabolism* 6:785-806.

431. Wene, J.D., Connor, W.E., and DenBesten, L. (1975): Development of essential fatty acid deficiency in healthy men fed fat-free diets intravenously or orally. *J. Clin. Invest.* 36:127-134.
432. Kinsell, L.W., Partridge, J.W., Boling, L.A., Margen, S., and Michaels, G. (1952): Dietary modification of serum cholesterol and phospholipid levels. *J. Clin. Endocrinol.* 12:909-913.
433. Kinsell, L.W., Michaels, G.D., Partridge, J.W., Boling, L.A., Balch, H.E., and Cochrane, G.C. (1953): Effect upon serum cholesterol and phospholipids of diets containing large amounts of vegetable fat. *J. Clin. Nutr.* 1:224-231.
434. Ahrens, E.H., Jr., Blankenhorn, D.H., and Tsaltas, T.T. (1954): Effect on human serum lipids of substituting plant for animal fat in diet. *Proc. Soc. Exp. Biol. Med.* 86:872-878.
435. Beveridge, J.M.R., Connell, W.F., and Meyer, G.A. (1956): Dietary factors affecting the level of plasma cholesterol in humans: the role of fat. *Canadian J. Biochem. & Physiol.* 34:441-455.
436. Bronte-Stewart, B., Antonis, A., Eales, L., and Brock, J.F. (1956): Effects of feeding different fats on serum cholesterol level. *Lancet* 1:521-527.
437. Keys, A. Anderson, J.T., and Grande, F. (1957): "Essential" fatty acids, degree of unsaturation, and the effect of corn (maize) oil on the serum cholesterol in man. *Lancet* 1:66-68.
438. Malmros, H., and Wigand, G. (1957): The effect on serum cholesterol of diets containing different fats. *Lancet* 2:1-7.
439. Brown, H.B., and Page, I.H. (1958): Lowering blood lipid levels by changing food patterns. *J. Am. Med. Assoc.* 168:1989-1995.
440. Grundy, S.M., and Ahrens, E.H., Jr. (1970): The effects of unsaturated dietary fats on absorption, excretion, synthesis, and distribution of cholesterol in man. *J. Clin. Invest.* 49:1135-1152.
441. Frantz, I.D., Jr., Dawson, E.A., Kuba, K., Brewer, E.R., Gatewood, L.C., and Bartach, C.E. (1975): The Minnesota Coronary Survey: effect of diet on cardiovascular events and deaths. *Circulation* 51 & 52: (suppl. II) p. 4.
442. Ahrens, E.H., Jr., Insull, W., Jr., Hirsch, J., Stoffel, W., Peterson, M.L., Farquhar, J.W., Miller, T., and Thomasson, H.J. (1959): The effect on human serum lipids of a dietary fat, highly unsaturated, but poor in essential fatty acids. *Lancet* 1:115-119.
443. Keys, A., Anderson, J.T., and Grande, F. (1965): Serum cholesterol response to changes in diet. IV. Particular saturated fatty acids in the diet. *Metabolism* 14:776-87.
444. Hegsted, D.M., McGandy, R.B., Myers, M.L., and Stare, F.J. (1965): Quantitative effects of dietary fat on serum cholesterol in man. *Am. J. Clin. Nutr.* 17:231-295.
445. Hashim, S.A., Arteaga, A., and VanItallie, T.B. (1960): Effect of a saturated medium-chain triglyceride on serum lipids in man. *Lancet* 1:1105-1108.
446. Grande, F., Anderson, J.T., and Keys, A. (1961): The influence of chain length of the saturated fatty acids on their effect on serum cholesterol concentration in man. *J. Nutrition* 74:420-428.
447. Keys, A., Anderson, J.T., and Grande, F. (1958): Effect on serum cholesterol in man of mono-ene fatty acid (oleic acid) in the diet. *Proc. Soc. Exp. Biol. Med.* 98:387-91.
448. Anderson, J.T., Grande, F., and Keys, A. (1961): Hydrogenated fats in the diet and lipids in the serum of man. *J. Nutrition* 75:388-394.
449. Ahrens, E.H., Jr., Chairman. (1969): Mass Field Trials of the Diet-Heart Question. Their Significance, Timeliness, Feasibility, and Applicability. Report of the Diet-Heart Review Panel of the National Heart Institute. American Heart Association Monograph, Number Twenty-Eight. American Heart Association, New York.
450. Task Force on Arteriosclerosis. National Heart and Lung Institute (1971): Report. Vol. 1. June. National Heart and Lung Institute. Bethesda, Md.

451. Watkin, D.M. (1978): Logical bases for action in nutrition and aging. *J. Am. Geriatric Soc.* 26:193-202.
452. Cantarow, A., and Schepartz, B. (1962): *Biochemistry, Third Edition.* W. B. Saunders Company. Philadelphia. p. 559.
453. Cohn, C. and Joseph, D. (1960): Role of rate of ingestion of diet on regulation of intermediary metabolism ("meal eating" vs. "nibbling"). *Metabolism* 9:492-500.
454. Cohn, C., and Joseph, D. (1960): Effects on metabolism produced by the rate of ingestion of the diet. "Meal eating" vs. "nibbling." *Am. J. Clin. Nutrition* 8:682-690.
455. Cohn, C. (1961): Meal eating, nibbling, and body metabolism. *J. Am. Dietet. Assoc.* 38:433-436.
456. Cohn, C., Pick, R., and Katz, L.N. (1961): Effect of meal eating compared to nibbling upon atherosclerosis in chickens. *Circulation Res.* 9:139-145.
457. Cohn, C., Joseph, D., and Allweiss, M.D. (1962): Nutritional effects of feeding frequency. *Am. J. Clin. Nutrition* 11:356-361.
458. Cohn, C. (1962): Meals? *Nutrition Rev.* 20:321-323.
459. Pyke, M., and Harrison R., Holmes, S., and Chamberlain, K. (1947): Nutritional value of diets eaten by old people in London. *Lancet* 2:461-464.
460. Vinther-Paulsen, N. (1950): Investigations of the actual food intake of elderly, chronically hospitalized patients. *J. Gerontology* 5:331-338.
461. Ohlson, M.A., Jackson, L., Boek, J., Cedarquist, D.C., Brewer, M.D., Brown, E.G., Traver, J., Lett, M.M., Mayhew, M., Dunsing, D., and Tobey, H. (1950): Nutrition and dietary habits of aging women. *Am. J. Public Health* 40:1101-1108.
462. Schlenker, E.D., Feurig, J.S., Stone, L.H., and Ohlson, M.A. (1973): Nutrition and health of older people. In: *Symposium on Nutrition and Aging, Part II* edited by D.M. Watkin and G.V. Mann. *Am J. Clin. Nutrition* 26:1111-1119.
463. Todhunter, E.N. (1976): Life style and nutrient intake of the elderly. In: *Nutrition and Aging,* edited by M. Winick. John Wiley & Sons, New York. pp. 119-127.
464. Abraham, S., Carroll, M.D., Dresser, C.M., and Johnson, C.L. (1977): Dietary intake of persons 1-74 years of age in the United States. Advance Data from Vital & Health Statistics of the National Center for Health Statistics. No. 6. March 30, 1977. Health Resources Administration, Public Health Service, Rockville, Md.
465. Rensberger, B. (1977): No health benefits seen in saccharin. Experts say diabetics and dieters do not need the chemical — 'sweet tooth' blamed. *New York Times,* March 27. p. 32.
466. Cummings, J.H. (1976): What is fiber? In: *Fiber in Human Nutrition,* edited by G.A. Spiller, and R.J. Amen. Plenum Press, New York. pp. 1-30.
467. Spiller, G.A., and Amen, R.J. (1975): Plant fibers in nutrition: need for better nomenclature. *Am. J. Clin. Nutrition* 28:675-676.
468. Huntgate, R.T. (1976): Microbial activities related to mammalian digestion and absorption of food. In: *Fiber in Human Nutrition,* edited by G.A. Spiller, and R.J. Amen. Plenum Press, New York. pp. 131-142.
469. Page, L., and Friend, B. (1974): Levels of uses of sugar in the United States. In: *Sugars in Nutrition.* Nutrition Foundation, New York. pp. 93-107.
470. Pederson, P.O. (1938): Investigations into dental conditions of about 3000 ancient and modern Greenlanders. A preliminary report. *Dental Rec.* 58:191-198.
471. McGregor, A.B. (1963): Changing diet and its effects on caries prevalence in Ghana. *J. Dental Res.* 42:1086-1087.
472. Fry, A.J., and Grenby, T.H. (1972): The effects of reduced sucrose intake on the formation and composition of dental plaque in a group of men in the Antarctic. *Arch. Oral Biol.* 17:873-882.
473. Breese, F. (1934): Diet and the teeth. *Brit. Dental J.* 56:120-124, 147-148.
474. Gustafsson, B.E., Quensel, C.-E., Lanke, L.S., Lundquist, C., Grahnén, H., Bonow, B.E., and Krasse, B. (1954): Vipeholm dental caries study: effect of different levels of carbohydrate intake on caries activity in 436 individuals observed for five years. *Acta Odon, Scandinav.* 11:232-364.

475. Grenby, T.H., Powell, J.M., and Gleeson, M.J. (1974): Effect of sweets made with and without sucrose on the dental plaque and the correlation between the extent of plaque and human dental caries experience. *Arch. Oral Biol.* 19:217-224.
476. Gibbons, R.J., and Socransky, S.S. (1962): Intracellular polysaccharide storage by organisms in dental plaques. Its relation to dental caries and the microbiology of the oral cavity. *Arch. Oral Biol.* 7:73-79.
477. Madsen, K.O. (1975): Frequency of eating and dental health. *Food and Nutrition News* 46:(4), 1,2,4.
478. Yudkin, J. (1967): Evolutionary and historical changes in dietary carbohydrates. *Amer. J. Clin. Nutrition* 20:108-115.
479. Cohen, A.M. (1963): Fats and carbohydrate as factors in atherosclerosis and diabetes in Yemenite Jews. *Amer. Heart J.* 65:291-293.
480. Stare, F.J. (1967): Dietary fats and carbohydrates, blood lipids, and coronary disease. *Amer. J. Clin. Nutrition* 20:149-151.
481. Connor, W.E., and Connor, S.J. (1976): Sucrose and carbohydrate. In *Present Knowledge in Nutrition, Fourth Edition.* The Nutrition Foundation. New York. pp. 33-42.
482. American Medical Association (1977): Statement of the American Medical Association submitted to the Select Committee on Nutrition and Human Needs of the United States Senate *re Dietary Goals for the United States,* April 18. American Medical Association, Chicago.
483. Harper, A.E. (1978): Dietary goals — a skeptical view. *Amer. J. Clin. Nutrition* 31:310-321.
484. White, P.L. (1977): The realism of dietary goals. *Nutrition Notes* 13:(2)4-5.
485. Harper, A.E. (1977): Editor's note. Nutrition Notes 13:(2)5.
486. Sorenson, A.W., Woolley, F.R., Wyse, B.W., and Hansen, R.G. (1978): Dietitians: contributing members of the health care team. *Family & Comm. Hlth.* 1:91-100.
487. Fredrickson, D.S., Goldstein, J.L., and Brown, M.S. (1978): The familial hyperlipoproteinemias. In: *The Metabolic Basis of Inherited Disease, Fourth Edition,* edited by J.B. Stanbury, J.B. Wyngaarden, and D.S. Fredrickson. McGraw-Hill Book Co., New York. pp. 604-655.
488. Stamler, J. (1977): Quoted in *Dietary Goals for the United States, Second Edition.* U.S. Government Printing Office, Washington, D.C.. Committee Print 98-364 0. p. 14.
489. Watkin, D.M. (1969): Diabetes mellitus in an internist: a vignette. *Arch. Opthal.* 81:115-123.
490. Williams, C.D. (1933): Nutritional disease of childhood associated with maize diet. *Arch. Dis. Childhood* 8:423-433.
491. Williams, C.D. (1935): Kwashiorkor, a nutritional disease of children associated with a maize diet. *Lancet* 2:1151-1152.
492. Brock, J.F., and Autret, M. (1952): Kwashiorkor in Africa. Nutrition Studies No. 8. Food and Agriculture Organization, Rome.
493. Viteri, F., Béhar, M., and Arroyave, G. (1964): Clinical aspects of protein malnutrition. In: *Mammalian Protein Metabolism, Vol. II* edited by H.M. Munro and J.B. Allison. The Academic Press, New York. pp. 523-568.
494. Béhar, M. (1977): Protein-Calorie deficits in developing countries. In: *Food and Nutrition in Health and Disease,* edited by N.H. Moss and J. Mayer. *Ann. N.Y. Acad. Sci.* 300:176-187.
495. Health Services and Mental Health Administration, DHEW (1972): Ten State Nutrition Survey, 1968-1970. III. Clinical, Anthropometry, Dental. DHEW Publication No. (HSM) 72-8131. U.S. Government Printing Office, Washington, D.C.
496. Abraham, S., Lowenstein, F.W., and O'Connell, M.A. (1975): Preliminary findings of the first health and nutrition examination survey, United States. 1971-1972. Anthropometric and clinical findings. DHEW Publication No. (HRA) 75-1229. U.S. Government Printing Office, Washington, D.C.
497. Passmore, R., and Swindells, Y.E. (1963): Observations on the respiratory quo-

tient and weight gain of man after eating large quantities of carbohydrate. *Brit. J. Nutrition* 17:331-339.

498. Passmore, R., Strong, J.A., Swindells, Y.E., and el Din, N. (1963): The effect of overfeeding on two fat young women. *Brit. J. Nutrition* 17:373-383.
499. Passmore, R. (1964): Carbohydrates, the Cinderella of nutrition. In: *Diet and Bodily Constitution,* edited by G.E.W. Wolstenholme and M. O'Connor. J. & A. Churchill, Ltd., London. pp. 59-68.
500. Anonymous (1963): Personal papers: obesity and sugar addiction. *Lancet* 1:768.
501. Yudkin, J. (1963): Nutrition and palatability with special reference to obesity, myocardial infarction, and other diseases of civilization. *Lancet* 1:1335-1338.
502. Corn Refiners Association, Inc. (1976): *Nutritive Sweeteners from Corn.* Corn Refiners Association, Inc. Washington, D.C. pp. 15-16.
503. Finch, C.A., Miller, L.R., Inamdar, A.R., Person, R., Seiler, K., and Mackler, B. (1976): Iron deficiency in the rat. Physiological and biochemical studies of muscle dysfunction. *J. Clin. Invest.* 58:447-453.
504. Macdougall, L.G., Anderson, R., McNab, G.M., and Katz, J. (1975): The immune response in iron-deficient children: impaired cellular defense mechanisms with altered humoral components. *J. Pediatr.* 86:833-843.
505. Ulmer, D.L. (1977): Current concepts: trace elements. *New Engl. J. Med.* 297:318-321.
506. Widdowson, E.M., McCance, R.A., and Spray, C.M. (1951): Chemical composition of the human body. *Clin. Sci.* 10:113-125.
507. Leitch, I. (1964): Calcium and phosphorus. In: *Nutrition: a Comprehensive Treatise, Vol. 1: Macronutrients and Nutrient Elements,* edited by G.H. Beaton and E.W. McHenry. The Academic Press, New York. p. 269.
508. Neuman, W.F., and Neuman, M.W. (1958): *The Chemical Dynamics of Bone Mineral.* University of Chicago Press, Chicago.
509. Needleman, H.L. (1977): Exposure to lead: sources and effects. *New Engl. J. Med.* 297:943-945.
510. Feldman, R.G. (1978): Urban lead mining: lead intoxication among deleaders. *New Engl. J. Med.* 298:1143-1145.
511. Gershon, S., and Shopsin, B. Editors (1973): *Lithium — Its Role in Psychiatric Research and Treatment.* Plenum Press, New York.
512. Johnson, F.N., Editor (1974): *Lithium Research and Therapy.* Academic Press, New York.
513. Dahl. L.K. (1958): Salt intake and salt need. *New Engl. J. Med.* 258:1152-1157; 1205-1208.
514. U.S. Department of Agriculture. Agricultural Research Service (1969): Food Intake and nutritive value of diets of men, women and children in the United States, spring, 1965. USDA Publication No. ARS-62-18. U.S. Government Printing Office, Washington, D.C.
515. Abraham, S., Carroll, M.D., Dresser, C.M., and Johnson, C.L. (1977): Dietary intake findings, 1971-1974, Health and Nutrition Examination Survey. DHEW Publication No. (HRA) 77-1647. U.S. Government Printing Office, Washington, D.C.
516. Food and Nutrition Board. National Academy of Sciences — National Research Council (1968): *Recommended Dietary Allowances. Seventh Edition. 1968.* National Academy of Sciences, Washington, D.C.
517. Schroeder, H.A., and Balassa, J.J. (1961): Abnormal trace metals in man: cadmium. *J. Chronic Dis.* 14:236-258.
518. Schroeder, H.A., Balassa, J.J., and Vinton, W.H., Jr. (1965): Chromium, cadmium and lead in rats: effects on life span, tumors and tissue levels. *J. Nutrition* 86:51-66.
519. Perry, H.M., Jr., and Perry, E.F. (1976): Cadmium and hypertension. In: *The Biomedical Role of Trace Elements in Aging,* edited by J.M. Hsu, R.L. Davis and R.W. Neithamer. Eckerd College Gerontology Center, St. Petersburg, Florida. p.203.
520. Crawford, M.D., unpublished data quoted by Perry, H.M., Jr., and Perry, E.F. (1976): Cadmium and hypertension. In: *The Biomedical Role of Trace Ele-*

ments in Aging, edited by J.M. Hsu, R.L. Davis, and R.W. Neithamer. Eckerd College Gerontology Center, St. Petersburg, Florida. p. 194.

521. Perry, H.M., Tipton, I.M., Schroeder, H.A., Steiner, R.L., and Cook, M.J. (1961): Variations in the concentrations of cadmium in human kidney as a function of age and geographic origin. *J. Chronic Dis.* 14:259-271.

522. Ohanian, E.V., and Dahl, L.K. (1976): Acute effects of intra-arterial cadmium injection on blood pressure in hypertension-sensitive and resistant rats. *Federation Proc.* 35:555.

523. White, M.G., and Fetner, C.D. (1975): Treatment of the syndrome of inappropriate secretion of anti-diuretic hormone with lithium carbonate. *New Engl. J. Med.* 292:390-392.

524. Rothstein, G., Clarkson, D.R., Larsen, W., Grosser, B.I., and Athens, J.W. (1978): Effect of lithium on neutrophil mass and production. *New Engl. J. Med.* 298:178-180.

525. Prockop, L.D. (1976): Lithium: research and therapeutic profile in affective disorders. In: *The Biomedical Role of Trace Elements in Aging,* edited by J.M. Hsu, R.L. Davis and R.W. Neithamer. Eckerd College Gerontology Center, St. Petersburg, Florida. p. 217.

526. Kline, N.S. (1974): *From Sad to Glad: Kline on Depression.* G.P. Putman's Sons, New York.

527. Fieve, R.R. (1975): *Moodswing: the Third Revolution in Psychiatry.* William Morrow & Company, New York.

528. Food and Nutrition Board. National Academy of Sciences — National Research Council (1964): *Recommended Dietary Allowances. Sixth Edition, 1964.* National Academy of Sciences, Washington, D.C.

529. Adler, P. (1970): Fluorides and dental health. In: *Fluorides and Human Health,* World Health Organization Monograph Series, No. 59. World Health Organization, Geneva. pp. 323-354.

530. Bernstein, D., Sadowsky, N., Hegsted, D.M., Guri, C., and Stare, F.J. (1966): Prevalence of osteoporosis in high- and low-fluoride areas of North Dakota. *J. Amer. Med. Assoc.* 198:499-504.

531. Rose, G.A. (1965): a study of the treatment of osteoporosis with fluoride therapy. *Proc. Royal Soc. Med.* 58:436-440.

532. Life Sciences Research Office, Federation of American Societies for Experimental Biology (1974): A review of the significance of untoward reactions to iodine in foods. FDA Contract No. FDA 71 - 294, Division of Nutrition, Food and Drug Administration, Washington, D.C.

533. Eddy, T.P. (1968): The problem of retaining vitamins in hospital food. In: *Vitamins for the Elderly,* edited by A.N. Exton-Smith and D.L. Scott. John Wright & Sons, Ltd. Bristol, United Kingdom.

534. Watkin, D.M. (1978): The Limited Use Supplemental Food (LUSF) case: Can rational nutrition succeed? *Proceedings of the XI International Congress of Nutrition,* Rio de Janeiro. Sociedade Brasileira de Nutrição, Rio de Janeiro, RJ, Brazil.

535. Hegsted, D.M., Moscoso, I., and Collazos Ch., C. (1952): A study of the minimum calcium requirements of adult men. *J. Nutrition* 46:181-201.

535a. Instituto de Nutrición de Centro América y Panamá (INCAP) and the Interdepartmental Committee on Nutrition for National Defense (ICNND) (1972): Nutritional evaluation of the population of Central America and Panama. DHEW Publication No. (HSM) 72-8120. U.S. Government Printing Office, Washington, D.C.

536. Prasad, A.S., Halsted, J.A., and Nadimi, M. (1961): Syndrome of iron deficiency anemia, hepato-splenomegaly, hypogonadism, dwarfism and geophasia. *Amer. J. Med.* 31:532-546.

537. Ohlson, M.A., Roberts, P.H., Joseph, S.A., and Nelson, P.M. (1948): Dietary practices of 100 women from 40 to 75 years of age. *J. Amer. Dietetic Assoc.* 24:286-291.

538. Roberts, P.H., Kerr, C.H., and Ohlson, M.A. (1948): Nutritional status of older women. Nitrogen, calcium, phosphorus retentions in nine women. *J. Amer. Dietetic Assoc.* 24:292-299.

539. Ackermann, P.G., and Toro, G. (1953): Calcium and phosphorus balance in elderly men. *J. Gerontol.* 8:289-300.
540. Bogdonoff, M.D., Shock, N.W., and Nichols, M.P. (1953): Calcium, phosphorus, nitrogen and potassium balance studies in the aged male. *J. Gerontol.* 8:272-288.
541. Malm, O. (1958): *Calcium Requirement and Adaptation in Adult Men,* Oslo University Press, Oslo.
542. Harrison, H.H. (1959): Factors influencing calcium absorption. *Federation Proc.* 18:1085-1096.
543. Nordin, B.E.C. (1962): Calcium balance and calcium requirement in spinal osteoporosis. *Amer. J. Clin. Nutrition* 10:384-390.
544. Lutwak, L. (1969): Nutritional aspects of osteoporosis. *J. Amer. Geriatrics Soc.* 17:115-119.
545. Rich, C., and Ivanovich, P. (1965): Response to sodium fluoride in severe osteoporosis. *Ann. Internal Med.* 63:1069-1074.
546. Bernstein, D.S., and Cohen, P. (1967): Use of sodium fluoride in the treatment of osteoporosis. *J. Clin. Endo. Metab.* 27:197-210.
547. Jowsey, J. (1976): Prevention and treatment of osteoporosis. In: *Nutrition and Aging,* edited by M. Winick. John Wiley and Sons, New York.
548. Shorr, E., and Carter, A.C. (1952): The usefulness of strontium as an adjuvant to calcium in the remineralization of the skelton in man. *Bull. Hosp. Jt. Dis.* 13:59-66.
549. Reinfenstein, E.C., Jr., and Albright F. (1947): The metabolic effects of steroid hormones in osteoporosis. *J. Clin. Invest.* 26:24-56.
550. Garn. S.M., Rohmann, C.G., and Wagner, B. (1967): Bone loss as a general phenomenon in man. *Federation Proc.* 26:1729-1736.
551. Garn, S.M. (1970): *The Earlier Gain and Later Loss of Cortical Bone in Nutritional Perspective.* Charles C. Thomas, Springfield, Illinois.
552. Exton-Smith, A.N. (1972): Physiological aspects of aging: relation to nutrition. In: *Symposium on Nutrition and Aging, Part I,* edited by D.M. Watkin, *Amer. J. Clin. Nutrition* 25:853-859.
553. Garn. S.M., Rohmann, C.G., and Nolan, P. (1964): The developmental nature of bone changes during aging. In: *Relations of Development and Aging,* edited by J.E. Birren. Charles C. Thomas, Springfield, Illinois.
554. Hegsted, D.M. (1973): Major minerals: Section A, calcium and phosphorus. In: *Modern Nutrition in Heath and Disease, Fifth Edition,* edited by R.S. Goodhart and M.E. Shils. Lea & Febiger, Philadelphia. pp. 273-282.
555. Malm, O. *Calcium Requirement and Adaptation in Adult Men.* Oslo University Press, Oslo, 1958.
556. Henry, K.M., and Kon, S.K. (1953): Relationship between calcium retention and body stores of calcium in the rat. *Brit. J. Nutrition* 7:147-159.
557. Boda, J.M., and Cole, H.H. (1956): Studies on parturient paresis in cattle. *Ann. N.Y. Acad. Sci.* 64:370-374.
558. Smith, R.W., Jr., Rizek, J., and Frame, B. (1964): Determinants of serum antirachitic activity. Special reference to involutional osteoporosis. *Amer. J. Clin. Nutrition* 14:98-108.
559. Calkins, E., quoted by Watkin, D.M. (1973): Nutrition for the aging and the aged. In: *Modern Nutrition in Health and Disease, Fifth Edition,* edited by R.S. Goodhart and M.E. Shils. Lea & Febiger, Philadelphia. p. 698.
560. Watkin, D.M., and Steinfeld, J.L. (1964): Metabolic relationships between tumor and host during massive doses of prednisone in human neoplastic disease. *J. Nat'l. Cancer Inst.* 33:149-191.
561. Roe, D.A. (1976): *Drug-Induced Nutritional Deficiencies.* The AVI Publishing Company, Westport, Connecticut.
562. Albanese, A.A. (1977): *Bone Loss: Causes, Detection and Therapy.* Alan R. Liss, New York.
563. Albanese, A.A., Edelson, A.H., Lorenze, E.H., Jr., Woodhull, M.L., and Wein, E.H. (1975): Problems of bone health in the elderly: ten year study. *N.Y. State J. Med.* 75:326-336.

564. Krook, L., Lutwak, L., Henrikson, P.-A., Kallfelz, F., Hirsch, C., Romanus, B., Bélanger, L.F., Marier, J.R., and Sheffy, B.E. (1971): Reversibility of nutritional osteoporosis: Physicochemical data on bones from our experimental study in dogs. *J. Nutrition* 101:233-246.
565. Lutwak, L. (1969): Nutritional aspects of osteoporosis. *J. Amer. Geriatrics Soc.* 17:115-119.
566. Lutwak, L., Krook, L., Henrikson, P.-A., Uris, R., Whalen, J., Coulston, A., and Lesser, G. (1971): Calcium deficiency and human periodontal disease. *Israel J. Med. Sci.* 7:504-505.
567. Lutwak, L. (1977): Nutrition and metabolic bone disease. In: *Proceedings of the 1977 Clinical Nutrition Update Symposium,* edited by L. Lutwak. Institute of Continuing Medical Education, Akron City Hospital, Akron, Ohio.
568. Bayless, T.M., and Christopher, N.L. (1969): Perspectives in nutrition: Disaccharidase deficiency. *Amer. J. Clin. Nutrition* 22:181-190.
569. Bayless, T.M., and Paige, D.M. (1972): Disaccharide intolerance in feeding programs. *Proceedings of the Western Hemisphere Nutrition Congress III, Miami Beach, 1971.* Futura Publishing Company, Mount Kisco, New York. pp. 188-193.
570. Newcomer, A.D., Hodgson, S.F., McGill, D.B., and Thomas, P.J. (1978): Lactase deficiency: prevalence in osteoporosis. *Ann. Internal Med.* 89:218-220.
571. Birge, S.J., Jr., Keutmann, H.T., Cualtrecasas, P., and Whedon, G.W. (1967): Osteoporosis, intestinal lactase deficiency and low dietary calcium intake. *New Engl. J. Med.* 276:445-448.
572. Scrimshaw, N.S. (1972): In: Questions and comments on disaccharide intolerance in feeding programs, moderated by A.I. Mendeloff. *Proceedings of the Western Hemisphere Nutrition Conference III, Miami Beach, 1971.* Futura Publishing Company, Mount Kisco, New York. pp. 193-195.
573. Fletcher, R.F., Jones, J.H., and Morgan, D.B. (1963): Bone disease in chronic renal failure. *Quart. J. Med.* 32:321-339.
574. Lotz, M., Zisman, E., and Bartter, F.C. (1968): Evidence for a phosphorus depletion syndrome in man. *New Engl. J. Med.* 278:409-415.
575. Harris, R.S. (1959): Discussion of a paper by C.W. Vermeulen entitled Effects of high calcium intakes on urine in animals. *Federation Proc.* 18:1100-1102.
576. Goldsmith, R.S., Woodhouse, C.F., Ingbar, S.H., and Segal, D. (1967): Effect of phosphate supplements in patients with fractures. *Lancet* 1:687-690.
577. Epstein, F. H. (1968): Editorial comment. *Year Book of Medicine, 1968.* Year Book Medical Publishers, Chicago, pp. 427-428.
578. Ettinger, B. (1976): Recurrent nephrolithiasis: Natural history and effect of phosphate therapy: Double-blind controlled study. *Amer. J. Med.* 61:200-206.
579. Slatopolsky, E., and Bricker, N.S. (1973): Role of phosphorus restriction in prevention of secondary hyperparathyroidism in chronic renal disease. *Kidney Int.* 4:141-145.
580. Gray R.W., Wilz, D.R., Caldas, A.E., and Lemann, J., Jr. (1977): Importance of phosphate in regulating 1,25$(OH)_2$-vitamin D_3 levels in humans: Studies in healthy subjects, in calcium stone formers and in patients with primary hyperparathyroidism. *J. Clin. Endocrinol. Metab.* 45:299-306.
581. Fleisch, H., Bisaz, S., Care, A.D., Mühlbauer, R.C., and Russell, R.G.G. (1970): A review of the effects of phosphonates on calcium metabolism. In: *Proceedings of an International Symposium on Calcitonin and the C-Cells,* edited by S. Taylor. Springer-Verlag, New York. pp. 409-417.
582. Mühlbauer, R.C., Russell, R.G.G., Williams, D.A., and Fleisch, H. (1971): The effects of diphosphonates, polyphosphates, and calcitonin on "immobilization osteoporosis" in rats. *Europ. J. Clin. Invest.* 1:336-344.
583. Cabanela, M.E., and Jowsey, J. (1971): The effect of diphosphonate on phosphate-induced bone loss and soft-tissue calcification. *Mayo Clinic Proc.* 46:492-495.
584. Jowsey, J., Riggs, B.L., Kelly, P.J., Hoffman, D.L., and Bordier, P. (1971): The treatment of osteoporosis with disodium ethane-1-hydroxy-1, 1 diphosphonate. *J. Lab. Clin. Med.* 78:574-584.

585. Smith, R., Russell, R.G.G., and Bishop, M. (1971): Diphosphonates and Paget's disease of bone. *Lancet* 1:945-947.
586. Hosking, D.J., Bijvoet, O.L.M., van Aken, J., and Will, E.J. (1976): Paget's disease of bone treated with diphosphonate and calcitonin. *Lancet* 1:615-617.
587. Chase, L.R., and Slatopolsky, E. (1974): Secretion and metabolic efficacy of parathyroid hormone in patients with severe hypomagnesemia. *J. Clin. Endocrinol. Metab.* 38:363-371.
588. Gamble, J.L. (1950): *Chemical Anatomy, Physiology and Pathology of Extracellular Fluid.* Harvard University Press, Cambridge.
589. Ellis, F.P. (1972): Mortality from heat illness and heat-aggravated illness in the United States. *Environ. Res.* 5:1-58.
590. Fox, R.H., Woodward, P.M., Exton-Smith, A.N., Green, M.F., Donnison, D.V., and Wicks, M.H. (1973): Body temperatures in the elderly: A national study of physiological, social, and environmental conditions. *Brit. Med. J.* 62:200-206.
591. Knochel, J.P., and Caskey, J.H. (1977): Mechanism for hypophosphatemia in acute heat stroke. *J. Amer. Med. Assoc.* 238:425-426.
592. Freis, E.D. (1974): The clinical spectrum of essential hypertension. *Arch. Internal Med.* 133:982-987.
593. Leaf, A. (1962). Clinical and physiologic significance of the serum sodium concentration. *New Engl. J. Med.* 267:24-30; 77-83.
594. Bondy, P.K. (1963): Editorial comment. *Year Book of Medicine, 1963-1964 Series.* Year Book Publishers, Chicago. p. 680.
595. Schultze, R.G. (1973): Recent advances in the physiology and pathophysiology of potassium excretion. *Arch. Internal Med.* 131:885-897.
596. Meneely, G.R., and Battarbee, H.D. (1976): Sodium and potassium. In: *Nutrition Reviews' Present Knowledge in Nutrition, Fourth Edition,* edited by D.M. Hegsted, C.O. Chichester, W.J. Darby, K.W. McNutt, R.J. Stalvey, and E.H. Stotz. The Nutrition Foundation, Inc. New York and Washington, pp. 259-279.
597. McQuarrie, I, Thompson, W.H., and Anderson, J.A. (1936): Effects of excessive ingestion of sodium and potassium salts on carbohydrate metabolism and blood pressure in diabetic children. *J. Nutrition* 11:77-101.
598. Priddle, W.W. (1931): Observations on the management of hypertension. *Canad. Med. Assoc. J.* 25:5-8.
599. Meneely, G.R., Ball, C.O.T., and Youmans, J.B. (1957): Chronic sodium chloride toxicity: the protective effect of added potassium chloride. *Ann. Internal Med.* 44:263-273.
600. Meneely, G.R., and Ball, C.O.T. (1958): Experimental epidemiology of chronic sodium chloride toxicity and the protective effect of potassium chloride. *Amer. J. Med.* 25:713-725.
601. Kempner, W. (1945): Compensation of renal metabolic dysfunction. Treatment of kidney disease and hypertensive vascular disease with rice diet. *North Carolina Med. J.* 6:61-87.
602. Sasaki, N. (1962): High blood pressure and salt intake of the Japanese. *Japanese Heart J.* 3:313-324.
603. Shohl, A.T. (1937): The effect of the acid-base content of the diet upon the production and cure of rickets with special reference to citrates. *J. Nutrition* 14:69-83.
604. Finch, C.A. (1977): Iron nutrition. In: *Food and Nutrition in Health and Disease,* edited by H.N. Moss and J. Mayer, *Ann. N.Y. Acad. Sci.* 300:221-227.
605. Jacobs, P., Bothwell, T.H., and Charlton, R.W. (1964): Role of hydrochloric acid in iron absorption. *J. Applied Physiol.* 19:187-188.
606. Elwood, P.C., Newton, D., Eakins, J.D., and Brown, D.A. (1968): Absorption of iron from bread. *Amer. J. Clin. Nutrition* 21:1162-1169.
607. Cook, J.D., Minnick, V., Moore, C.V., Rasmussen, A., Bradley, W.B., and Finch, C.A. (1973): Absorption of fortification iron in bread. *Amer. J. Clin. Nutrition* 26:861-872
608. Crosby, W.H. (1977): Who needs iron? *New Engl. J. Med.* 297:543-545.

609. Cook, J.D., Lipschitz, D.A., Miles, L.E.M., and Finch, C.A. (1974): Serum ferritin as a measure of iron stores in normal subjects. *Amer. J. Clin. Nutrition* 27:681-687.
610. Finch, C.A. (1976): Iron metabolism. In: *Nutrition Reviews' Present Knowledge of Nutrition,* edited by D.M. Hegsted, C.O. Chichester, W.J. Darby, K.W. NcNutt, R.M. Stalvey, and E.H. Stotz. The Nutrition Foundation, Inc. New York and Washington. pp. 280-289.
611. Mertz, W. (1969): Chromium occurrence and function in biological systems. *Physiol. Rev.* 49:163-239.
612. Mertz, W. (1976): Effects and metabolism of glucose tolerance factor. In: *Nutrition Reviews' Present Knowledge of Nutrition, Fourth Edition,* edited by D.M. Hegsted, C.O. Chichester, W.J. Darby, K.W. McNutt, R.M. Stalvey, and E.H. Stotz. The Nutrition Foundation, Inc. New York and Washington. pp. 365-375.
613. Schroeder, H.A., Balassa, J.J., and Tipton, I.H. (1962): Abnormal trace metals in man — chromium. *J. Chronic Dis.* 15:941-964.
614. Canfield, W.K., and Doisy, R.J. (1976): Chromium and diabetes in the aged. In: *Biomedical Role of Trace Elements in Aging,* edited by J.M. Hsu, R.L. Davis, and R.W. Neithamer. Eckerd College Gerontology Center, St. Petersburg, Florida. pp 119-128.
615. Levine, R.A., Streeten, D.H.P., and Doisy, R.J. (1968): Effects of oral chromium supplementation on the glucose tolerance of elderly human subjects. *Metabolism* 17:114-125.
616. Glinsmann, W.H., and Mertz, W. (1966): Effect of trivalent chromium on glucose tolerance. *Metabolism* 15:510-515.
617. Hopkins, L.L., Jr., and Price, M.G. (1969): Effectiveness of chromium (III) in improving the impaired glucose tolerance of middle-aged Americans. *Proceedings: Western Hemisphere Nutrition Congress II — San Juan, Puerto Rico, 1968.* American Medical Association, Chicago, pp. 235-236.
618. Doisy, R.J., Streeten, D.H.P., Freiberg, J.M., and Schneider, A.J. (1976): Chromium metabolism in man and biochemical effects. In: *Trace Elements in Human Health and Disease, Volume 2,* edited by A.S. Prasad. Academic Press, New York. pp. 79-104.
619. Hambridge, K.M. (1971): Chromium nutrition in the mother and growing child. In: *The Newer Trace Elements in Nutrition,* edited by W. Mertz and W.E. Cornatzer. Marcel Dekker, New York. pp. 169-194.
620. Cartwright, G.E., and Wintrobe, M.M. (1964): The question of copper deficiency in man. *Amer. J. Clin. Nutrition* 15:94-110.
621. Cartwright, G.E., and Wintrobe, M.M. (1964): Copper metabolism in normal subjects. *Amer. J. Clin. Nutrition* 14:224-232.
622. Denny-Brown, D., and Porter, H. (1951): The effect of BAL (2,3-dimercaptopropanol) on hepatolenticular degeneration (Wilson's disease). *New Engl. J. Med.* 245:917-925.
623. Cumings, J.N. (1951): The effect of BAL on hepatolenticular degeneration. *Brain* 74:10-22.
624. Walshe, J.M. (1956): Penicillamine, a new oral therapy for Wilson's disease. *Amer. J. Med.* 21:487-495.
625. Deiss, A., Lynch, R.E., Lee, G.R., and Cartwright, G.E. (1971): Long-term therapy for Wilson's disease. *Ann. Internal Med.* 75:57-65.
626. Bearn, A.G. (1961): Genetic considerations in Wilson's disease. In: *Wilson's Disease, Some Current Concepts,* edited by J.M. Walshe and J.N. Cumings. Blackwell, Oxford. pp. 118-123.
627. Bearn, A.G. (1972): Wilson's disease. In: *The Metabolic Basis of Inherited Disease,* edited by J.B. Stanbury, J.B. Wyngaarden and D.S. Fredrickson. The Blakiston Division, McGraw-Hill Book Company, New York. pp. 761-779.
628. Graham, G.G., and Cordano, A. (1969): Copper depletion and deficiency in malnourished infants. *Johns Hopkins Med. J.* 124:139-150.
629. Shahidi, N.T., Diamond, L.K., and Schwachman, H. (1961): Anemia associated with protein deficiency. A study of two cases with cystic fibrosis. *J. Pediat.* 59:533-542.

630. Stransky, E., Dauis-Lawas, D.T., and Lawas, I.L. (1952): On serum copper level and its importance in childhood. *Ann. Paediat.* 179:1-11.

631. Lahey, M.E., Béhar, M., Viteri, F., and Scrimshaw, N.S. (1958): Values for copper, iron and iron-binding capacity in the serum in kwashiorkor. *Pediatrics* 22:72-79.

632. Edozien, J.C., and Udeozo, I.O. (1960): Serum copper, iron and iron-binding capacity in kwashiorkor. *J. Trop. Pediat.* 6:60-64.

633. MacDonald, I., and Warren, P.J. (1961): The copper content of the liver and hair of African children with kwashiorkor. *Brit. J. Nutrition* 15:593-596.

634. Schubert, W.K., and Lahey, M.E. (1959): Copper and protein depletion complicating hypoferric anemia in infancy. *Pediatrics* 24:710-733.

635. Sturgeon, P., and Brubaker, C. (1956): Copper deficiency in infants. A syndrome characterized by hypocupremia, iron deficiency anemia and hypoproteinemia. *American (A.M.A.) J. Dis. Child.* 92:254-265.

636. Munch-Petersen, S. (1950): On the copper content in urine in proteinuria. *Scandinav. J. Clin. & Lab. Invest.* 2:337-340.

637. Cartwright, G.E., Gubler, C.J., and Wintrobe, M.M. (1954): Studies on copper metabolism. XI. Copper and iron metabolism in the nephrotic syndrome. *J. Clin. Invest.* 33:685-698.

638. Butterworth, C.E., Jr., Gubler, C.J., Cartwright, G.E., and Wintrobe, M.M. (1958): Studies on copper metabolism. XXVI. Plasma copper in patients with tropical sprue. *Proc. Soc. Exper. Biol. & Med.* 98:594-597.

639. Cartwright, G.E. (1955): The relationship of copper, cobalt and other trace elements to hemopoiesis. *Amer. J. Clin. Nutrition* 3:11-17.

640. Gross, P.A., Embree, L.J., Bally, P., Shipp, J.C., and Thorn, G.W. (1960): Hypoalbuminemia (with anasarca) due to hypercatabolism, serum protein exudation into the gastrointestinal tract, increased capillary permeability and hypoanabolism. The unusual occurrence of increased capillary permeability temporarily reversed by human growth hormone therapy. *Amer. J. Med.* 29:386-404.

641. Holman, H., Nickel, W.F., Jr., and Sleisenger, M.H. (1959): Hypoproteinemia antedating intestinal lesions, and possibly due to excessive serum protein loss in the intestine. *Amer. J. Med.* 27:963-975.

642. Waldmann, T.A., Steinfeld, J.L., Dutcher, T.F., Davidson, J.D., and Gordon, R.S., Jr. (1961): The role of the gastrointestinal system in "ideopathic hypoproteinemia." *Gastroenterology* 41:197-207.

643. Jeffries, G.H., Holman, H.R., and Sleisenger, M.H. (1962): Plasma proteins and the gastrointestinal tract. *New Engl. J. Med.* 266:652-660.

644. Graham, G.G, and Cordano, A. (1976): Copper deficiency in human subjects. In: *Trace Elements in Human Health and Disease, Volume 1,* edited by A.S. Prasad. Academic Press, New York. pp. 363-372.

645. Harris, E.D., and O'Dell, B.L. (1974): Copper and amine oxidases in connective tissue metabolism. In: *Protein-Metal Interaction*, edited by M. Freidman. *Advances in Experimental Medicine and Biology*, 48:267-284. Plenum Press, New York.

646. O'Dell, B.L. (1976): Biochemistry and physiology of copper in vertebrates. In: *Trace Elements in Human Health and Disease, Volume 1,* edited by A.S. Prasad. Academic Press, New York. pp. 391-413.

647. Gallagher, C.H., and Reeve, V.E. (1971): Copper deficiency in the rat. Effect on synthesis of phospholipids. *Aust. J. Exp. Biol. Med. Sci.* 49:21-31.

648. Klevay, L.M. (1973): Hypercholesterolemia in rats produced by an increase in the ratio of zinc to copper ingested. *Amer. J. Clin. Nutrition* 26:1060-1068.

649. Murthy, L., Klevay, L.M., and Petering, H.G. (1974): Interrelations of zinc and copper nutriture in the rat. *J. Nutrition* 104:1458-1465.

650. Klevay, L.M. (1975): Coronary heart disease: the zinc/copper hypothesis. *Amer. J. Clin. Nutrition* 28:764-774.

651. Reinhold, J.G., Faradji, B., Abadi, P., and Ismail-Beigi, F. (1976): Binding of zinc to fiber and other solids of wholemeal bread. In: *Trace Elements in Human Health and Disease, Volume 1,* edited by A.S. Prasad. Academic Press, New York. pp. 163-180.

652. Wester, P.O. (1965): Trace elements in human myocardial infarction determined by neutron activation analysis. *Acta. Med. Scand.* 178:765-788.
653. Schroeder, H.A., Nason, A.P., Tipton, I.H., and Balassa, J.J. (1966): Essential trace elements in man: copper. *J. Chron. Dis.* 19:1007-1034.
654. White, H.S. (1969): Inorganic elements in weighed diets of girls and young women. *J. Amer. Dietetic Assoc.* 55:38-43.
655. Price, N.O., Bunce, G.E., and Engel, R.W. (1970): Copper, manganese and zinc balance in preadolescent girls. *Amer. J. Clin. Nutrition* 23:258-260.
656. Evans, G.W. (1973): Copper homeostasis in the mammalian system. *Physiol. Rev.* 53:535-570.
657. Department of Health, Education and Welfare, Public Health Service, Bureau of State Services, Division of Dental Public Health (1956): Present status of controlled fluoridation in the United States. *Public Health Reports* 71:963-966.
658. Arnold, F.A., Jr., Dean, H.T., Jay, P., and Knutson, J.W. (1956): Effect of fluoridated public water supplies on dental caries prevalence. *Public Health Reports* 71:652-658.
659. American Academy of Pediatrics, Committee on Nutrition (1972): Fluoride as a nutrient. *Pediatrics* 49:456-460.
660. Morrey, L.W. (1962): Aid for the aging: more comprehensive dental services (editorial). *J. Amer. Dental Assoc.* 64:578.
661. Rich, C., and Ensinck, J. (1961): Effect of sodium fluoride on calcium metabolism of human beings. *Nature (London)* 191:184-185.
662. Rich, C., Ensinck, J., and Ivanovich, P. (1964): The effect of sodium fluoride on calcium metabolism of subjects with metabolic bone disease. *J. Clin. Invest.* 43:545-555.
663. Cohen, P., and Gardner, F.H. (1964): Induction of subacute skeletal fluorosis in a case of multiple myeloma. *New Engl. J. Med.* 271:1129-1133.
664. Rich, C., and Ivanovich, P. (1965): Response to sodium fluoride in severe primary osteoporosis. *Ann. Internal Med.* 63:1068-1074.
665. Cohen, P., and Gardner, F.H. (1966): Induction of skeletal fluorosis in two common demineralizing disorders. *J. Amer. Med. Assoc.* 195:962-963.
666. Higgins, B.A., Nassim, J.R., Alexander, R., and Hilb, A. (1965): Effect of sodium fluoride on calcium, phosphorus and nitrogen balance in patients with Paget's disease. *Brit. Med. J.* 1:1159-1161.
667. Rich, C. (1966): Osteoporosis and fluoride therapy. In: Questions and Answers. *J. Amer. Med. Assoc.* 196:1165.
668. Spencer, H., Osis, D., Wiatrowski, E., and Samachson, J. (1970): Availability of fluoride from fish protein concentrate and from sodium fluoride in man. *J. Nutrition* 100:1415-1424.
669. Spencer, H., Samachson, J., Fowler, J., and Kulka, M.J. (1971): Availability in man of protein and minerals from fish protein concentrate. *Amer. J. Clin. Nutrition* 24:311-317.
670. Greer, M.A. (1962): The natural occurrence of goitrogenic agents. *Recent Progress in Hormone Research* 18:187-219.
671. Van Etten, C.H., and Wolff, I.A. (1973): Natural sulfur compounds. In: *Toxicants Occurring Naturally in Foods, Second Edition.* Committee on Food Protection, Food and Nutrition Board, National Research Council, National Academy of Sciences, Washington, D.C. pp. 210-234.
672. Beckers, C. (1969): Pathophysiology of nontoxic goiter. In: *Endemic Goiter*, edited by J.B. Stanbury. Pan-American Health Organization Scientific Publication No. 193. Pan-American Health Organization, Washington, D.C. pp. 30-48.
673. Food and Nutrition Board, National Research Council. (1970): *Iodine nutriture in the United States.* National Academy of Sciences, Washington, D.C.
674. Department of Health, Education and Welfare, Center for Disease Control, Atlanta, Georgia. (1972): *Highlights: Ten-State Nutrition Survey, 1968-1970.* U.S. Government Printing Office, Washington, D.C. p. 12, DHEW Publication No. (HSM) 72-8134.

675. Marine, D., and Kimball, O.P. (1920): Prevention of simple goiter in man. *Arch. Internal Med.* 25:661-672.

676. Marine, D., and Kimball, O.P. (1921): The prevention of simple goiter in man. *J. Amer. Med. Assoc.* 77:1068-1070.

677. Kimball, O.P. (1922): The prevention of simple goiter in man. *Amer. J. Med. Sci.* 163:634-649.

678. Braverman, L.E., Woeber, K.A., and Ingbar, S.H. (1969): Induction of myxedema by iodide in patients euthyroid after radioiodine or surgical treatment of diffuse toxic goiter. *New Engl. J. Med.* 281:816-821.

679. Wolff, J. (1969): Iodide goiter and the pharmacological effects of excess iodide. *Amer. J. Med.* 47:101-124.

680. Cavalieri, R.R. (1973): Trace elements. Section A. Iodine. In: *Modern Nutrition in Health and Disease, Fifth Edition*, edited by R.S. Goodhart and M.E. Shils. Lea & Febiger, Philadelphia. pp. 362-371.

681. Stadtman, T.C. (1977): Biological function of selenium. *Nutrition Rev.* 35:161-166.

682. Underwood, E.J. (1977): *Trace Elements in Human and Animal Nutrition, Fourth Edition.* Academic Press, New York.

683. Schwartz, K., and Foltz, C.M. (1957): Seleium as an integral part of factor 3 against dietary necrotic liver regeneration. *J. Amer. Chem. Soc.* 79:3292-3293.

684. Patterson, E.L., Milstrey, R., and Stokstad, E.L.R. (1957): Effect of selenium in preventing exudative diathesis in chicks. *Proc. Soc. Exper. Biol. Med.* 95:617-620.

685. Smith, M.I. (1941): Chronic endemic selenium poisoning. *J. Amer. Med. Assoc.* 116:562-567.

686. Smith, M.I., Franke, K.W., and Westfall, B.B. (1936): The selenium problem in relation to public health. A preliminary survey to determine the possibility of selenium intoxication in the rural population living on seleniferous soil. *Pub. Health Reports* 51:1496-1505.

687. Smith, M.I., and Westfall, B.B. (1937): Further field studies on the selenium problem in relation to public health. *Public Health Reports* 52:1375-1384.

688. Hadjimarkos, D.M., and Bonhorst, C.W. (1958): The trace element selenium and its influence on dental caries susceptibility. *J. Pediat.* 52:274-278.

689. Tappel, A.L. (1965): Free radical lipid peroxidation damage and its inhibition by vitamin E and selenium. *Federation Proc.* 24:73-78.

690. Rotruck, J.T., Pope, A.L., Ganther, H.E., Swanson, A.B., Hafeman, D.G., and Hoekstra. W.G. (1973): Selenium: biochemical role as a component of glutathione peroxidase. *Science* 179:588-590.

691. Hartley, W.J., and Grant, A.B. (1961): A review of selenium-responsive diseases in New Zealand livestock. *Federation Proc.* 20:679-688.

692. Ganther, H.E., Hafeman, D.G., Lawrence, R.A., Serfass, R.E., and Hoekstra, W.G. (1976): Selenium and glutathione peroxidase in health and disease: a review. In: *Trace Elements in Human Health and Disease, Volume 2*, edited by A.S. Prasad. Academic Press, New York. pp. 165-234.

693. Thompson, C.D., Rea, H.M., Robinson, M.F., and Chapman, O.W. (1977): Low blood selenium concentrations and glutathione peroxidase activities in elderly people. *Proc. Univ. Otago Med. Sch.* 55:18-19.

694. Li, T.-K., and Vallee, B.L. (1973): The biochemical and nutritional role of trace elements. In: *Modern Nutrition in Health and Disease, Fifth Edition*, edited by R.S. Goodhart and M.E. Shils. Lea & Febiger, Philadelphia. p. 392.

695. Morris, V.C., and Levander, O.A. (1970): Selenium content of foods. *J. Nutrition* 100:1383-1388.

695a. Johnson, R.A., Baker, S.S., Fallon, J.T., Maynard, E.P., III, Ruskin, J.N., Wen, Z., Ge, K. and Cohen, H.J. (1981): An Occidental case of cardiomyopathy and selenium deficiency. *New Engl. J. Med.* 304:1210-1212.

695b. Collipp, P.J., and Chen, S.Y. (1981): Cardiomyopathy and selenium deficiency in a two-year-old girl (a letter to the editor). *New Engl. J. Med.* 304:1304-1305.

695c. Aaseth, J., Thomassen, Y., Alexander, J., and Norheim, G. (1980): Decreased serum selenium in alcoholic cirrhosis. *New Engl. J. Med.* 303:944-945.

695d. Goldman, I.S., and Kantrowitz, N.E. (1981): Cardiomyopathy associated with selenium deficiency (a letter to the editor). *New Engl. J. Med.* 305:701.
695e. Dock, W. (1966): How some hearts age. *J. Amer. Med. Assoc.* 195:442-444.
695f. Burch, G., and Giles, T. (1971): Senile cardiomyopathy. *J. Chronic Dis.* 24:1-3.
695g. Dock, W. (1972): Cardiomyopathies of the senescent and the senile. *Cardiovasc. Clin.* 4:362-73.
695h. Dock, W. (1972): Cardiomyopathies of the senescent and the senile. In: *Cardiomyopathy*, edited by G.E. Burch. F.A. Davis Company, Philadelphia. pp. 361-374.
696. Hopkins, L.L., Jr., and Mohr, H.E. (1971): The biological essentiality of vanadium. In: *Newer Trace Elements in Nutrition*, edited by W. Mertz and W.E. Cornatzer. Marcel Dekker, New York. pp. 195-213.
697. Strasia, C.A. (1971): Vanadium: essentiality and toxicity in the laboratory rat. Ph.D. Thesis. University Microfilms, Ann Arbor, Michigan.
698. Schwarz, K., and Milne, D.B. (1971): Growth effects of vanadium in the rat. *Science* 174:426-428.
699. Miller, W.J., and Neathery, M.W. (1977): Newly recognized trace mineral elements and their role in animal nutrition. *Bioscience* 27:674-679.
700. Curran, G.L. (1954): Effect of certain transition elements on hepatic synthesis of cholesterol in the rat. *J. Biol. Chem.* 210:765-770.
701. Curran, G.L., and Azarnoff, D.L. (1957): Site of vanadium inhibition of cholesterol biosynthesis. *J. Amer. Chem. Soc.* 79:2968-2969.
702. Curran, G.L., and Costello, R.L. (1956): Reduction of excess cholesterol in rabbit aorta by inhibition of endogenous synthesis. *J. Exper. Med.* 103:49-56.
703. Curran, G.L., Azarnoff, D.L., and Bolinger, R.E. (1959): Effect of cholesterol synthesis inhibition in normocholesterolemic young men. *J. Clin. Invest.* 38:1251-1261.
704. Hopkins, L.L., Jr., and Mohr, H.E. (1971): Effect of plasma vanadium deficiency on plasma cholesterol of chicks. *Federation Proc.* 30:462 Abs.
705. Nielsen, F.H., and Ollerich, D.A. (1973): Studies on a vanadium deficiency in chicks. *Federation Proc.* 32:929 Abs.
706. Hopkins, L.L., Jr., and Mohr, H.E. (1974): Vanadium as an essential nutrient. *Federation Proc.* 33:1773-1775.
707. Curran, G.L., and Burch, R.E. (1967): Biological and health effects of vanadium. In: *Proceedings of the First Annual Conference on Trace Substances in Environmental Health*, edited by D.D. Hemphill. Environmental Health Center and Extension Division, University of Missouri, Columbia. pp. 96-104.
708. Schroeder, H.A., Balassa, J.J., and Tipton, I.H. (1963): Abnormal trace elements in man: vanadium. *J. Chron. Dis.* 16:1047-1071.
709. Dimond, E.G., Caravaca, J., and Benchimol, A. (1963): Vanadium: excretion, toxicity, lipid effect in man. *Amer. J. Clin. Nutrition* 12:49-53.
710. Schroeder, H.A. (1968): Serum cholesterol levels in rats fed thirteen trace elements. *J. Nutrition* 94:475-480.
711. Hafez, Y., and Kratzer, F.H. (1976): The effects of dietary vanadium on fatty acid and cholesterol synthesis and turnover in the chick. *J. Nutrition* 106:249-257.
712. Söremark, R., Üllberg, S., and Appelgren, L.-E. (1962): Autoradiographic localization of vanadium pentoxide ($^{48}V_2O_5$) in developing teeth and bones of rats. *Acta Odontol. Scand.* 20: 225-232.
713. Söremark, R., Üllberg, S. (1962): Distribution and kinetics of $^{48}V_2O_5$ in mice. In: *The Use of Radioisotopes in Animal Biology and in the Medical Sciences*, edited by N. Fried. Academic Press, New York. p. 103.
714. Schwarz, K. (1974): Recent dietary trace element research, exemplified by tin, fluorine and silicon. *Federation Proc.* 33:1748-1757.
715. Underwood, E.J. (1971): *Trace Elements in Human and Animal Nutrition, Third Edition.* Academic Press, New York.
716. Schroeder, H.A., Mitchener, M., and Nason, A.P. (1970): Zirconium, niobium, antimony, vanadium and lead in rats: life term studies. *J. Nutrition* 100:59-68.
717. Walford, R.L., quoted by Blinsky, G. (1976): Science is on the trail of the fountain of youth. *Fortune* 94:134-140.

718. Schroeder, H.A., and Nason, A.P. (1976): Interactions of trace metals in mouse and rat tissues: zinc, chromium, copper and manganese with 13 other elements. *J. Nutrition* 106:198-203.
719. Muhler, J.C. (1957): The effect of vanadium pentoxide, fluorides and tin compounds on the dental caries experience in rats. *J. Dental Res.* 36:787-794.
720. Todd, W.R., Elvehjem, C.A., and Hart, E.B. (1934): Zinc nutrition in the rat. *Amer. J. Physiol.* 107:146-156.
721. Prasad, A.S., Halsted, J.A., and Nadimi, M. (1961): Syndrome of iron deficiency anemia, hepatosplenomegaly, hypogonadism, dwarfism and geophasia. *Amer. J. Med.* 31:532-546.
722. Prasad, A.S., Miale, A., Jr., Farid, Z., Schulert, A., and Sandstead, H.H. (1963): Zinc metabolism in patients with the syndrome of iron deficiency anemia, hepatosplenomegaly, dwarfism and hypogonadism. *J. Lab. & Clin. Med.* 61:537-549.
723. Prasad, A.S., Miale, A., Jr., Farid, Z., Sandstead, H.H., and Darby, W.J. (1963): Biochemical studies on dwarfism, hypogonadism and anemia. *Arch. Internal Med.* 111:407-428.
724. Sandstead, H.H., Prasad, A.S., Schulert, A.R., Farid, Z., Miale, A., Jr., Bassilly, S., and Darby, W.J. (1967): Human zinc deficiency, endocrine manifestations and response to treatment. *Amer. J. Clin. Nutrition* 30:422-442.
725. Halsted, J.A., Ronaghy, H.A., Ababi, P., Haghshenass, M., Amirhakimi, G.H., Barakat, R.M., and Reinhold, J.G. (1972): Zinc deficiency in man: The Shiraz experiment. *Amer. J. Med.* 53:277-284.
726. Poires, W.J., Henzel, J.H., Rob, C.C., and Strain, W.H. (1967): Acceleration of wound healing in man with zinc sulfate given by mouth. *Lancet* 1:121-124.
727. Henkin, R.I. (1976): Taste loss in aging. In: *The Biomedical Role of Trace Elements in Aging*, edited by J.M. Hsu, R.L. Davis and R.W. Neithamer. Eckerd College Gerontology Center, St. Petersburg, Florida. pp. 221-236.
728. Watkin, D.M., Chairman (1975): Cooperative study of orally administered zinc sulfate in the management of pressure ulcers. Cooperative Studies Program, Department of Medicine and Surgery, Veterans Administration, Washington, D.C.
729. Prasad, A.S. (1976): Zinc in human nutrition. In: *The Biomedical Role of Trace Elements in Aging*, edited by J.M. Hsu, R.L. Davis, and R.W. Neithamer. Eckerd College Gerontology Center, St. Petersburg, Florida. pp. 15-33.
730. Prasad, A.S., and Oberleas, D. (1973): Ribonuclease and deoxyribonuclease activity in zinc-deficient tissues. *J. Lab. & Clin. Med.* 82:461-466.
731. Prasad, A.S., and Oberleas, D. (1974): Thymidine kinase activity and incorporation of thymidine into DNA in zinc deficient tissue. *J. Lab. & Clin. Med.* 83:634-639.
732. Terhune, M.W., and Sandstead, H.H. (1972): Decreased RNA polymerase activity in mammalian zinc deficiency. *Science* 177:68-69.
732a. Watkin, D.M. (1978): The Limited Use Supplemental Food (LUSF) case: Can rational nutrition succeed? In: *Resumos Temas Livres*, Publição da Commissão, Executiva do XI Congresso Internacional de Nutrição, Rio de Janeiro, RJ, Brasil. p. 437.
732b. Watkin, D.M. (1980): Better nutrition for those already old: The challenges of the eighties. *Aging*, September-October, 1980. pp. 21-28.
732c. Watkin, D.C. (1981): Aging and the food service industry: Effects upon consumers, employees and executives. *Proceedings of the 36th Conference: The Food Service Industry in the 1980's — A More Complex Environment, San Antonio, Texas, November 6-8, 1980.* The Society for the Advancement of Food Service Research, Fort Wayne, Indiana. pp. 31-40.
733. Hansen, R.G. (1973): An index of food quality. *Nutrition Reviews* 31:1-17.
734. Hansen, R.G., and Wyse, B.W. (1979): Planning for the inevitable: Snack foods in the diet. *Family and Community Health* 1:31-39.
735. Sorenson, A.W., and Lyon, J.L. (1979): Nutritional epidemiology: A research approach. *Family and Community Health* 1:69-82.
736. Watkin, D.M. (1979): Nutrition, health and aging. In: *Nutrition and the World Food Problem*, edited by M. Rechcigl. Karger, Basel. pp. 20-62.

737. Hansen, R.G., Wyse, B.W., and Sorenson, A.W. (1979): *Nutritional Quality Index of Foods.* The AVI Publishing Co., Inc. Westport, CT.
738. Weg, R.B. (1978): *Nutrition and the Later Years.* The University of Southern California Press, Los Angeles. pp. 38, 48, 55, 57, 66, 109, 131, 133.
739. Interdepartmental Committee on Nutrition for National Defense (1963): *Manual for Nutrition Surveys, Second Edition.* U.S. Government Printing Office, Washington, DC.
740. U.S. Department of Health, Education and Welfare (1972): *Ten-State Nutrition Survey, 1968-1970: I — Historical Developments.* DHEW Publication No. (HSM) 72-8130. U.S. Government Printing Office, Washington, D.C. pp. I-1 — I-121.
741. Bauernfeind, J.C., and Cort, W.M. (1974): Nutrification of foods with added vitamin A. In: *CRC Critical Reviews in Food Technology*, edited by T.E. Furia. CRC Press, Cleveland. pp. 337-375.
742. Alexander, B., Lorenzen, E., Hoffman, R., and Garfinkel, A. (1947): The effect of ingested mineral oil on plasma carotene and vitamin A. *Proc. Soc. Exper. Biol. Med.* 65:275-28.
743. Levy, R.I., Fredrickson, D.S., Stone, N.J., Bilheimer, D.W., Brown, W.V., Glueck, C.J., Gotto, A.M., Herbert, P.N., Kwiterovich, P.O., Langer, T., LaRosa, J., Lux, S.E., Rider, A.K., Shulman, R.S., and Sloan, M.D. (1973): Cholestyramine in type II hyperlipoproteinemia: a double blind trial. *Ann. Internal Med.* 79:51-58.
744. Danhof, I.E. (1966): Effects of cholestyramine on fecal excretion of ingested radioiodinated lipids. *Amer. J. Clin. Nutrition* 18:343-349.
745. Hofmann, A.F., and Poley, J.R. (1969): Cholestyramine treatment of diarrhea associated with ileal resection. *New England J. Med.* 281:397-402.
746. Hofmann, A.F., and Poley, J.R. (1972): Role of bile acid malabsorption in pathogenesis of diarrhea and steatorrhea in patients with ileal resecton: I. Response to cholestyramine or replacement of dietary long-chain triglyceride by medium-chain triglyceride. *Gastroenterology* 69:918-934.
747. Ingelfinger, F.L. (1967): Editorial comment. *Year Book of Medicine, 1967-1968 Series.* Year Book Medical Publishers, Inc. Chicago. p. 378.
747a. DeLuca, L.M. (1978): Vitamin A. In: *The Fat-Soluble Vitamins, Handbook of Lipid Research, 2*, edited by H.F. DeLuca. Plenum Press, New York. pp. 1-67.
748. Wald, G. (1968): Molecular basis of visual excitation. *Science* 162:230-239.
749. Hodges, R.E., Sauberlich, H.E., Canham, J.E., Wallace, D.L., Rucker, R.B., Mejia, L.A., and Mohanran, M. (1978): Hematopoietic studies in vitamin A deficiency. *Amer. J. Clin. Nutrition* 31:876-885.
750. Watkin, D.M., Ferencz, C., Reh, E., Weswig, P., Pearson, W., Chichester, C., Kocher, R., and Sheehy, R. (1967): Encuesta de Nutrición, Republica del Paraguay, Mayo-Agosto de 1965. Programa de Nutrición, Centro Nacional para el control de Enfermedades Crónicas, Servicio de Salud Pública, Departmento de Salud, Educación y Bienstar de las EUA, Bethesda, Maryland. pp. 1-482.
751. Mejia, L.A., Hodges, R.E., Arroyave, G., Viteri, F., and Torun, B. (1977): Vitamin A deficiency and anemia in Central American children. *Amer. J. Clin. Nutrition* 30:1175-1184.
752. Rodahl, K., and Moore, T., (1943): The vitamin A content and toxicity of polar bear and seal liver. *Biochem. J.* 37:166-168.
753. Moore, T. (1967): Pharmacology and toxicology of vitamin A. In: *The Vitamins: Chemistry, Physiology, Pathology, Methods, Second Edition, Vol. 1*, edited by W.H. Sebrell, Jr. and R.S. Harris. Academic Press, New York, pp. 280-294.
753a. Hillman, R.W. (1965): Hypervitaminosis A: experimental induction in the human subject. *Amer. J. Clin. Nutrition* 4:603-608.
754. Smith, F.R. and Goodman, D.S. (1976): Vitamin A transport in human vitamin A toxicity. *New England J. Med.* 294:805-808.
755. Kirk, E. and Chieffi, M. (1948): Vitamin studies in middle-aged and old individuals. I. The vitamin A, total carotene and alpha and beta carotene concentrations in plasma. *J. Nutr.* 36:315-322.
756. Yiengst, M.J. and Shock, N.W. (1949): Effect of oral administration of vitamin A on plasma levels of vitamin A and carotene in aged males. *J. Geront.* 4:205-211.

757. Birren, J.E., Bick, M.W., and Fox, C. (1948): Age changes in the light threshold of the dark-adapted eye. *J. Geront.* 3:267-271.
758. Birren, J.E., Bick, M.W., and Yiengst, M. (1950): The relation of structural changes of the eye and vitamin A to elevation of the light threshold in later life. *J. Exp. Psychol.* 40:260-266.
759. Bergen, S.J., Jr. and Roels, O.A. (1965): Hypervitaminosis A: report of a case. *Amer. J. Clin. Nutrition* 16:265-269.
760. Schütte, D. (1824): Beobachtungen über den Nutzen des Berger Leberthrans. (Oleum jecoris Aselli, von Gadus Asellus L.). *Arch. Med. Erfahrung,* Jahrgang Juli, Aug., pp. 79-92.
761. Palm, T.A. (1890): The geographical distribution and etiology of rickets. *The Practitioner* 45:270-279; 321-342.
762. McCollum, E.V., Simonds, N., Becker, J.E., and Shipley, P.G. (1922): Studies on experimental rickets. XXI. An experimental demonstration of the existence of a vitamin which promotes calcium deposition. *J. Biol. Chem.* 53:293-312.
763. McCollum, E.V., Simonds, N., Becker, J.E., and Shipley, P.G. (1922): Studies on experimental rickets. XXI. An experimental demonstration of the existence of a vitamin which promotes calcium deposition. *Bull. Johns Hopkins Hosp.* 33:229.
764. Steenbock, H. and Black, A. (1924): Fat-soluble vitamins. XVII. The induction of growth-promoting and calcifying properties in a ration by exposure to ultra-violet light. *J. Biol. Chem.* 61:405-422.
765. Steenbock, H. (1924): The induction of growth promoting and calcifying properties in a ration by exposure to light. *Science* 60:224-225.
766. Blunt, J.W., DeLuca, H.F., and Schnoes, H.K. (1968): 25-hydroxycholecalciferol: a biologically active metabolite of vitamin D_3. *Biochemistry* 7:3317-3322.
767. DeLuca, H.F. and Schnoes, H.K. (1976): Metabolism and mechanism of action of vitamin D. *Ann. Rev. Biochem.* 45:631-666.
768. DeLuca, H.F. (1976): Vitamin D endocrinology. *Ann. Internal Med.* 85-367-377.
769. DeLuca, H.F. (1976): Recent advances in our understanding of the metabolism of vitamin D and its regulation. *Clin. Endocrin.* suppl. 5, pp. 97s-108s.
770. DeLuca, H.F. (1976): Metabolism of vitamin D: current status. *Amer. J. Clin. Nutrition* 29:1258-1270.
771. Proscal, D.A., Okamura, W.H., and Norman, A.W. (1976): Vitamin D, its metabolites and analogs: a review of the structural requirements for biological activity. *Amer. J. Clin. Nutrition* 29:1271-1282.
772. Haussler, M.R. and McCain, J.A. (1977): Basic and clinical concepts related to vitamin D metabolism and action. *New Engl. J. Med.* 297:974-983; 1041-1051.
773. Brickman, A.S., Hartenbower, D.L., Norman, A.W., and Coburn, J.W. (1977): Actions of 1 alpha-hydroxy-vitamin D_3 on mineral metabolism. *Amer. J. Clin. Nutrition* 30:1064-1069.
773a. DeLuca, H.F. (1978): Vitamin D. In: *The Fat-Soluble Vitamins, Handbook of Lipid Research, 2,* edited by H.F. DeLuca. Plenum Press, New York. pp. 69-132.
773b. DeLuca, H.F. (1979): The vitamin D system in the regulation of calcium and phosphorus metabolism. Eleventh Annual W.O. Atwater Memorial Lecture sponsored by the Science and Education Administration, U.S. Department of Agriculture, given at the Annual Meeting of the American Institute of Nutrition, Dallas, Texas, April 2, 1979. *Nutrition Reviews* 37:161-193.
774. Avioli, L.V., and Haddad, J.G. (1977): Vitamin D: more and more measured better and better. *New Eng. J. Med.* 207:1006-1007.
775. Stamp, T.C.B. (1974): Intestinal absorption of 25-hydrocholecalciferol. *Lancet* 2:121-122.
776. Gray, R.W., Wilz, D.R., Caldas, A.E., and Lemann, J., Jr. (1977): The importance of phosphate in regulating plasma 1,25-$(OH)_2$-vitamin D_3 levels in humans: studies in healthy subjects, in calcium-stone formers and in patients with primary hyperparathyroidism. *J. Clin. Endocrinol. Metab.* 45:299-306.
777. Rosen, J.F., Fleischman, A.R., Finberg, S., Eisman, J., and DeLuca, H.F. (1977): 1,25-dihydroxycholecalciferol: its use in the long-term management of

idiopathic hyperparathyroidism in children. *J. Clin. Endocrinol. Metab.* 45:457-468.
778. DeLuca H.F., Personal communication.
779. Albanese, A.A. (1975): Nutritional aspects of bone loss. Parts I and II. *Food Nutr. News* 47: no. 1, pp. 1, 4; No. 2, pp. 1, 4.
780. Davies, D.G. and Shock, N.W. (1950): Age changes in glomerular filtration rate, effective renal plasma flow, and tubular excretory capacity in adult males. *J. Clin. Invest.* 29:496-507.
781. Watkin, D.M. and Shock, N.W. (1955): Agewise standard values for C_{In}, C_{PAH}, and Tm_{PAH} in adult males. (Abstract). *J. Clin. Invest.* 34:969.
782. Oliver, J. (1954): Anatomic changes of normal senescence. In: *Geriatric Medicine: Medical Care of Later Maturity, Third Edition,* edited by E.J. Stieglitz. Lippincott, Philadelphia, pp. 44-63.
783. Pitt, M.J. and Haussler, M.R. (1977): Vitamin D: biochemistry and clinical applications. *Skelet. Radiol.* 1:191-208.
784. Werner, E., Mallache, H.H., and Kutschera, J. (1976): Intestinal calcium absorption and whole body calcium retention in various stages of renal insufficiency. *Calcif. Tiss. Res.* 21: suppl., pp. 210-215.
785. Haussler, M.R., Baylink, D.J, Hughes, M.R., Brumbaugh, P.F., Wergedal, J.W., Shen, F.H., Nielsen, R.L., Counts, S.J., Bursac, K.M., and McCain, T.A. (1976): The assay of 1-alpha,25-dihydroxy vitamin D_3: physiologic and pathologic modulation of circulating hormone levels. *Clin. Endocr.* suppl. 5, pp. 151s-165s.
786. Haussler, M.R., Hughes, M.R., Pike, J.W., and McCain, T.A. (1977): Radioligand receptor assay for 1,25-dihydroxyvitamin D_3: biochemical, physiologic and clinical applications. In: *Vitamin D: Biochemical, Chemical, and Clinical aspects related to Calcium Metabolism,* edited by A.W. Norman, K. Schaefer, J.W. Coburn, H.F. DeLuca, D. Fraser, H.G. Grigoleit, and D.V. Merrath. Walter de Gruyter, Berlin, pp. 473-482.
787. Brickman, A.S., Coburn, J.W., Friedman, G.R., Okamura, W.H., Massry, S.G., and Norman, A.N. (1976): Comparison of effects of 1-alpha-hydroxy-vitamin D_3 and 1,25-dihydroxy-vitamin D_3 in man. *J. Clin. Invest.* 57:1540-1547.
788. Davie, M.W.J., Chalmers, T.M., Hunter, J.O., Pelc, B., and Kodicek, E. (1976): 1-alpha-hydroxycholecalciferol in chronic renal failure: studies of the effects of oral doses. *Ann. Internal Med.* 84:281-285.
789. Gallagher, J.C., Riggs, B.L., Eisman, J., Arnaud, S.B., and DeLuca, H.F. (1976): Impaired production of 1,25-dihydroxy vitamin D_3 in postmenopausal osteoporosis. *Clin. Res.* 24:580A.
790. Yendt, E.R., DeLuca, H.F., Garcia, D.A., and Cohanim, M. (1969): Clinical aspects of vitamin D. In: *Fat Soluble Vitamins,* edited by H.F. DeLuca and G.W. Suttie. U. of Wisconsin Press, Madison, pp. 125-158.
791. Freeman, S., Rhoads, P.S., and Yeager, L.B. (1946): Toxic manifestations following large doses of Ertron (R). *J. Lab. Clin. Med.* 31:480-481.
792. Bauer, J.M. and Freyberg, R.H. (1946): Vitamin D intoxication with metastatic calcification. *J. Amer. Med. Assoc.* 130:1208-1215.
793. Donegan, C.K., Messer, A.L., and Orgain, E.S. (1949): Vitamin D intoxication due to Ertron (R): report of two cases. *Ann. Internal Med.* 30:429-435.
794. Farrell, P.M. and Bieri, J.G. (1975): Megavitamin E supplementation in man. *Amer. J Clin. Nutrition* 28:1381-1386.
795. Expert panel on Food Safety and Nutrition and Committee on Public Information, Institute of Food Technologists (1977): Special report: vitamin E, a scientific status summary. *Nutrition Rev.* 35:57-62.
796. Herbert, V. (1977): Letter to the editor: Vitamin E report. *Nutrition Rev.* 36:158.
797. Hays, K.C. and Hegsted, D.M. (1973): Toxicity of the vitamins. In: *Toxicants Occurring Naturally in Foods,* edited by the Committee on Food Protection, Food and Nutrition Board, National Research Council. National Academy of Sciences, Washington, D.C., pp. 235-253.
798. Corrigan, J.J. and Marcus, F.I. (1974): Coagulopathy associated with vitamin E ingestion. *J. Am. Med. Ass.* 230:1300-1301.
799. Briggs, M.H. (1974): Vitamin E in clinical medicine. *Lancet* 1:220.

800. Scott, M.L. (1978): Vitamin E. In: *The Fat-Soluble Vitamins, Handbook of Lipid Research, 2.* Plenum Press, New York, pp. 133-210.
801. Tsai, A.C., Kelley, J.J., Peng, B., and Cook, N. (1978): Study on the effect of megavitamin E supplementation in man. *Amer. J. Clin. Nutrition* 31:831-837.
802. Hillman, R.W. (1957): Tocopherol excess in man. Creatinuria associated with prolonged ingestion. *Amer. J. Clin. Nutrition* 5:597-600.
803. Cohen, H.M. (1973): Fatigue caused by vitamin E. *Calif. Med.* 119:No. 1 (July), 72.
804. Briggs, M. (1974): Vitamin E supplements and fatigue. *New England J. Med.* 290:579-580.
805. Dahl, S. (1974): Vitamin E in clinical medicine. *Lancet* 1:465.
806. Horwitt, M.K. (1976): Vitamin E: a reexamination. *Amer. J. Clin. Nutrition* 29:569-578.
807. Tappel, A.L. (1973): Vitamin E. *Nutrition Today* 8:4-12.
808. Vogelsang, A. and Shute, E.V. (1946): Effect of vitamin E in coronary heart disease. *Nature* 157:772.
808a. Vogelsang, A. (1970): Twenty-four years of using alpha-tocopherol in degenerative cardiovascular disease. *Angiology* 21:275-279.
809. Toone, W.M. (1973): Effects of vitamin E: good and bad. *New England J. Med.* 289:979-980.
810. Uracchio, J.F. and Calenda, D.G. (1953): Treatment of angina pectoris. *New England J. Med.* 249:689-698.
811. Anderson, T.W. (1974): Vitamin E in angina pectoris. *Can. Med. Assoc. J.* 101:401-406.
811a. Anderson, T.W. and Reid, D.B.W. (1974): A double-blind trial of vitamin E in angina pectoris. *Amer. J. Clin. Nutrition* 27:1174-1178.
812. Gillilan, R.E., Mondell, B., and Warbasse, J. R. (1977): Quantitative evaluation of vitamin E in the treatment of angina pectoris. *Amer. Heart J.* 93:444-449.
813. Vessby, B., Lithell, H., and Boberg, J. (1977): Supplementation with vitamin E in hyperlipidemic patients treated with diet and clofibrate. Effects on serum lipoprotein concentrations, plasma fatty acid composition and adipose tissue lipoprotein lipase activity. *Amer. J. Clin. Nutrition* 30:517-522.
814. Leonhardt, E.T.G. (1978): Effects of vitamin E on serum cholesterol and triglycerides in hyperlipidemic patients treated with diet and clofibrate. *Amer. J. Clin. Nutrition* 31:100-105.
815. Benson, H. and McCallie, D.P. (1979): Angina pectoris and the placebo effect. *New England J. Med* 300:1424-1429.
816. Olson, R.E. (1973): Vitamin E and its relation to heart disease. *Circulation* 48:179-184.
817. Anonymous (1974): Editorial: Vitamin E in clinical nutrition. *Lancet* 1:18.
818. Clein, L.J., Williams, H.T.G., and Macbeth, R.A. (1962): The use of tocopherol in the treatment of intermittent claudication. *Can. Med. Asoc. J.* 86:215-216; 87:538-541.
819. Boyd, A.M. and Marks, J. (1963): Treatment of intermittent claudication — reappraisal of the value of alpha-tocopherol. *Angiology* 14:198-208.
820. Williams, H.T., Fenna, D., and Macbeth, R.A. (1971): Alpha tocopherol in the treatment of intermittent claudication. *Surgery Gynec. Obstet* 132:662-666.
821. Haeger, K. (1974): Long-time treatment of intermittent claudication with vitamin E. *Amer. J. Clin. Nutrition* 27:1179-1181.
822. Young, J.R. and deWolfe, V.G. (1978): Diseases of the peripheral arteries and veins. In: *The Heart, Arteries and Veins,* edited by J.W. Hurst, R.B. Logue, R.C. Schlant, and N.K. Wenger. Blakiston Division, McGraw-Hill, New York, p. 1865.
824. Tappel, A.L. (1970): Biological antioxidant protection against lipid peroxidation damage. *Amer. J. Clin. Nutrition* 23:1137-1139.
825. Csallany, A.S. and Ayaz, K.L. (1976): Quantitative determination of organic solvent soluble lipofuscin pigments in animal tissues. *Lipids* 11:412-417.
826. Csallany, A.S., Ayaz, K.L., and Su, L-C (1977): Effect of dietary vitamin E and aging on tissue lipofuscin pigment concentration in mice. *J. Nutrition* 107:1792-1799.

827. Grinna, L.S. (1976): Effect of dietary alpha tocopherol on liver microsomes and mitochondria of aging rats. *J. Nutrition* 106:918-929.
828. Jager, F.C. (1972): Long-term dose response effects of vitamin E in rats. *Nutr. Metab.* 14:1-7.
829. Tappel, A., Fletcher, B., and Deamer, D. (1973): Effects of antioxidants and nutrients on lipid peroxidation fluorescent products and aging parameters in the mouse. *J. Geront.* 28:415-424.
830. Horwitt, M.K. (1962): Interrelations between vitamin E and polyunsaturated fatty acids in adult men. *Vitamin. Horm.* 20:541-558.
831. Bieri, J.G. and Evarts, R.P. (1973): Tocopherols and fatty acids in American diets. The recommended allowance for vitamin E. *J. Am. Diet. Assoc.* 62:147-151.
832. Horwitt, M.K. (1974): Status of human requirements of vitamin E. *Amer. J. Clin. Nutrition.* 27:1182-1193.
833. Dam, H. (1935a): The antihaemorrhagic vitamin of the chick: occurrence and chemical nature. *Nature* 135:652-653.
833a. Dam, H. (1935b): CLIV. The antihaemorrhagic factor of the chick. *Biochem. J.* 29:1273-1285.
834. Dam, H. (1934): Haemorrhages in chicks reared on artificial diets: a new deficiency disease, *Nature* 133:909-910.
835. International Union of Pure and Applied Chemistry — International Union of Biochemistry (IUPAC-IUB), Commission on Biochemical Nomenclature (1966): Tentative rules: nomenclature of quinones with isoprenoid side chains. *J. Biol. Chem.* 241:2989-2291.
836. Olson, R.E. (1973): Section C. Vitamin K. In: *Modern Nutrition in Health and Disease, Fifth Edition,* edited by R.S. Goodhart and M.E. Shils. Lea and Febiger, Philadelphia, p. 172.
837. Rietz, P., Gloor, U., and Wiss, O. (1970): Menachione aus menschlicher Leber und Faulschlamm. *Internat. Z. Vitaminforsch.* 40:351-362.
838. McCollum, E.B. and McCollum, E.V. (1959): Vitamins A,D,E,K. In: *Food: The Yearbook of Agriculture 1959,* The United States Department of Agriculture. The United States Government Printing Office, Washington, D.C., p. 138.
839. Aggeler, P.M., Lucia, S.P., and Fishbon, H.M. (1942): Purpura due to vitamin K deficiency in anorexia nervosa. *Am. J. Dig. Dis.* 9:227-229.
840. Kark, R. and Lozner, E.L. (1939): Nutritional deficiency of vitamin K in man. *Lancet* 2:1162-1164.
841. Hazell, K. and Baloch, K.H. (1970): Vitamin K deficiency in the elderly. *Gerontol. Clin.* 12:10-17.
842. Watkin, D.M., Van Itallie, T.B., Logan, W.B., Geyer, R.P., Davidson, C.S., and Stare, F.J. (1951): The treatment of dicumarol-induced hypoprothrombinemia in man with emulsified vitamin K administered intravenously. *J. Lab. Clin. Med.* 37:269-271.
843. Dam, H. (1966): Historical survey and inroduction. In: International Symposium on Recent Advances in Research on Vitamins K and Related Quinones (Vitamins K, Ubiquinones or Coenzymes Q, Plastoquinones) in Honor of Professor Henrik Dam. *Vitamins Hormones* 24:295-306.
844. Douglas, A.S. and Brown, A. (1952): Effect of vitamin K preparations on hypoprothrombinaemia induced by dicoumarin and tromexan. *Brit. Med. J.* 1:412-415.
845. Jeffries, G.H. (1975): Section eleven. Diseases of the Liver. In: *Textbook of Medicine, Fourteenth Ed.,* edited by P.B. Beeson and W. McDermott. W.B. Saunders Company, Philadelphia p. 1333.
846. Frick, P.G., Riedler, G., and Brögli, H. (1976): Dose response and minimal daily requirement for vitamin K in man. *J. Appl. Physiol.* 23:387-389.
847. Doisy, E.A. (1971): Vitamin K in human nutrition. In: *The Biochemistry, Assay, and Nutritional Value of Vitamin K and Related Compounds,* Association of Vitamin Chemists, Chicago, pp. 79-92.
848. O'Reilly, R.A. (1971): Vitamin K in hereditary resistance to oral anticoagulant drugs. *Am. J. Physiol.* 221:1327-1330.
849. Ramasarma, T. (1968): Lipid quinones. *Adv. Lipid Res.* 6:107-180.

850. Brodie, A.F. and Watanabe, T. (1966): Mode of action of vitamin K in microorganisms. *Vitamins Hormones* 24:447-463.
851. Gel'man, N.S., Lukoyanova, M.A., and Ostrovskii, D.N. (1967): *Respiration and Phosphorylation of Bacteria*. Plenum, New York.
852. Stenflo, J. (1976): A new vitamin K-dependent protein: purification from bovine plasma and preliminary characterization. *J. Biol. Chem.* 251:355-363.
853. Anonymous (1979): Osteocalcin: a vitamin K-dependent calcium-binding protein in bone. *Nutrition Rev.* 37:54-57.
854. Lian, J.B., Hauschka, P.V., and Gallop, P.M. (1978): Properties and biosynthesis of a vitamin K-dependent calcium binding protein in bone. *Fed. Proc.* 37:2615-2620.
855. American Academy of Pediatrics, Committee on Nutrition (1971): Vitamin K supplementation for infants receiving milk substitute infant formulas and for those with fat malabsorption. *Pediatrics* 48:483-497.
855a. Herbert, V. (1979): Pangamic acid ("vitamin B_{15}"). *Amer. J. Clin. Nutrition* 32:1534-1540.
855b. Herbert, V. (1979): Laetrile: the cult of cyanide. Promoting poison for profit. *Amer. J. Clin. Nutrition* 32:1121-1158.
856. Horwitt, M.K., Liebert, E., Kreisler, O., and Wittman, P. (1948): Investigations of human requirements for B-complex vitamins. National Research Council Bull. No. 116, National Academy of Sciences, Washington D.C.
857. Lossy, F.T., Goldsmith, G.A., and Sarett, H.P. (1951): A study of test dose excretion of five B-complex vitamins in man. *J. Nutrition* 45:213-224.
858. Schmidt, V. (1951): The excretion of pantothenic acid in the urine of young and old individuals. *J. Geront.* 6:132-134.
859. Schmidt, V. (1951): The excretion of pantothentic acid in patients with amitochondria and alopecia. *J. Geront.* 6:369-371.
860. Exton-Smith, A.N. and Scott, D.L. (1968): *Vitamins in the elderly.* Rep. Proc. Symp. Royal College of Physicians, London, 1968. John Wright and Sons, Bristol.
861. Eddy, T.P. (1968): The problem of retaining vitamins in hospital food. In: *Vitamins in the elderly.* Rep. Proc. Symp. Royal College of Physicians, London, 1968, edited by A.N. Exton-Smith and D.L. Scott. John Wright and Sons, Bristol, pp. 86-92.
862. Roe, D.A. (1976): *Drug-induced Nutritional Deficiencies.* AVI Publishing, Westport, Conn.
863. Murphy, F., Srivastava, P.C., Varadi, S., and Elwis, A. (1969): Screening of psychiatric patients for hypovitaminosis B_{12}. *Brit. Med. J.* 3:559-560.
864. Batata, M., Spray, G.H., Bolton, F.G., Higgins, G., and Wollner, L. (1967): Blood and bone marrow changes in elderly patients, with special reference to folic acid, vitamin B_{12}, iron, and ascorbic acid. *Brit. Med. J.* 2:667-669.
865. Stephenson, W., Penton, C., and Korenchevsky, V. (1941): Some effects of vitamins B and C on senile patients. *Brit. Med. J.* 2:839-844.
866. Wexberg, E. (1941): Neurometabolic deficiency in old age (senile encephalomyelosis). *Am. J. Psychiat.* 97:1406-1418.
867. Jollife, N. (1941): Treatment of neuropsychiatric disorders with vitamins. *J. Amer. Med. Assoc.* 117:1496-1500.
868. Overholser, W. and Fong, T.C.C. (1954): Mental diseases. In: *Geriatric Medicine, Third Ed.*, edited by E. J. Stieglitz. Lippincott, Philadelphia, pp. 257-270.
869. Rafsky, H.A. and Newman, B. (1941): Vitamin C studies in aged. *Amer. J. Med. Sci.* 201:749-756.
870. Rafsky, H.A. and Newman, B. (1943): Vitamin B_1 excretion in the aged. *Gastroenterology* 1:737-742.
871. Rafsky, H.A. and Newman, B. (1947): Nutritional aspects of aging. *Geriatrics* 2:101-104.
872. Ranke, E., Tauber, S.A., Horonick, A., Ranke, B., Goodhart, R.S., and Chow, B.F. (1960): Vitamin B_6 deficiency in the aged. *J. Geront.* 15:41-44.
873. Hamfelt, A. (1964): Age variations of vitamin B_6 metabolism in man. *Clin. Chim. Acta* 10:48-54.
874. Jacobs, A., Cavill, I.A.J., and Hughes, J.N.P. (1968): Erythrocyte transaminase

activity. Effect of age, sex and vitamin B_6 supplementation. *Amer. J. Clin. Nutrition* 21:502-507.

875. Lumeng, L. and Li, T.K. (1974): Vitamin B-6 metabolism in chronic alcohol abuse. *J. Clin. Invest.* 53:693-704.
876. Rose, C.S., György, P., Butler, M., Andres, R., Norris, A.H., Shock, N.W., Tobin, J., Brin, M., and Spiegel, H. (1976): Age differences in vitamin B_6 status of 617 men. *Amer. J. Clin. Nutrition* 29:847-853.
877. Oldham, H.G. (1962): Thiamine requirements of women. *Ann. N.Y. Acad. Sci.* 98:542-549.
878. Hodges, R.E., Bean, W.B., Ohlson, M.A., and Bleiler, R. (1959): Human pantothenic acid deficiency produced by omega-methyl pantothenic acid. *J. Clin. Invest.* 38:1421-1425.
879. Leevy, C.M., Baker, H., Tenhove, W., Frank, O., and Chjerrick, G.R. (1965): B-complex vitamins in liver disease of the alcoholic. *Amer. J. Clin. Nutrition* 16:338-346.
880. Syndenstricke, V.P., Singal, S.A., Briggs, A.P., DeVaughn, N.M., and Isbell, H. (1942): Observations of the "egg white injury" in man and its cure with a biotin concentrate. *J. Amer. Med. Assoc.* 118:1199-1200.
881. Williams, R.H. (1943): Clinical biotin deficiency. *New Engl. J. Med.* 288:247-252.
882. Baugh, C.M., Malone, J.H., and Butterworth, C.E., Jr. (1968): Human biotin deficiency. A case history of biotin deficiency induced by raw egg consumption in a cirrhotic patient. *Amer. J. Clin. Nutrition* 21:173-182.
883. Oppel, T.W. (1942): Studies of biotin metabolism in man; excretion of biotin in human urine; relationship between biotin content of diet and its ouput in urine and feces; excretion of 2 biotin-like substances in urine. *Amer. J. Med. Sci.* 204:856-875.
884. Pauling, L.C. (1970): *Vitamin C and the Common Cold.* Freeman, San Francisco.
885. Cameron, E. and Pauling, L.C. (1976): Supplemental ascorbate in the supportive treatment of cancer. Prolongation of survival times in terminal human cancer. *Proc. Nat. Acad. Sci. USA* 73:3685-3689.
886. Wilson, C.W.M. (1975): Colds, ascorbic acid metabolism, and vitamin C. *J. Clin. Pharmacol.* 15:570-578.
887. Chalmers, T.C. (1975): Effects of ascorbic acid on the common cold. An evaluation of the evidence. *Amer. J. Med.* 58:532-536.
888. Rhead. W.J. and Schrauzer, G.N. (1971): Risks of long-term ascorbic acid overdosage. *Nutrition Rev.* 29:262-263.
889. Jaffe, R.M., Kasten, B., Young, P.S., and MacLowry, J.D. (1975): False negative stool occult blood tests caused by ingestion of ascorbic acid (vitamin C). *Ann. Intern. Med.* 83:824-826.
890. Herbert, V. and Jacob, E. (1974): Destruction of vitamin B_{12} by ascorbic acid. *J. Amer. Med. Assoc.* 230:241-242.
891. Jacob, E., Scott, J., Brenner, L., and Herbert, V. (1973): Apparent low serum vitamin B_{12} levels in paraplegic veterans taking ascorbic acid. In: *Proc. 16th Ann. Meet. Amer. Soc. Hemat., Chicago, 1973.*
892. Hines, J.D. (1975): Ascorbic acid and vitamin B_{12} deficiency. *J. Amer. Med. Assoc.* 234:24.
893. Newmark, H.L., Scheiner, J., Marcus, M., and Prabhudesai, M. (1976): Stability of vitmin B_{12} in the presence of ascorbic acid. *Amer. J. Clin. Nutrition* 29:645-649.
894. Herbert, V., Jacob, E., Wong, K.-T.J., Scott, J., and Pfeffer, R.D. (1978): Low serum vitamin B_{12} levels in patients receiving ascorbic acid in megadoses: studies concerning the effect of ascorbate on radioisotope B_{12} assay. *Amer. J. Clin. Nutrition.* 31:253-258.
895. Carmel, R., Rosenberg, A.H., Lau, K.S., Streiff, R.R., and Herbert, V. (1969): Vitamin B_{12} uptake by human small bowel homogenate and its enhancement by intrinsic factor. *Gastroenterology* 56:548-555.
896. Allen, R.H., Seetharam, B., Allen, N.C., Podell, E., and Alpers, D.H. (1977): Cobalamin malabsorption in pancreatic insufficiency is due to an inability to partially degrade R-type cobalamin-binding protein. *Blood* 50: suppl. 1, p. 88.
897. Stein, H.B., Hasan, A., and Fox, I.H. (1976): Ascorbic acid-induced uricosuria: a consequence of megavitamin therapy. *Ann. Intern. Med.* 84:385-388.

897a. Smith, L.H. (1978): Risk of oxalate stones from large doses of vitamin C. *N. Engl. J. Med.* 298:856.

898. Mengel, C.A. and Greene, H.L. (1976): Ascorbic acid effects on erythrocytes. *Ann. Intern. Med.* 84:490.

899. Campbell, G.D., Steinberg, M.H., and Bower, J.D. (1975): Ascorbic acid-induced hemolysis in G-6-PD deficiency. *Ann. Intern. Med.* 82:810.

900. Burr, M.L., Elwood, P.C., Hole, D.J., Hurley, R.J., and Hughes, R.E. (1974): Plasma and leukocyte ascorbic acid levels in the elderly. *Amer. J. Clin. Nutrition* 27:144-151.

901. Kaplan, L., Landes, J.H., and Pincus, J. (1955): The nutritional status of noninstitutionalized aged persons. *Geriatrics* 10:287-290.

902. Chope, H.D., Breslow, L. (1956): Nutritional status of the aging. *Amer. J. Pub. Health* 46:61-67.

903. United States Department of Health, Education and Welfare (1972): *Ten State Nutrition Survey, 1968-1970: IV - Biochemical.* DHEW Publication No. 72-8132, United States Government Printing Office, Washington, D.C.

904. Davidson, C.S., Livermore, J., Anderson, P., and Kaufman, S. (1962): The nutrition of a group of apparently healthy aging persons. *Amer. J. Clin. Nutrition* 10:181-199.

905. Hankin, J.H., and Antonmattei, J.C. (1960): Survey of food service practices in nursing homes. *Amer. J. Public Health* 50:1137-1144.

906. LeBovit, C. (1965): The food of older persons living at home. *J. Amer. Diet. Assoc.* 46:285-289.

907. Andrews, J., Brook, M., and Allen, M.A. (1966): Influence of abode and vitamin C status of the elderly. *Geront. Clin.* 8:257-266.

908. Andrews, J. (1973): Vitamin C status of elderly long-stay hospital patients. *Geront. Clin.* 15:221-226.

909. Griffith, L.L., Brocklehurst, J.C., Scott, D.L., Marks, J., and Blackley, J. (1967): Thiamine and ascorbic acid levels in the elderly. *Geront. Clin* 9:1-10.

910. Milne, J.S., Lonergan, M.E., Williamson, J., Moore, F.M.L., McMaster, R., and Percy, N. (1971): Leukocyte ascorbic acid levels and vitamin C intake in older people. *Brit. Med. J.* 4:383-386.

911. Bates, C.J. (1977): Proline and hydroxyproline excretion and vitamin C status in elderly human subjects. *Clin. Sci. Mol. Med.* 52:535-543.

912. Brin, M. and Bauernfeind, J.C. (1978): Vitamin needs of the elderly. In: *Symp. on Nutrition of the Elderly*, edited by A.A. Albanese. *Postgrad. Med.* 63:155-163.

913. Krumdieck, C. and Butterworth, C.E. (1974): Ascorbate-cholesterol-lecithin interactions: factors of potential importance in the pathogenesis of atherosclerosis. *Amer. J. Clin Nutrition* 27:866-876.

914. Ginter, E. (1973): Cholesterol: vitamin C controls its transformation to bile acids. *Science* 179:702-704.

915. Ginter, E. (1976): Vitamin C and plasma lipids. *N. Engl. J. Med.* 294:559-560.

916. Ginter, E. (1979): Decline of coronary mortality in the United States and vitamin C. *Amer. J. Clin. Nutrition* 32:511-512.

917. Bates, C.J., Mandal, A.R., and Cole, T.J. (1977): H.D.L. cholesterol and vitamin-C status. *Lancet* 2:611.

918. Knox, E.G. (1973): Ischaemic heart disease mortality and dietary intake of calcium. *Lancet* 1:1465-1467.

919. Irwin, M.I. and Hutchins, B.K. (1976): A conspectus of research on vitamin C requirements of man. *J. Nutrition* 106:821-879.

920. Kallner, A., Hartmann, D. and Hornig, D. (1979): Steady-state turnover and body pool of ascorbic acid in man. *Amer. J. Clin Nutrition* 32:530-539.

921. Kallner, A., Hartmann, D., and Hornig, D. (1977): On the absorption of ascorbic acid in man. *Internat. J. Vit. Nutrition Res.* 47:383-388.

921a. Monsen, E.R., Hallberg, L., Layrisse, M., Hegsted, D.M., Cook, J.D., Mertz, W., and Finch, C.A. (1978): Estimation of available dietary iron. *Amer. J. Clin Nutrition* 31:134-141.

922. Castle, W.B. (1961): The Gordon Wilson Lecture. A century of curiosity about pernicious anemia. *Trans. Amer. Clin. Climat. Assoc.* 73:54-80.

923. Wills, L., and Mehta, M.M. (1930): Studies in "pernicious anemia" of pregnancy. Part I. Preliminary report. *Indian J. Med. Res.* 17:777-792.
924. Wills, L., Clutterbuck, P.W., and Evans, B.D.F. (1937): A new factor in the production and cure of macrocytic anemias and its relation to other haematopoietic principles curative in pernicious anemia. *Biochem. J.* 31:2136-2147.
925. Watson, J., and Castle, W.B. (1946): Nutritional macrocytic anemia especially in pregnancy. Response to a substance in liver other than that effective in pernicious anemia. *Amer. J. Med. Sci.* 21:513-530.
926. Stokstad, E.L.R., Hutchings, B.L., and Subbarow, Y. (1948): The isolation of the *Lactobacillus casei* factor from liver. *J. Amer. Chem. Soc.* 70:3-5.
927. Mowat, J.H., Boothe, J.H., Hutchings, B.L., Stokstad, E.L.R., Waller, C.W., Angier, R.B., Semb, J., Cosulich, D.B., and Subbarow, Y. (1948): The structure of liver *L. casei* factor. *J. Amer. Chem. Soc.* 70:14-18.
928. Waller, C.W., Hutchings, B.L., Mowat, J.H., Stokstad, E.L.R., Boothe, J.H., Angier, R.B., Semb, J., Subbarow, Y., Cosulich, D.B., Fabrenbach, M.J., Hultquist, M.E., Kuh, E., Northcy, E.H., Seeger, D.R., Sickels, J.P., and Smith, J.M., Jr. (1948): Synthesis of pteroylglutamic acid (liver *L. casei* factor) and pteroic acid. *J. Amer. Chem. Soc.* 70:19-22.
929. Mitchell, H.K., Snell, E.E., and Williams, R.J. (1941): Concentration of "folic acid". *J. Amer. Chem. Soc.* 63:2284.
930. IUNS-AIN Committee on Nomenclature (1976): Nomenclature policy: Generic descriptors and trivial names for vitamins and related compounds. *J. Nutrition* 106:8-14.
931. Rodriguez, M.S. (1978): A conspectus on folacin requirements of man. *J. Nutrition* 108:1983-2075.
932. Butterworth, C.E., Jr., Santini, R., Jr., and Frommeyer, W.B., Jr. (1963): The pteroylglutamate composition of American diets as determined by chromatographic fractionation. *J. Clin. Invest.* 42:1929-1939.
933. Chanarin, I., Rothman, D., Perry, J., and Stratfull, D. (1968): Normal dietary folate, iron, and protein intake, with particular reference to pregnancy. *Brit. Med. J.* 2:394-397.
934. Hurdle, A.D.F., Barton, D., and Searles, I.H. (1968): A method for measuring folate in food and its application to a hospital diet. *Amer. J. Clin. Nutrition* 21:1202-1207.
935. Hurdle, A.D.F. (1968): The assessment of folate intake of elderly patients in the hospital. *Med. J. Australia* 55:101-104.
936. Perry, J. (1971): Folate analogues in normal mixed diets. *Brit. J. Haematol.* 21:435-441.
937. Moscovitch, L.F., and Cooper, B.A. (1973): Folate content of diets in pregnancy: Comparison of diets collected at home and diets prepared from dietary records. *Amer. J. Clin. Nutrition* 26:707-714.
938. Herbert, V. (1973): The five possible causes of all nutrient deficiency: illustrated by deficiencies of vitamin B_{12} and folic acid. *Amer. J. Clin. Nutrition* 26:77-88.
939. Grundy, W.E., Freed, M., Johnson, H.C., Henderson, C.R., and Berryman, G.H. (1947): The effect of phthalylsulfathiazole (sulfathalidine) on the excretion of B-vitamins by normal adults. *Arch. Biochem.* 15:187-194.
940. Hoffbrand, A.V., Tabaqchali, S., Booth, C.C., and Malin, D.L. (1971): Small intestinal bacterial flora and folate status in gastrointestinal disease. *Gut* 12:27-33.
941. Luckey, T.D. (1970): Vitamin metabolism in germ free animals: folic acid. In: *Nutrition: Proceedings of the Eighth International Congress, Prague, September 1969*, edited by J. Masek, K. Osancova, and D.P. Cuthbertson. International Congress Series No. 213. Excerpta Medica Foundation, Amsterdam. pp. 399-407.
942. Halsted, C.H., Robles, E.A., and Mezey, E. (1971): Decreased jejunal uptake of labeled folic acid (^{3}H-PGA) in alcoholic patients: roles of alcohol and nutrition. *New Engl. J. Med.* 285:701-706.
943. Deller, D.J., Kimber, C.L., and Ibbotson, R.N. (1965): Folic acid deficiency in cirrhosis of the liver. *Amer. J. Digest. Dis.* 10:35-42.
944. Wu, A., Chanarin, I., Slavin, G., and Levi, A.J. (1975): Folate deficiency in the

alcoholic — its relationship to clinical and haematological abnormalities, liver disease and folate stores. *Brit. J. Haematol.* 29:469-478.

945. Greene, H.L., Stifel, F.B., Herman, R.H., Herman, Y.F., and Rosenweig, N.S. (1974): Ethanol-induced inhibition of human intestinal enzyme activities: reversal by folic acid. *Gastroenterology* 67:434-440.
946. Porta, E.A., Koch, O.R., and Hartroft, W.S. (1972): Recovery from chronic hepatitis lesions in rats fed alcohol and a super solid diet. *Amer. J. Clin. Nutrition* 25:881-896.
947. Bertino, J.R., editor (1971): Folate antagonists as chemotherapeutic agents. *Ann. N.Y. Acad. Sci.* Vol. 186.
948. Stebbins, D., Scott, J., and Herbert, V. (1973): Drug induced megaloblastic anemias. *Semin. Hematol.* 10:235-251.
949. Herbert, V., and Tisman, G. (1973): Effects of deficiencies of folic acid and vitamin B_{12} on central nervous system function and development. *Biol. Brain Dysfunction* 1:373-392.
950. Ritland, S., Fausa, O., Gjone, E., Blomhoff, J.P., Skrede, S., and Lanner, A. (1975): Effect of treatment with a bile-sequestering agent (Secholex) on intestinal absorption, duodenal bile acids, and plasma lipids. *Scand. J. Gastroenterol.* 10:791-800.
951. West, R.J., and Lloyd, J.K. (1973): Use of cholestyramine in treatment of children with familial hypercholesterolaemia. *Arch. Dis. Child.* 48:370-374.
952. West, R.J., and Lloyd, J.K. (1975): The effect of cholestyramine on intestinal absorption. *Gut* 16:93-98.
953. Alter, H.J., Zvaifler, N.J., and Rath, C.E. (1971): Interrelationship of rheumatoid arthritis, folic acid, and aspirin. *Blood* 38:405-416.
954. Herbert, V. (1973): Section J: Folic acid and vitamin B_{12}. In: *Modern Nutrition in Health and Disease, Fifth Edition*, edited by R.S. Goodhart and M.E. Shils. Lea & Febiger, Philadelphia. pp. 221-244.
955. Hunter, R., Barnes, J., Oakeley, H.F., and Matthews, D.M. (1970): Toxicity of folic acid given in pharmacological doses to healthy volunteers. *Lancet* 1:61-63.
956. Hellström, L. (1971): Lack of toxicity of folic acid given in pharmacological doses to healthy volunteers. *Lancet* 1:59-61.
957. Richens, A. (1971): Toxicity of folic acid. *Lancet* 1:912.
958. Hoogstraten, B., Cuttner, J., and Natovitz, B. (1964): Sequence of recovery from multiple manifestations of folic acid deficiency. *J. Mt. Sinai Hosp.* 31:10-16.
959. Ch'ien, L.T., Krumdieck, C.L., Scott, C.W., and Butterworth, C.E., Jr. (1975): Harmful effects of megadoses of vitamins: Electroencephalogram abnormalities and seizures induced by intravenous folate in drug treated epileptics. *Amer. J. Clin. Nutrition* 28:51-58.
960. Lawson, D.H., Murray, R.M., and Parker, J.L.W. (1972): Early mortality in the megaloblastic anemias. *Quart. J. Med.* 41:1-14.
961. Heinle, R.W., and Welch, A.D. (1947): Folic acid in pernicious anemia. Failure to prevent neurologic relapse. *J. Amer. Med. Assoc.* 133:739-741.
962. Vilter, C.F., Vilter, R.W., and Spies, T.D. (1947): The treatment of pernicious anemia and related anemias with synthetic folic acid. I. Observation on the maintenance of a normal hematologic status and on occurrence of combined system disease at the end of one year. *J. Lab. Clin. Med.* 32:262-273.
963. Crosby, W. (1960): The danger of folic acid in multivitamin preparations. *Mil. Med.* 125:233-235.
964. Sheehy, T. (1961): How much folic acid is safe in pernicious anemia. *Amer. J. Clin. Nutrition* 9:703-714.
965. Katz, M. (1973): Potential danger of self-medication with folic acid. *New Engl. J. Med.* 289:1095.
966. Fox, J.H., Topel, J.L., and Huckman, M.S. (1975): Dementia in the elderly — a search for treatable illnesses. *J. Gerontol.* 30:557-564.
967. Hansen, H.A., Nordqvist, P., and Sourander, P. (1964): Megaloblastic anemia and neurological disturbances combined with folic acid deficiency. *Acta Med. Scand.* 176:243-251.

968. Hurdle, A.D.F., and Williams, P. (1966): Folic acid deficiency in elderly patients admitted to hospital. *Brit. Med. J.* 2:202-205.
969. Melamed, E., Reches, A., and Hershko, C. (1975): Reversible central nervous system dysfunction in folate deficiency. *J. Neurol. Sci.* 25:93-98.
970. Pincus, J.H., Reynolds, E.H., and Glaser, G.H. (1972): Subacute combined system degeneration with folate deficiency. *J. Amer. Med. Assoc.* 221:496-497.
971. Read, A.E., Gough, K.R., Pardoe, J.L., and Nicholas, A. (1965): Nutritional studies on the entrants to an old people's home, with particular reference to folic-acid deficiency. *Brit. Med. J.* 11:843-848.
972. Shaw, D.M., MacSweeney, D.A., Johnson, A.L., O'Keeffe, R., Naidoo, D., MacLeod, D.M., Jog, S., Preece, J.M., and Crowley, J.M. (1971): Folate and amine metabolites in senile dementia: a combined trial and biochemical study. *Physiol. Med.* 1:166-171.
973. Sneath, P., Chanarin, I., Hodkinson, H.M., McPherson, C.K., and Reynolds, E.H. (1973): Folate status in a geriatric population and its relation to dementia. *Age Ageing* 2:177-182.
974. Strachan, R.W., and Henderson, J.G. (1967): Dementia and folate deficiency. *Quart. J. Med.* 36:189-204.
975. Addison, T. (1855): *On the Constitutional and Local Effects of Disease of the Suprarenal Capsules.* S. Highley, London.
976. Biermer, A. (1872): Über progressive perniciöse Anämie. *Korrespondenzblatt schweiz. Aerzte.* 2:15.
977. Fenwick, S. (1880): *On atrophy of the stomach and on the nervous affections of the digestive organs.* J. & A. Churchill, London. pp. 1-204.
978. Whipple, G.H., Carrier, E.B., and Lee, F.W. (1922): Determinations of plasma and hemoglobin volumes after unit hemorrhages under controlled experimental conditions. *Amer. J. Physiol.* 61:138-148.
978a. Whipple, G.H., and Robscheit-Robbins, F.S. (1925): Blood regeneration in severe anemia: standard basal ration bread and experimental method. *Amer. J. Physiol.* 72:395-407.
978b. Whipple, G.H., and Robscheit-Robbins, F.S. (1925): Blood regeneration in severe anemia: influence of liver, heart and skeletal muscle in diet. *Amer. J. Physiol.* 72:408-418.
979. Minot, G.R., and Murphy, W.P. (1926): Treatment of pernicious anemia by special diet. *J. Amer. Med. Assoc.* 87:470-476.
980. Castle, W.B. (1929): Observations on the etiologic relationship of achylia gastrica to pernicious anemia. I. The effect of the administration to patients with pernicious anemia of the contents of the normal human stomach after the ingestion of beef muscle. *Amer. J. Med Sci.* 178:748-764.
980a. Castle, W.B., and Townsend, W.C. (1929): Observations on the etiologic relationship of achylia gastrica to pernicious anemia. II. The effect of the administration to patients with pernicious anemia of beef muscle after incubation with normal human gastric juice. *Amer. J. Med. Sci.* 178:764-777.
981. Castle, W.B., and Bowie, M.A. (1929): A domestic liver extract for use in pernicious anemia. Method of preparation. *J. Amer. Med. Assoc.* 92:1830-1832.
982. Sharp, E.A. (1929): An anti-anemic factor in desiccated stomach. *J. Amer. Med. Assoc.* 93:749.
983. Shorb, M.S. (1948): Activity of vitamin B_{12} for the growth of *Lactobacillus lactis. Science* 107:397-398.
984. Rickes, E.L., Brink, N.G., Koniuszy, F.R., Wood, T.R., and Folkers, K. (1948): Crystalline vitamin B_{12}. *Science* 107:396-397.
985. Smith, E.L, and Parker, L.F.J. (1948): Purification of anti-pernicious anemia factor. *Biochem. J.* 43:viii-ix.
986. Hodgkin, D.C., Pickworth, J., Robertson, J.H., Trueblood, K.N., Prosen, R.B., and White, J.G. (1955): Structure of vitamin B_{12}. The crystal structure of the hexacarboxylic acid derived from B_{12} and the molecular structure of the vitamin. *Nature* 176:325-328.
987. Bonnett, R. Cannon, J.R., Johnson, A.W., Sutherland, I., Todd, A.R., and Smith, E.L. (1955): The structure of vitamin B_{12} and its hexacarboxylic degradation product. *Nature* 176:328-330.

988. Kuehl, F.A., Shunk, C.H., and Folkers, K. (1955): Vitamin B_{12}. XXIV. DL-3,3-dimethyl-2,5-diox-4-hydroxypyrrolidine-4-propionic acid lactone and DL-3,3-dimethyl-2,5-dioxopyrrolidine-4-propionic acid, new degradation products. *J. Amer. Chem. Soc.* 77:251-252.

989. West, R. (1948): Activity of vitamin B_{12} in Addisonian pernicious anemia. *Science* 107:398.

990. Hodgkin, D.C., Kamper, J., Mackay, M., Pickworth, J., Trueblood, K.N., and White, J.G. (1956): Structure of vitamin B_{12}. *Nature* 178:64-66.

990a. Chow, B.F. (1964): The B vitamins: B_6, B_{12}, folic acid, pantothenic acid and biotin. In: *Nutrition: a Comprehensive Treatise, Volume II*, edited by G.H. Beaton and E.W. McHenry. Academic Press, New York. pp. 207-264.

991. Herbert, V. (1973): Section J. Folic acid and vitamin B_{12}. In: *Modern Nutrition In Health and Disease, Fifth Edition*, edited by R.S. Goodhart and M.E. Shils. Lea & Febiger, Philadelphia. pp. 221-244.

991a. Herbert, V. (1976): Vitamin B_{12}. In: *Nutrition Reviews' Present Knowledge in Nutrition, Fourth Edition*, edited by D.M. Hegsted, C.O. Chichester, W.J. Darby, K.W. McNutt, R.M. Stalvey, and E.H. Stotz. The Nutrition Foundation, New York and Washington. pp. 191-203.

992. Hall, C.A., and Finkler, A.E. (1965): The dynamics of transcobalamin II. A vitamin B_{12} binding substance in plasma. *J. Lab. & Clin. Med.* 65:459-468.

993. Hall, C.A., and Finkler, A.E. (1966): Measurement of the amounts of the individual vitamin B_{12} binding proteins in plasma. I. Studies of normal plasma. *Blood* 27:611-617.

994. Hall, C.A., and Finkler, A.E. (1966): Measurement of the amounts of the individual vitamin B_{12} binding proteins in plasma. II. Abnormalities in leukemia and pernicious anemia. *Blood* 27:618-622.

995. Gottlieb, C.W., Retief, F.B., Pratt, P.W., and Herbert, V (1966): Correlation of B_{12}-binding proteins with disorders of B_{12} metabolism: Relation to hypo- and hyper-leukocytic states and leukocyte turnover. (Abstract). *J. Clin. Invest.* 45:1016.

996. Mikkonen, L., Finkler, A.E., and Hall, C.A. (1967): A diagnostic test for chronic myelogenous leukemia based on abnormalities of B_{12}-binding. *Acta Med. Scandinav.* 181:591-596.

997. Hall, C.A., and Finkler, A.E. (1969): Vitamin B_{12}-binding protein in polycythemia vera plasma. *J. Lab. & Clin. Med.* 73:60-69.

998. Gräsbeck, R. (1969): Intrinsic factor and other vitamin B_{12} transport proteins. In: *Progress in Hematology, Volume VI*, edited by E.B. Brown and C.V. Moore. Grune & Stratton, New York. pp. 233-260.

999. Bloomfield, F.J., and Scott, J.M. (1972): Identification of a new vitamin B_{12} binder (transcobalamin III) in normal human serum. *Brit. J. Haematol.* 22:33-42.

1000. Carmel, R., and Herbert, V. (1972): Vitamin B_{12}-binding protein of leukocytes as a possible major source of the third vitamin B_{12}-binding protein of serum. *Blood* 40:542-549.

1001. Scott, J.M., Bloomfield, F.J., Stebbins, R., and Herbert, V. (1974): Studies in the derivation of transcobalamin III from granulocytes. Enhancement by lithium and elimination by fluoride of *in vitro* increments in vitamin B_{12}-binding capacity. *J. Clin. Invest.* 153:228-239.

1002. Burger, R.L., Mehlman, C.S., and Allen, R.H. (1975): Human plasma R-type vitamin B_{12}-binding proteins. I. Isolation and characterization of transcobalamin I, transcobalamin III, and the normal granulocyte vitamin B_{12}-binding protein. *J. Biol. Chem.* 250:7700-7706.

1003. Burger, R.L., Schneider, R.J., Mehlman, C.S., and Allen, R.H. (1975): Human plasma R-type vitamin B_{12}-binding proteins. II. The role of transcobalamin I, transcobalamin III, and the normal granulocyte vitamin B_{12}-binding protein in the plasma transport of vitamin B_{12}. *J. Biol. Chem.* 250:7707-7713.

1004. Gilbert, H.S. (1974): Proposal of a possible function for granulocyte B_{12}-binding proteins in host defense against bacteria. *Blood* 44:926.

1005. Watkin, D.M. (1959): Unpublished data.

1006. Mendelsohn, R.S., and Watkin, D.M. (1958): Serum B_{12} concentrations deter-

mined by *L. leichmannii* assay in patients with neoplastic disease. *J. Lab. & Clin. Med.* 51:860-866.
1007. Carmel, R. (1975): Extreme elevation of serum transcobalamin I in patients with metastatic cancer. *New Engl. J. Med.* 292:282-284.
1008. Watkin, D.M., Lang, C.A., Shock, N.W., and Chow, B.F. (1953): Agewise differences in the urinary excretion of vitamin B_{12} following intramuscular administration. *J. Nutrition.* 50:341-349.
1009. Boger, W.P., Wright, L.D., Strickland, S.C., Gylfe, J.S., and Ciminera, J.L. (1955): Vitamin B_{12}: Correlation of serum concentration and age. *Proc. Soc. Exper. Biol. Med.* 89:375-378.
1010. Chow, B.F., Wood, R., Horonick, A., and Okuda, K. (1956): Agewise variation of vitamin B_{12} serum levels. *J. Gerontol.* 11:142-146.
1011. Gaffney, G.W., Horonick, A., Okuda, K., Meier, P., Chow, B.F., and Shock, N.W. (1957): Vitamin B_{12} serum concentrations in 528 apparently healthy human subjects of ages 12-94. *J. Gerontol.* 12:32-38.
1012. Watkin, D.M., Barrows, C.H., Jr., Chow, B.F., and Shock, N.W. (1961): Renal clearance of intravenously administered vitamin B_{12}. *Proc. Soc. Exper. Biol. Med.* 107:219-221.
1013. Weinstein, I.B., Weissman, S.M., and Watkin, D.M. (1959): The plasma vitamin B_{12}-binding substance. I. Its detection in the seromucoid fraction of plasma of normal subjects and patients with chronic myelocytic leukemia. *J. Clin. Invest.* 38:1904-1914.
1014. Mollin, D.L., Anderson, B.B., and Burman, J.F. (1976): The serum vitamin B_{12} level: its assay and significance. *Clin. Haematol.* 5:521-546.
1015. Kolhouse, J.F., Kondo, H., Allen, N.C., Podell, A.B., and Allen, R.H. (1978): Cobalamin analogues are present in human serum and can mask cobalamin deficiency because current radioisotope dilution assays are not specific for true cobalamin. *New Engl. J. Med.* 299:785-792.
1016. Cooper, B.A., and Whitehead, V.M. (1978): Evidence that some patients with pernicious anemia are not recognized by radiodilution assay for cobalamin in serum. *New Engl. J. Med.* 299:816-818.
1017. Donaldson, R.M. (1978): "Serum B_{12}" and the diagnosis of cobalamin deficiency. *New Engl. J. Med.* 299:827-828.
1018. Cullen, R.W., and Oace, S.M. (1978): Methylmalonic acid and vitamin B_{12} excretion in rats consuming diets varying in cellulose and pectin. *J. Nutrition* 108:640-647.
1019. Noronka, J.M., and Silverman, M. (1962): On folic acid, vitamin B_{12}, methionine and formiminoglutamic acid metabolism. In: *Vitamin B_{12} and Intrinsic Factor, Second European Symposium,* edited by H.C. Heinrich. F. Enke Verlag, Stuttgart. p. 728.
1020. Herbert, V., and Zalusky, R. (1962): Interrelations of vitamin B_{12} and folic acid metabolism: folic acid clearance studies. *J. Clin. Invest.* 41:1263-1276.
1021. Vilter, R.W. (1968): The vitamins: folic acid. In: *Modern Nutrition in Health and Disease, Fourth Edition,* edited by M. G. Wohl and R.S. Goodhart. Lea & Febiger, Philadelphia. pp. 273-285.
1022. Vilter, R.W. (1968): The vitamins: vitamin B_{12}. In: *Modern Nutrition in Health and Disease, Fourth Edition,* edited by M.G. Wohl and R.S. Goodhart. Lea & Febiger, Philadelphia. pp. 285-296.
1023. Stokstad, E.L.R. (1976): Vitamin B_{12} and folic acid. In: *Nutrition Reviews' Present Knowledge in Nutrition,* Fourth Edition, edited by D.M. Hegsted, C.O. Chichester, W.J. Darby, K.W. McNutt, R.M. Stalvey, and E.H. Stotz. The Nutrition Foundation, New York and Washington. pp. 204-216.
1024. Berkow, R., Editor. (1977): Principles of fluid therapy. In: *The Merck Manual of Diagnosis and Therapy, Thirteenth Edition.* Merck Sharp & Dohme Research Laboratories, Rahway, N.J. pp. 1185-1186.
1025. McCay, C.M., Editor (1952): Nutritional aspects of aging. *J. Gerontol.* 7:448-451.
1026. McCay, C.M. (1955): Research areas in gerontology nutrition that are now neglected. In: *Ciba Foundation Colloquia on Aging, Volume I,* edited by G.E.W. Wolstenholme and M.P. Cameron. J. & A. Churchill, London. pp. 173-185.

1027. Ross, M.H., and Bras, G. (1974): Dietary preferences and diseases of age. *Nature* 250:263-265.
1028. Ross, M.H., Lustbader, E., and Bras, G. (1976): Dietary practices and growth responses as predictors of longevity. *Nature* 262:548-553.
1029. Ross, M.H. (1977): Dietary behavior and longevity. *Nutrition Rev.* 35:257-265.
1030. Berg, B.N., and Simms, H.S. (1960): Nutrition and longevity in the rat. II. Longevity and onset of disease with different levels of food intake. *J. Nutrition.* 71:255-263.
1031. Berg, B.N., Wolf, A., and Simms, H.S. (1962): Nutrition and longevity in the rat. IV. Food restriction and the radiculoneuropathy of aging rats. *J. Nutrition.* 77:439-442.
1032. Shock, N.W., Watkin, D.M., Yiengst, M.J., Norris, A.H., Gaffney, G.W., Gregerman, R.I., and Falzone, J.A. (1963): Age differences in the water content of the body as related to basal oxygen consumption in males. *J. Gerontol.* 18:1-8.
1033. Watkin, D.M., Das, J.B., and McCarthy, M.C. (1965): The influence of dietary protein and Calories on physiological performance during strenuous work in man. *Abstracts of Papers Presented at the XXIII International Congress of Physiological Sciences, Tokyo, September, 1965.* Science Council of Japan, Tokyo. p. 314.
1034. Andres, R. (1980): Influence of obesity on longevity in the aged. In: *Advances in Cancer Biology Series, Volume VII. Aging, Cancer and Cell Membranes,* edited by Borek, C. Stratton Intercontinental Medical Book Corporation, New York.
1035. Editorial (1979): Orphans. *The Washington Post,* September 24. p. 22.
1036. Administration on Aging (1976): Older Americans Act of 1965, as Amended, and Related Acts. DHEW Publication No. (OHD) 76-20170. U.S. Government Printing Office, Washington, D.C.
1037. Administration on Aging (1979): Older Americans Act of 1965, as Amended. History and Related Acts, DHEW Publication No. (OHDS) 79-20170. U.S. Government Printing Office, Washington, D.C.
1038. Watkin, D.M. (1979): Mutual relationships among aging, nutrition and health. In: *Human Nutrition, a Comprehensive Treatise, Volume IV. Nutrition: Metabolic and Clinical Applications,* edited by R.E. Hodges. Plenum Press, New York. pp. 219-240.
1039. National Institute on Aging (1977): *Proceedings of a Symposium on Exercise in the Elderly — Its Role in the Prevention of Physical Decline and in Rehabilitation.* National Institute on Aging, Bethesda, MD.
1040. Watkin, D.M. (1978): Personal responsibility: Key to effective and cost-effective health. *Family & Commun. Health* 1:1-7.
1040a. Watkin, D.M. (1977): Aging, nutrition and the continuum of health care. In: *Food and Nutrition in Health and Disease,* edited by N.H. Moss and J. Mayer, *Ann. N.Y. Acad. Sci.* 300:290-297.
1040b. Watkin, D.M. (1980): Maintenance — prevention — promotion: Changing public and private sector views of clients' responsibility for personal health. In: *Current Practice in Family Oriented Community Nursing, Volume II,* edited by A. M. Reinhardt and M.D. Quinn. C.V. Mosby Company, St. Louis.
1040c. Gastineau, C.F., Darby, W.J., and Turner, T.B., Editors (1979): *Fermented Food Beverages in Nutrition. A Monograph Series Publication of the Nutrition Foundation.* Academic Press, New York.
1040d. Watkin, D.M. (1979): Role of alcoholic beverages in gerontology. In: *Fermented Food Beverages in Nutrition. A Monograph Series Publication of The Nutrition Foundation.* Academic Press, New York. pp. 225-243.
1041. Ferguson, R.J., Petitclerc, R., Choquette, G., Chaniotis, L., Gauthier, P., Huot, R., Allard, C., Janowski, L., and Campeau, L. (1974): *Amer. J. Cardiology* 34:764-769.
1042. Holman, B.L. (1977): Promising new radiotracer technics for the diagnosis of coronary artery disease. *New Engl. J. Med.* 296:876-877.
1043. Borer, J.S. (1977): Computerization of radionucleotide imaging. In: *Proceedings of a Symposium on Exercise in the Elderly — Its Role in Prevention of Physical Decline and in Rehabilitation.* National Institute on Aging, Bethesda, MD.
1044. Watkin, D.M., and Mueller, P.S. (1959): Effects of exercise on nutrient and en-

ergy metabolism in adolescents with neoplastic disease. *Federation Proc.* 18:no. 1, part I, 167 (abstract).

1045. Watkin, D.M., Das, J.B., and McCarthy, M.C. (1963): Protein requirement as a function of work load. *Federation Proc.* 22: no. 2, part I, 260 (abstract).

1046. Christophe, J., and Mayer, J. (1958): Effect of exercise on glucose uptake in rats and men. *J. Appl. Physiol.* 13:269-272.

1047. Thompson, P.D., Stern, M.P., Williams, P., Duncan, K., Haskell, W.L., and Wood, P.D. (1979): Death during jogging and running. *J. Amer. Med. Assoc.* 24:1265-1267.

1048. Vaisrub, S. (1979): Exercise — a diagnostic virtuoso. *J. Amer. Med. Assoc.* 24:1292.

1049. Gsell, D. (1964): Evaluation of food consumption and nutritional status. Surveys on the mountain population of Switzerland. *Voeding.* 25:92-96.

1050. Belloc, N.B., and Breslow, L. (1972): Relationship of physical health status and health practices. *Preventive Med.* 1:409-421.

1051. Goldstein, M.S. (1961): Humoral nature of hypoglycemia in muscular exercise. *Amer. J. Physiol.* 200:67-70.

1052. Das, J.B. (1967): Body composition and work performance with respect to protein nutriture. Ph.D. dissertation. Massachusetts Institute of Technology.

1053. Kattus, A.A., Chairman, Committee on Exercise. (1972): *Exercise Testing and Training of Apparently Healthy Individuals: A Handbook for Physicians.* American Heart Association, Dallas.

1054. Kattus, A.A., Chairman, Committee on Exercise. (1975): *Exercise Testing and Training of Individuals with Heart Disease or at High Risk for its Development: A handbook for Physicians.* American Heart Association, Dallas.

1055. Weiner, D.A., Ryan, T.J., McCabe, C.H., Kennedy, J.W., Schloss, M., Tristani, F., Chaitman, B.R., and Fisher, L.D. (1979): Exercise stress testing: Correlations among history of angina, S-T segment response and prevalence of coronary artery disease in the coronary artery surgery study (CASS). *New Engl. J. Med.* 301:230-235.

1056. Epstein, S.E. (1979): Limitations of electrocardiographic exercise testing. *New Engl. J. Med.* 301:264-265.

1057. Rynearson, R.R., Roberts, J.W., and Stewart, W.L. (1979): Do physician athletes believe in pre-exercise examinations and stress tests? *New Engl. J. Med.* 301:792-793.

1058. Food and Nutrition Service, Department of Agriculture. (1978): Food Stamp Program. Implementing the Food Stamp Act of 1977. *Federal Register* 43:47846-47934.

1059. Davis, D.W., and McGeary, B.K. (1973): *Cooking for Two.* Food and Nutrition Service and Agricultural Research Service, U.S. Department of Agriculture. Stock Number 0100-02985, U.S. Government Printing Office, Washington, D.C.

1060. Office of Human Development Services, Department of Health, Education and Welfare. (1979): Notice of proposed rulemaking: Grants for State and Community Programs on Aging. *Federal Register.* 44:45032-45063.

1061. Office of Human Development Services, Department of Health, Education and Welfare. (1980): Rules. 45 CFR Parts 1320, 1321, 1324, 1326. Grants for State and Community Programs on Aging. *Federal Register* 45:21126-21166.

1062. Watkin, D.M. (1981): Policy on nutrition in contemporary America. In: *The Value of Aging,* a special issue of *Health Values: Achieving High Level Wellness,* edited by H.M. Garrity and E.A. Neilson. Charles B. Slack, Inc. Thorofare, N.J. 5:11-19.

Index

John H. Browe, M.D., M.P.H., Director (Ret.), Bureau of Nutrition, New York State Health Department, provided valuable advice and assistance in developing this index.

NUTRITION AND KILLER DISEASES

The Effects of Dietary Factors on Fatal Chronic Diseases

Edited by

John Rose

Blackburn College of Technology and Design, Blackburn, England
Hon. Director, The Institution of Environmental Sciences, London, England

This important, timely book provides a critical evaluation of the effects of dietary factors on the so-called "killer diseases"—cardiovascular disease, cancer, and diabetes. There is ample evidence to support the thesis that inadequate nutrition and dietary management contribute to the alarming increase in occurrence of these fatal chronic diseases.

Based partly on the proceedings of a National Conference on "Killer Diseases" held at the Royal Society of Medicine in London (U.K.), the book contains contributions by American and British experts who have provided a wealth of useful information and advice concerning diet, which may lead to a reduction in the incidence and gravity of killer diseases.

Cardiovascular disease and cancer are covered from a variety of nutritional viewpoints. Each of these diseases is of complex etiology, and cause and effect have been impossible to prove. However, since each of the diseases has a nutritional component in its etiology or treatment, and because nutrition is a variable which can be altered, the evidence for nutritional patterns associated with the diseases is reviewed here. In diabetes, particular attention is directed to the role of diet and dietary management.

This book will be of great practical value to the medical profession and nutritionists. It is also a basic reference volume for medical, scientific, nursing, nutrition and biology libraries.

CONTENTS

ISBN 0-8155-0902-2 (1982) **185 pages**

Other Noyes Publications

HANDBOOK OF GERIATRIC NUTRITION

Principles and Applications for Nutrition and Diet in Aging

Edited by

Jeng M. Hsu, D.V.M., Ph.D. **Robert L. Davis, Sc.D.**

Veterans Administration Medical Center
Bay Pines, Florida

with a Foreword by
Hon. Claude Pepper, Chairman
Select Committee on Aging
U.S. House of Representatives

This important and timely new book presents and comprehensively reviews current pertinent information on the practical and applied aspects of nutrition and diet of the elderly. The many **contributions from leading researchers and workers in various areas of Gerontology research**–medicine, biology, psychology, economics, nutrition, and sociology–provide the basis for a rational approach to the triad of nutrition, health, and aging.

The various chapters in the Handbook discuss:

1) The present status of scientific knowledge and the relationship of major nutrients and other food components to aging and disease.
2) How nutritional regimens and needs of the elderly must be modified to take into account their various medical, surgical, economic, and psychological problems.
3) How to improve the nutrition of aged persons.
4) Nutrition misinformation, fads, and folkore of the elderly.

An excellent reference and essential volume for all those interested in geriatric nutrition and gerontology. A must for professional workers and researchers in Gerontology, Nutrition, Geriatric Medicine, as well as medical, biological, nutrition, and scientific libraries.

ISBN 0-8155-0880-8 (1981) **372 pages**

DATE DUE

MY 15 '95			
DEC 20	1997		